ON CALL

Neurology

4th Edition

STEPHAN A. MAYER, MD, FCCM

William T. Gossett Chair of Neurology
Co-Director, Neuroscience Institute
Henry Ford Health System
Professor of Neurology
Wayne State University School of Medicine
Detroit, Michigan

RANDOLPH S. MARSHALL, MD, MS

Elisabeth K Harris Professor of Neurology
Chief, Stroke Division
Department of Neurology
Columbia University Irving Medical Center
New York, New York

ELSEVIER

Elsevier
3251 Riverport Lane
St. Louis, Missouri 63043

ON CALL NEUROLOGY, FOURTH EDITION   ISBN: 978-0-323-54694-2

Notices

Practitioners and researchers must always rely on their own experience and knowledge in evaluating and using any information, methods, compounds or experiments described herein. Because of rapid advances in the medical sciences, in particular, independent verification of diagnoses and drug dosages should be made. To the fullest extent of the law, no responsibility is assumed by Elsevier, authors, editors or contributors for any injury and/or damage to persons or property as a matter of products liability, negligence or otherwise, or from any use or operation of any methods, products, instructions, or ideas contained in the material herein.

Library of Congress Control Number: 2019955977

Content Strategist: Marybeth Thiel
Content Development Specialists: Caroline Dorey-Stein/
  Kevin Travers
Publishing Services Manager: Shereen Jameel
Senior Project Manager: Umarani Natarajan
Design Direction: Amy Buxton

Printed in India
Last digit is the print number: 9 8 7 6 5 4 3 2

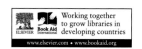

ON CALL

Neurology

Be ON CALL with confidence!

Successfully managing on-call situations requires a masterful combination of speed, skills, and knowledge. Rise to the occasion with **ELSEVIER's On Call Series!** These pocket-size resources provide you with immediate access to the vital, step-by-step information you need to succeed!

Other Titles in the ON CALL Series

Adams & Bresnick: **On Call Surgery**
Bernstein, Poag, & Rubinstein: **On Call Psychiatry**
Marshall & Ruedy: **On Call Principles & Protocols**
Nocton & Gedeit: **On Call Pediatrics**

To the New York-Presbyterian residents, past and present,
who have helped us teach and learn.

Contributors

CIGDEM AKMAN, MD
Chief, Child Neurology
Director, Pediatric Epilepsy
Department of Neurology
Columbia University Irving
    Medical Center
New York, NY, United States
Chapter 27: Pediatric Neurology

NEERAJ BADJATIA, MD, MSc
Professor and Vice Chair
Department of Neurology
University of Maryland School of
    Medicine
Baltimore, MD, United States
Chapter 9: Head Injury

MICHELLE BELL, MD
Assistant Professor
Department of Neurology
Columbia University Irving
    Medical Center
New York, NY, United States
Chapter 10: Focal Mass Lesions

COMANA CIORIOU, MD
Assistant Professor
Department of Neurology
Columbia University Irving
    Medical Center
New York, NY, United States
Chapter 18: Pain Syndromes

JAN CLAASSEN, MD, PhD
Associate Professor of Neurology
    and Neurosurgery
Department of Neurology
Columbia University Irving
    Medical Center
New York, NY, United States
**Chapter 4: Acute Seizures and
    Status Epilepticus**

**NEHA DANGAYACH, MD,
    MSCR**
Assistant Professor
Departments of Neurosurgery and
    Neurology
Icahn School of Medicine at
    Mount Sinai
Co-Director, Neurosciences ICU
Mount Sinai Health System
New York, NY, United States
**Chapter 16: Neuromuscular
    Respiratory Failure**

**ERROL LLOYD GORDON, Jr.,
    MD**
Associate Professor
Department of Internal
    Medicine
University of Oklahoma College of
    Medicine, School of
    Community Medicine
Tulsa, OK, United States
Chapter 19: Brain Death

LAWRENCE HONIG, MD, PhD
Professor of Neurology
Director, Center of Excellence for
    Alzheimer's Disease
Department of Neurology, Taub
    Institute, and Sergievsky Center
Columbia University Irving
    Medical Center
New York, NY, United States
Chapter 28: Dementia

FABIO IWAMOTO, MD
Assistant Professor
Deputy Director, Division of
    Neuro-Oncology
Department of Neurology
Columbia University Irving
    Medical Center
New York, NY, United States
Chapter 23: Neurooncology

JULIE KROMM, BMSc, MD,
    FRCPC
Postdoctoral Clinical Fellow
Department of Neurological
    Critical Care
Columbia University Irving
    Medical Center
New York, NY, United States
Chapter 4: Acute Seizures and
    Status Epilepticus

ELAN D. LOUIS, MD
Professor of Neurology
Director, Movement Disorders
Department of Neurology
Yale University School of
    Medicine
Professor of Epidemiology
Yale University School of Public
    Health
New Haven, CT, United States
Chapter 25: Movement Disorders

JEREMY J. MOELLER, MD,
    FRCPC
Associate Professor
Department of Neurology
Yale University School of
    Medicine
New Haven, CT, United States
Chapter 26: Epilepsy and Seizure
    Disorders

JAMES M. NOBLE, MD, MS
Associate Professor of Neurology
Department of Neurology
Taub Institute
Columbia University Irving
    Medical Center
New York, NY, United States
Chapter 8: Delirium and
    Amnesia

ASHWINI K. RAO, OTR/L,
    EdD
Associate Professor
Department of Rehabilitation and
    Regenerative Medicine
    (Physical Therapy)
G.H. Sergievsky Center
Columbia University Irving
    Medical Center
New York, NY, United States
Chapter 11: Gait Failure

CLAIRE RILEY, MD
Assistant Professor of Neurology
Director, Multiple Sclerosis
    Center
Department of Neurology
Columbia University Irving
    Medical Center
New York, NY, United States
Chapter 21: Demyelinating and
    Inflammatory Disorders
    of the CNS

KIRK ROBERTS, MD
Associate Professor
Department of Neurology
Columbia University Irving
    Medical Center
New York, NY, United States
**Chapter 14: Dizziness and
    Vertigo**

JANET C. RUCKER, MD
Bernard A. and Charlotte Marden
    Professor of Neurology
Departments of Neurology and
    Opthalmology
New York University School of
    Medicine, NYU Langone
    Medical Center
New York, NY, United States
**Chapter 12: Acute Visual
    Disturbances**

HIRAL SHAH, MD
Assistant Professor
Department of Neurology
Columbia University Irving
    Medical Center
New York, NY, United States
Chapter 11: Gait Failure

TINA T. SHIH, MD
Associate Professor
Department of Neurology
University of California at San
    Francisco, San Francisco
San Francisco, CA, United States
Chapter 17: Syncope

KIRAN THAKUR, MD
Winifred M. Pitkin Assistant
    Professor
Department of Neurology
Columbia University Irving
    Medical Center
New York, NY, United States
**Chapter 22: Infections of the
    CNS**

**NATALIE WEATHERED, MD,
    MS**
Assistant Professor of Neurology
Department of Neurology
Weill Cornell Medicine
New York, NY, United States
**Chapter 7: Spinal Cord
    Compression**

LOUIS WEIMER, MD
Professor
Department of Neurology
Columbia University Irving
    Medical Center
New York, NY, United States
**Chapter 20: Nerve and Muscle
    Diseases**

**MARIANNA SHNAYDERMAN
    YUGRAKH, MD**
Assistant Professor
Department of Neurology
Columbia University
New York, NY, United States
Chapter 15: Headache

Preface

In 1997 we published the first edition of *On Call: Neurology*. The book was meant to serve as a pocket reference for students, trainees, advanced practice providers and physicians who care for neurological patients in the hospital and clinic. The goal was to provide the reader with accessible, highly structured protocols for the assessment and management of neurologic disorders in the emergency room, intensive care unit, hospital floor, or outpatient setting.

Long thought of as primarily a diagnostic specialty, in 1997 neurology was just beginning to enter a new era of advances in therapeutics. Tissue plasminogen activator had only recently been approved for acute ischemic stroke, a new generation of disease-modifying biological treatments for multiple sclerosis had just been introduced, and an explosion of new antiepileptic medications were starting to move through the pipeline, just to name a few. It was an exciting time, and we felt that to some extent the neurological literature had not kept up. Traditionally there was too much of a focus on diagnosis rather than treatment, and on complexity rather than simplicity.

With *On Call: Neurology* we sought to modernize the traditional clinical pocket guide by emphasizing therapeutics (for instance, all medications with dosages were type set in bold) and by walking the reader through the focused and goal-directed thought processes of an experienced clinical neurologist. Designed to be broad in scope, the book by necessity was limited in depth, with the suggested management protocols intending to serve as a starting point for action. It was our hope that the protocols presented in the book would stimulate students of neurology (whether a medical student or an attending neurologist) to research the literature, analyze the available data, and reach independent conclusions regarding optimal patient care.

Happily, this turned out to be the case, and it is safe to make the argument that *On Call: Neurology* is a classic of the neurology pocket guide genre. Ubiquitous in resident call rooms, nursing stations, and white coat pockets around the world, over the past 20 years the book has introduced an entire generation of young doctors and nurses to neurology. We are now thrilled to present a new fourth edition of the book, fully updated to reflect the most recent advances in neurological diagnostics and therapeutics. We wrote the first edition entirely by ourselves, but as neurology has grown in complexity and because of the sheer number of therapeutic options available, *On Call: Neurology* now has a completely multiauthor format, allowing true experts to impart their wisdom.

We are grateful to our patients, colleagues, and teachers at The Neurological Institute of New York at New York-Presbyterian Hospital who encouraged and inspired us to write the first edition of *On Call: Neurology*. In particular, we would like to thank J.P. Mohr, John Brust, and Matthew Fink, and we would like to honor the memory of Lewis P. "Bud" Rowland, who was truly one of the great academic neurologists of the 20th century. Their voices can be heard in many of the pages of this text, and their dedication to teaching and education has served as an inspiration to us, as well as countless other neurologists.

Stephan A. Mayer
Randolph S. Marshall

Contents

Structure of the Book

This book is divided into four main sections:

The first section, **Introduction**, provides an overview of the clinical approach to the neurologic patient, including the neurologic examination, neuroanatomic localization, and neurodiagnostic testing.

The second section, **Patient-Related Problems: The Common Calls**, is a symptom-oriented approach to chief complaints that frequently require neurologic consultation in the emergency department, clinic, or hospital floor. Each problem is approached from its inception, beginning with relevant questions that should be asked over the phone, temporary orders that should be given, and the major life-threatening disorders that should be considered as one approaches the bedside.

PHONE CALL

Questions
Pertinent questions to assess the urgency of the situation.

Orders
Urgent orders to stabilize the patient and gain additional information before you arrive at the bedside.

Inform RN
RN to be informed of the time the house staff anticipates arrival at the bedside.

ELEVATOR THOUGHTS

The differential diagnoses to be considered while the house staff is on the way to assess the patient (i.e., while in the elevator).

MAJOR THREAT TO LIFE

Neurologic emergencies that can lead to death or neurologic devastation unless immediate action is taken.

BEDSIDE

Quick Look Test

The quick look test is a rapid visual assessment to place the patient into one of three categories: well, sick, or critical. This helps determine the necessity of immediate intervention.

Vital Signs

Which vital sign abnormalities to look out for.

Selective History and Chart Review

Including pertinent negatives and neurologic review of systems.

Selective Physical and Neurologic Examination

A rapid, focused neurologic examination designed to assess the extent and degree of neurologic dysfunction.

MANAGEMENT

Provides guidelines for neurodiagnostic testing and gives access to indicated medications and dosages. When applicable, checklists and specific management protocols are provided.

The third section, **Selected Neurologic Disorders**, provides an overview of important neurologic diseases and their management not covered comprehensively in the "common calls" section, such as central nervous system infections, multiple sclerosis, neuromuscular diseases, movement disorders, and brain tumors.

The fourth section, the **Appendices**, provides neuroanatomic references and other materials helpful for managing neurologic patients.

Finally, the **On-Call Formulary** is a compendium of medications commonly used to treat neurologic disorders. Drug indications, mechanisms of action, dosages, routes of administration, side effects, and comments for optimal use are provided.

Commonly Used Abbreviations

ABG	arterial blood gas
ACA	anterior cerebral artery
ACE	angiotensin-converting enzyme
ACTH	adrenocorticotropic hormone
AFB	acid-fast bacillus
AIDS	acquired immunodeficiency syndrome
AION	anterior ischemic optic neuropathy
ALS	amyotrophic lateral sclerosis
AMN	adrenomyeloneuropathy
ANA	antinuclear antibody
ANCA	antineutrophil cytoplasmic antibody
APD	afferent pupillary defect
aPTT	activated partial thromboplastin time
AV	arteriovenous
AVM	arteriovenous malformation
BAER	brain stem auditory evoked response
BID	two times a day
BP	blood pressure
BUN	blood urea nitrogen
CAA	cerebral amyloid angiopathy
CBC	complete blood cell count
CBF	cerebral blood flow
CHF	congestive heart failure
CIDP	chronic inflammatory demyelinating polyneuropathy
CK	creatine kinase
CMAP	compound muscle action potential
CMV	cytomegalovirus
CN	cranial nerve
CNS	central nervous system
CPAP	continuous positive airway pressure
CPK	creatine phosphokinase
CPP	cerebral perfusion pressure
CPR	cardiopulmonary resuscitation
CRAO	central retinal artery occlusion

CSF	cerebrospinal fluid
CT	computed tomography
D50W	50% dextrose in water
D5W	5% dextrose in water
D5WNS	5% dextrose in normal saline
DDAVP	desmopressin acetate
DIC	disseminated intravascular coagulation
DVT	deep vein thrombosis
DWI	diffusion-weighted imaging
EBV	Epstein-Barr virus
ECG	electrocardiogram
EEG	electroencephalography
EMG	electromyography
EP	electrophysiologic
ER	emergency room
ESR	erythrocyte sedimentation rate
EtOH	ethanol
FDA	Food and Drug Administration
FFP	fresh frozen plasma
FNF	finger-nose-finger
GBM	glioblastoma multiforme
GBS	Guillain-Barré syndrome
GCS	Glasgow Coma scale
GI	gastrointestinal
GU	genitourinary
hCG	human chorionic gonadotropin
HEENT	head, eyes, ears, nose, throat
HIV	human immunodeficiency virus
HKS	heel-knee-shin
HR	heart rate
HSE	herpes simplex encephalitis
HSV-1	herpes simplex virus 1
HTLV-1	human T-cell lymphotropic virus type 1
Hz	Hertz
ICA	internal carotid artery
ICH	intracerebral hemorrhage
ICP	intracranial pressure
ICU	intensive care unit
IgG	immunoglobulin G
IM	intramuscular
IMV	intermittent mandatory ventilation
INO	internuclear ophthalmoplegia
INR	international normalized ratio
ION	ischemic optic neuropathy
IV	intravenous

IVIG	intravenous immunoglobulin
IVP	intravenous push
KVO	keep the vein open
LCM	lymphocytic choriomeningitis
LFT	liver function test
LP	lumbar puncture
MABP	mean arterial blood pressure
MAO	monoamine oxidase
MCA	middle cerebral artery
MELAS	mitochondrial encephalomyopathy, lactic acidosis, and stroke
MI	myocardial infarction
MLD	metachromatic leukodystrophy
MLF	median longitudinal fasciculus
MMN	multifocal motor neuropathy
MMSE	Mini-Mental State Examination
MRI	magnetic resonance imaging
MS	multiple sclerosis
MSA	multiple-system atrophy
NCS	nerve conduction study
NCV	nerve conduction velocity
NPO	nil per os (nothing by mouth)
NS	normal saline
NSAID	nonsteroidal antiinflammatory drug
NSE	neuron-specific enolase
OCB	oligoclonal band
OKN	opticokinetic nystagmus
ON	optic neuritis
PCA	posterior cerebral artery
PCNSL	primary central nervous system lymphoma
P$_{CO_2}$	partial pressure of carbon dioxide
PCR	polymerase chain reaction
PE	pulmonary embolism
PEEP	positive end-expiratory pressure
PET	positron emission tomography
PLED	periodic lateralizing epileptiform discharge
PML	progressive multifocal leukoencephalopathy
PNET	primitive neuroectodermal tumor
PO	per os (by mouth)
P$_{O_2}$	partial pressure of oxygen
PPD	purified protein derivative
PPRF	paramedian pontine reticular formation
PRN	as needed
PT	prothrombin time
PTT	partial thromboplastin time

PVS	persistent vegetative state
QD	every day
qhs	every day at nighttime
QID	four times a day
RA	rheumatoid arthritis
RAM	rapid alternating movement
RBC	red blood cell
RF	rheumatoid factor
RPR	rapid plasmin reagin
SAH	subarachnoid hemorrhage
SBP	systolic blood pressure
SC	subcutaneous
SFEMG	single-fiber electromyogram
SIADH	syndrome of inappropriate antidiuretic hormone
SIMV	synchronized intermittent mandatory ventilation
SL	sublingual
SLE	systemic lupus erythematosus
SMA	spinal muscular atrophy
SMP	sympathetically maintained pain
SPECT	single-photon emission computed tomography
SPEP	serum protein electrophoresis
SSEP	somatosensory evoked potential
SSPE	subacute sclerosing panencephalitis
TCA	tricyclic antidepressant
TCD	transcranial Doppler
TENS	transcutaneous electric nerve stimulation
TFT	thyroid function test
TGA	transient global amnesia
TIA	transient ischemic attack
TID	three times a day
TMB	transient monocular blindness
tPA	tissue plasminogen activator
VDRL	Venereal Disease Research Laboratory
VEP	visual evoked potential
VER	visual evoked response
WBC	white blood cell

Introduction

Approach to the Neurologic Patient On Call: History Taking, Differential Diagnosis, and Anatomic Localization

It is in the early morning hours. You get a call from a resident in the emergency room (ER). A 48-year-old teacher has headache, neck pain, and urinary incontinence, and, as of this morning, is no longer able to hold a pen in his right hand. How do you proceed? What do you tell the ER resident? What tests should be ordered? How urgent is this situation?

Neurology, perhaps more than any other field in medicine, demands familiarity with a wide spectrum of anatomic details and diagnostic studies. Electrophysiologic, serologic, genetic, pathologic, and a host of imaging techniques have enabled diagnoses to be made with a higher degree of accuracy and certainty than ever before. Yet all diagnostic puzzles, simple or complex, begin with the presentation of a symptom by a patient to a doctor.

It is often said that 90% of the neurologic diagnosis comes from the patient's history. Indeed, it is the exception when a diagnosis is stumbled on after a "shotgun" approach of ordering diagnostic studies unguided by the patient's initial complaints. In the type of encounter for which this book was written, namely a rapid response to an acute complaint, the single most important factor in the encounter is the initial interview with the patient. This book aims to guide you through a logical, focused, and effective approach to diagnosis and management of your patient's acute problem. This fourth edition has updated chapters in all aspects of emergency neurologic care, including the latest pharmacologic and diagnostic options. After a discussion of general principles of managing patients on call, this chapter covers some key points about neurologic history taking along with principles of differential diagnosis and anatomic localization. The neurologic physical examination is outlined in Chapter 2. The basics of the most important initial diagnostic studies are covered in Chapter 3.

PRINCIPLES OF MANAGING PATIENTS WHEN ON CALL

1. **Obtain adequate information from the initial phone contact.**
   Establish the nature of the complaint, understand its acuteness and its severity, and learn what has been done so far. (Have vital signs been checked? Has any labwork been sent?)

2. **Establish a working differential diagnosis before you see the patient.**
   Some preparatory thought will produce a more efficient and directed interview and examination of the patient. Prioritize your diagnoses by placing the most potentially dangerous diagnoses at the top of the list, followed by the most likely diagnoses.

3. **Be focused in your bedside assessment.**
   Unlike the comprehensive examination that you perform when admitting a patient to the hospital or when seeing a patient for the first time in the clinic, your history taking and examination of the patient when you are on call needs to be focused and efficient.

4. **Know when to call for additional consultation.**
   Examples would be an ophthalmologic consultation for branch retinal artery occlusion versus anterior ischemic optic neuropathy, or a neurosurgical consultation to place an intracranial pressure monitor.

5. **Be accurate and concise in your documentation of the encounter.**
   Although it will be your responsibility to solve the clinical problem as completely as possible, many times you will be unable to make a diagnosis or complete a treatment during the time you are involved with the patient. You must document the patient's history and physical examination as precisely as possible. Make sure you date and time your note. If there was a delay in arriving at the bedside because of another emergency, then document this. Include relevant laboratory data in your note. Your evaluation and formulation of the problem should be well integrated and transparent. The recommendations for treatment should be stated clearly and should be concordant with what was written in the orders. If discussions with family members took place, then the content and outcome of the discussions should be documented.

PRINCIPLES OF HISTORY TAKING IN NEUROLOGY

Key features of the neurologic history include the following:

1. **Patient's demographics: age, gender, and race-ethnicity, if relevant**

   Age is often crucial in the initial consideration of the differential diagnosis. Disorders causing ataxia, for instance, would include multiple sclerosis and viral cerebellitis in patients under 45 years of age, whereas cerebral infarction and alcoholic cerebellar degeneration would be higher on the differential diagnosis list for the same syndrome in older patients. Gender-specific neurologic conditions include benign intracranial hypertension and multiple sclerosis, which are more common in women.

   Race ethnicity differences include the higher incidence of intracranial atherosclerosis in African American and Hispanic patients, whereas in Caucasians, extracranial atherosclerosis tends to develop with higher frequency.

2. **Temporal course of the disease**

   The temporal pattern of your patient's symptoms is one of the most important pieces of history that you will obtain. Many neurologic disorders can be differentiated by their temporal course. Precipitous onset suggests a vascular or epileptic etiology across a wide spectrum of complaints. Onset over minutes to hours suggests a toxic or infectious cause. Subacute or chronic progression of symptoms prompts investigation of metabolic, neoplastic, or degenerative disorders.

   The subsequent pattern of symptoms is also important. Symptoms that follow a paroxysmal course lead to a limited differential diagnosis: transient ischemic attack, migraine, and seizure are often considered when paroxysmal episodes are relatively short-lived. Myasthenia gravis, multiple sclerosis, and periodic paralysis have a fluctuating or recurrent course as well but typically with less rapid cycles.

3. **Characterization of the symptoms**

   It may seem excessive or inefficient to obtain a detailed description of your patient's symptoms, yet the initial disqualification of untenable diagnoses can be accomplished with confidence only when you are sure of the symptoms being reported. The mode of onset, prior occurrences, surrounding events, and character of the complaint (including what makes it better or worse) are important in establishing an initial differential diagnosis. You may need to ask more than once or use alternative terminology to elicit the details of a particular symptom. Notoriously ambiguous symptom descriptions in neurology include "heavy," which may mean weak, numb, or clumsy; "numb," which may mean decreased sensation or paresthesias; "dizzy," which may mean vertiginous, lightheaded, or confused; and "confused," which may mean disoriented, agitated, aphasic, or even sleepy. Also be wary of actual diagnoses that are presented in lieu of symptoms. The patient who keeps getting "seizures" in the arm or the one who presents with "trauma" should be redirected to a vocabulary of symptoms alone.

4. **Medical history**

Although a detailed medical history is not necessary in every interview, you will need to obtain information about any disease that could contribute to the patient's present complaint. For example, it is crucial to be aware of cerebrovascular risk factors including cardiac disease, hypertension, diabetes mellitus, and smoking if stroke is in the differential diagnosis. A history of carcinoma would be important if metastasis or paraneoplastic disease is considered. Some systemic illnesses, such as sarcoidosis, systemic lupus erythematosus, and diabetes mellitus, may be associated with a spectrum of neurologic complaints. Information regarding current medications should be elicited in every case. Travel and occupational history may be relevant, for example, when toxic and infectious etiologies are under consideration. If the patient cannot provide the necessary information, you may need to interview a family member or caretaker or review the patient's medical record.

ESTABLISHING THE INITIAL DIFFERENTIAL DIAGNOSIS

Neurologic complaints lend themselves to categorization of the differential diagnosis based on **anatomic localization.** Acute visual dysfunction, for example, may be divided into unilateral loss of vision (suggesting pathology in the retina or optic nerve), binocular visual field defects (implying disease in the optic tracts or radiations), or diplopia (suggesting either neuromuscular or brain stem dysfunction). Other neurologic complaints are best categorized initially by the **rate of onset.** The likely diagnoses related to acute ataxia, for instance, are different from those associated with chronic or subacute gait failure. The differential diagnosis for many neurologic complaints, however, contains a wide variety of disorders that are not easily sorted until more information is obtained from the history and physical examination. For these complaints, we suggest that you develop a standard method of considering the differential diagnosis. One mnemonic, which appears in many of our patient complaint chapters, may be useful: VITAMINS, representing vascular, infectious, traumatic, autoimmune, metabolic/toxic, iatrogenic/idiopathic or hereditary, neoplastic, and seizure/psychiatric/structural etiologies.

Anatomic Localization

The neurologic examination is presented in Chapter 2. Certain principles of anatomic localization warrant emphasis here because establishing the correct diagnosis in neurology is often dependent on localization of the lesion. Listed here in Boxes 1.1 to 1.4 are general principles of localization of lesions from the brain to the periphery. Most of these localizations are discussed within the pertinent chapters on **patient-related problems.**

BOX 1.1	**Localization in the Upper Motor Neuron (Pyramidal) System** *Principle: Tone Is Increased, Causing Spasticity and Hyperreflexia*	
Site	**Symptoms**	**Signs**
Cortex	• Differential weakness of limbs and face • Sensory symptoms • Language, visual, or attentional alterations	• Fractionated weakness (e.g., arm greater than face and leg) • Aphasia, hemianopia, or hemineglect • Cortical and primary sensory loss • Cognitive dysfunction
Corona radiata	• Differential weakness of limbs and face	• Fractionated weakness • Primary sensory loss
Internal capsule	• Weakness only	• Face, arm, and leg affected equally and densely
Brain stem	• Unilateral or bilateral weakness • Diplopia, vertigo, dysarthria, or weakness	• Dense hemiparesis • Ocular or oropharyngeal dysphagia • Motor posturing
Spinal cord	• Difficulty with gait • Difficulty walking • Urinary incontinence	• No face involvement • Spastic quadriparesis (cervical) or paraparesis (thoracic) • Sensory level

BOX 1.2	Localization in the Lower Motor Neuron System *Principle: Tone Is Decreased, Causing Flaccidity and Hyporeflexia*

Site	Symptoms	Signs
Anterior horn	• Progressive flaccid weakness	• Wasting, weakness, fasciculations • No sensory loss
Root/plexus	• Single-limb weakness and sensory loss • Pain in the neck, back, or limb	• Weakness in radicular/plexus distribution • EMG shows denervation in affected muscles
Nerve	• Focal weakness (mononeuritis) • Distal weakness (polyneuropathy)	• Focal or distal weakness • Atrophy in affected distribution • Fasciculations • Hyporeflexia • Slowing or low amplitude on conduction studies; denervation on EMG
Neuromuscular junction	• Fluctuating weakness • Diplopia	• Positive edrophonium test • Decremental response with repetitive stimulation on EMG
Muscle	• Proximal weakness • Difficulty climbing stairs and brushing hair • Muscle aches	• Proximal weakness • Polyphasic, low-amplitude motor units on EMG

EMG, Electromyogram.

BOX 1.3	Localization Within the Brain Stem **Principle: Specific Cranial Nerve Involvement Guides Localization (Fig. 1.1)**

Site	Signs and Symptoms
Midbrain	• Impaired vertical gaze • CN 3 palsy (plus contralateral abduction nystagmus suggests ipsilateral INO) • CN 4 palsy • Contralateral motor signs (hemiparesis suggests Weber syndrome; ataxia suggests Claude syndrome; tremor or chorea suggests Benedikt syndrome) • Alterations in consciousness, perception, or behavior (peduncular hallucinosis)
Pons	• Dysarthria and dysphagia • Contralateral hemiparesis or hemisensory loss • Ipsilateral facial sensory loss (CN 5) • Ipsilateral gaze palsy (PPRF) or one-and-a-half syndrome (PPRF and MLF) • Locked-in syndrome (bilateral basis pontis; associated with ocular bobbing) • Horizontal nystagmus (often brachium pontis) • Ataxia
Pontomedullary junction	• Vertigo (CN 8) • Dysarthria • Horizontal or vertical nystagmus • Contralateral hemisensory loss and hemiparesis
Lateral medulla (Wallenberg syndrome)	• Ipsilateral Horner syndrome • Ipsilateral limb ataxia • Ipsilateral face and contralateral body numbness • Gait ataxia • Vertigo, dizziness, nausea (CN 8) • Dysphagia (CN 9–CN 12 palsies)
Medial medulla (rare)	• Contralateral hemiplegia • Contralateral posterior column sensory loss • Ipsilateral tongue weakness (CN 12 palsy)

INO, Internuclear ophthalmoplegia; *MLF*, median longitudinal fasciculus; *PPRF*, paramedian pontine reticular formation

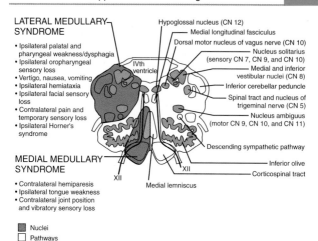

LATERAL MEDULLARY SYNDROME

- Ipsilateral palatal and pharyngeal weakness/dysphagia
- Ipsilateral oropharyngeal sensory loss
- Vertigo, nausea, vomiting
- Ipsilateral hemiataxia
- Ipsilateral facial sensory loss
- Contralateral pain and temporary sensory loss
- Ipsilateral Horner's syndrome

MEDIAL MEDULLARY SYNDROME

- Contralateral hemiparesis
- Ipsilateral tongue weakness
- Contralateral joint position and vibratory sensory loss

Hypoglossal nucleus (CN 12)
Medial longitudinal fasciculus
Dorsal motor nucleus of vagus nerve (CN 10)
Nucleus solitarius (sensory CN 7, CN 9, and CN 10)
Medial and inferior vestibular nuclei (CN 8)
Inferior cerebellar peduncle
Spinal tract and nucleus of trigeminal nerve (CN 5)
Nucleus ambiguus (motor CN 9, CN 10, and CN 11)
Descending sympathetic pathway
Inferior olive
Corticospinal tract
Medial lemniscus
IVth ventricle
XII

Nuclei
Pathways

FIG. 1.1 Brain stem sections at the level of the medulla.

BOX 1.4	**Localization in the Spinal Cord** *Principle: Localization Is Assisted by the* *Combination of Tracts Involved*

Site	Signs and Symptoms	Common Causes
Hemicord (Brown-Séquard syndrome)	• Ipsilateral hemiparesis • Contralateral spinothalamic sensory loss • Ipsilateral dorsal column sensory loss • Sphincter dysfunction	• Penetrating trauma • Extrinsic cord compression
Anterior cord	• Upper and lower motor paralysis • Spinothalamic sensory loss • Sphincter dysfunction • Sparing of posterior columns	• Anterior spinal artery infarction (often involves T4–T8)

Continued

BOX 1.4	Localization in the Spinal Cord—cont'd	

Site	Signs and Symptoms	Common Causes
Central cord	• Paraparesis • Lower motor paralysis; wasting and fasciculations in arms • Sensory loss in "shawl" distribution (if in cervical region)	• Syringomyelia • Neck flexion-extension injury • Intrinsic tumor
Posterior cord	• Proprioceptive and vibratory sensory loss • Segmental tingling and numbness • Sensation of constricting "bands"	• Vitamin B_{12} deficiency • Demyelination (multiple sclerosis) • Extrinsic compression
Foramen magnum	• Spastic quadriparesis • Neck pain and stiffness • C2–C4 and upper facial numbness • Ipsilateral Horner syndrome • Ipsilateral tongue and trapezius muscle weakness	• Tumor (meningioma, chordoma) • Atlantoaxial subluxation
Conus medullaris	• Lower sacral saddle sensory loss (S2–S5) • Sphincter dysfunction; impotence • Aching back or rectal pain • L5 and S1 motor deficits (ankle and foot weakness)	• Intrinsic tumor • Extrinsic cord compression
Cauda equina	• Sphincter dysfunction • Paraparesis with weakness in the distribution of multiple roots • Sensory loss in multiple bilateral dermatomes	• Extrinsic tumor • Carcinomatous meningitis • Arachnoiditis • Spinal stenosis

The Neurologic Examination

Clinical examination is of primary importance in the practice of neurology, even with the availability of advanced neuroimaging techniques. **This is because the neurologic examination provides critical information that no other test can provide, such as whether the patient's nervous system is working normally.** Unfortunately, many clinicians never master the neurologic examination because it is taught in a way that makes it seem time-consuming, excessively complicated, and of questionable relevance. In real on-call situations, however, expert neurologists almost never perform the type of comprehensive, top-to-bottom examination that is taught in medical school; rather, they focus on the problem at hand, eliminate those parts of the examination that are not relevant, and actively test hypotheses suggested by the history.

The intent of this chapter is to acquaint (or reacquaint) the physician with the basic components of the neurologic examination. Suggested problem-oriented examinations for specific clinical presentations (e.g., coma, back pain, acute weakness) are provided in later chapters.

The Neurologic Examination

The components of the neurologic examination are shown in Box 2.1.

MENTAL STATUS

The importance of the mental status examination cannot be over-emphasized. In patients with suspected intracranial pathology (e.g., in those experiencing sudden severe headache), a change in mental status signals that the problem is more than just one of pain: it indicates that the brain is not working correctly. The implications for further workup and management are significant.

BOX 2.1	Components of the Neurologic Examination

- For the beginner, even remembering all of the components of the neurologic exam can be difficult. Memorizing the first letter of the seven main sections of the exam (M C M C R S G) may be helpful for avoiding omissions when first learning the examination:
  - Mental status
  - Cranial nerves
  - Motor
  - Coordination
  - Reflexes
  - Sensory
  - Gait and station

Human mentation is extraordinarily complex, and students of neurology frequently have difficulty with the mental status (see Box 2.1) examination because they are taught to evaluate a "laundry list" of mental functions (Table 2.1) without emphasis on how to integrate the findings. To simplify the mental status examination, we advocate a five-step approach that emphasizes five basic elements: (1) alertness and attention; (2) confusion, disorientation, or abnormal behavior; (3) language; (4) memory; and (5) other higher cortical functions.

- **Step One: Examination of level of consciousness, attention, and concentration**

  As illustrated schematically in Fig. 2.1, the brain's arousal and attention mechanism (mediated by the diffuse cortical projections of the reticular activating system of the brain stem) serves as the foundation of all higher cognitive function. Level of consciousness, attention, and mental concentration can be conceptualized as three levels of a pyramid because dysfunction at a more basic level (depressed level of consciousness) almost guarantees that functions at the top of the pyramid (attention and concentration) will be abnormal. Similarly, if a patient cannot remain alert or attend or concentrate, normal functioning of memory, language, or other higher functions cannot be expected. *Delirium* is characterized by severe attentional deficits in a patient with relatively preserved alertness (mildly lethargic to hyperalert).

  1. **Level of consciousness.** *Is the patient alert, lethargic, stuporous, or comatose? Lethargy* resembles sleepiness but with one important difference: the patient cannot be fully and permanently awakened. *Stupor* can be operationally defined by the requirement for painful stimuli to obtain the patient's best verbal or motor response. *Coma* indicates lack of responsiveness even to painful stimuli.

TABLE 2.1	Mental Status: Emotional and Higher Cognitive Functions
Behavior	Is the patient's behavior appropriate, hostile, or bizarre?
Abstract reasoning	Can the patient judge similarities and interpret proverbs? Poor abstract reasoning results in "concrete thinking."
Insight	Does the patient have an appropriate understanding of the current medical problem?
Judgment	Is the patient's judgment impaired? Ask what the patient would do if he or she found a wallet or smelled smoke in a theater.
Calculations	Can the patient add, subtract, and multiply?
Visuospatial ability	Can the patient copy figures, draw a clock face, or bisect a line?
Praxis	Does the patient have apraxia, which is the inability to imitate or mime simple motor tasks, such as brushing your teeth (ideomotor apraxia), or conceptualize, plan, and execute a sequence of tasks, such as folding a letter and sealing in an envelope (ideational apraxia) in the absence of a comprehension, sensory, or motor deficit? Apraxia typically localizes to the dominant frontal or parietal lobe.
Affect	Is the patient's affect (an immediately expressed and observed emotion) depressed, euphoric, restricted, flat, or inappropriate?
Mood	What is the patient's long-term emotional disposition?
Thought form	Does the patient display loosening of associations, flight of ideas, tangentiality, circumstantiality, or incoherence? When seen in the absence of impaired level of consciousness, attention, memory, or language, thought disorders are characteristic of psychiatric illness.
Thought content	Is the patient's thought content characterized by paranoia, delusions, compulsions, obsessions, phobias, or derealization?
Perceptions	Does the patient have hallucinations or illusions?

2. **Attention.** *Is the patient attentive to you?* Global attention is impaired in patients who are lethargic or encephalopathic. A normally attentive patient looks at you and responds to questions and commands immediately. Inattention is characterized by impaired visual fixation and pursuit, delayed verbal responses requiring multiple prompts, and motor impersistence. *Spatial hemineglect* results from large hemispheric lesions and is almost always associated with impaired global attention as well (see Fig. 2.1).

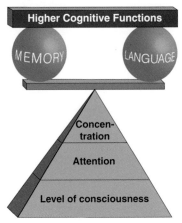

FIG. 2.1 Schematic representation of the basic elements of human cognition. Arousal mechanisms (level of consciousness, attention, and concentration) serve as the foundation of all mental activity. Language and memory are anatomically localized, highly developed basic cognitive modalities. All other higher cognitive functions depend on normal function of these three basic elements.

3. **Concentration.** *Can the patient count from 20 to 1 and recite the months in reverse?* These are relatively overlearned tasks and are less susceptible to the effects of prior education than are serial sevens. Abnormal responses include long pauses, omissions, and reversals.

- **Step Two: Assessment for disorientation, confusion, or a behavioral abnormality**

    This step is initially based on observation during history taking. *Behavior* should be assessed in terms of psychomotor activity (agitation versus abulia) and emotional responses (elation, sadness, anger, or flattening).

    1. **Formally test orientation to name, place, time (date, day of week, month, and year), and situation.** Disorientation reflects abnormal *integrative functioning* of the brain. Unlike abnormalities of arousal, memory, or language, disorientation has no implications regarding anatomic localization; there is no "orientation center" in the brain. *Remember that disorientation typically follows a sequential pattern, first involving situation, then time, place, and name.* Hence, a patient who is oriented to time and place but who does not know his or her own name probably has a psychiatric problem.

- **Step Three: Language testing**

   Focal lesions of the dominant hemisphere may lead to *aphasia,* which is defined as abnormal language production or comprehension. Four essential components of language should always be tested:

   1. **Fluency.** *Is the rate and flow of the patient's speech production normal?* Dysfluency is defined by reduction in the rate of speech production. Speaking with effort, finding words with difficulty, losing normal grammar and syntax, giving perseverative responses, and making spontaneous paraphasic errors are characteristic.

   2. **Comprehension.** *Can the patient perform one- and two-step commands?* If the patient is attentive, inability to follow commands implies impaired auditory comprehension.

   3. **Naming.** *Can the patient name a watch, a pen, and glasses?* Check for *anomia* and *paraphasic errors.* Listen for *phonemic paraphasias* (substitution of one phoneme for another, e.g., "tadle" for "table") and *semantic paraphasias* (substitution of one semantically related word for another, e.g., "door" for "window").

      Repetition. *Can the patient repeat "The train was an hour late" and "Today is a sunny day"?* Intact repetition in the presence of serious deficits in fluency or comprehension is diagnostic of *transcortical aphasia,* which implies a good prognosis for recovery. With the preceding information, fluency, comprehension, naming, and repetition, you can diagnose and classify any aphasia (Table 2.2). Asking the patient to read aloud is also a sensitive screening test

TABLE 2.2	Classification of Aphasias			
	Fluency	**Comprehension**	**Naming**	**Repetition**
Broca aphasia (motor)	0	+	0	0
Wernicke aphasia (sensory)	+	0	0	0
Transcortical motor aphasia	0	+	0	+
Transcortical sensory aphasia	+	0	0	+
Global aphasia	0	0	0	0
Conduction aphasia	+	+	0	0
Anomic aphasia	+	+	0	+

0, Abnormal; *+,* normal.

for aphasia and alexia. *Broca aphasia* (localized to the dorsolateral dominant frontal lobe) results in nonfluent, effortful speech and is usually associated with hemiparesis. *Wernicke aphasia* (localized to the posterior superior temporal lobe) leads to fluent, nonsensical speech with impaired comprehension, and in most cases, the patient is unaware of the problem (anosognosia). If an aphasia is present and more precise characterization of the deficit is desired, check reading and writing in detail. Do not confuse aphasia with *dysarthria,* which is a motor disorder.

- **Step Four: Memory testing**

    Memory is classified as **immediate, short term,** and **long term.** In neurologic patients, impaired immediate recall is usually caused by attentional deficits rather than by pure amnesia. Short-term memory can be tested by asking the patient to recall three words (e.g., "Jane, red, elephant") in 3 to 5 minutes. Long-term (remote) memory is best tested by asking about famous public figures (e.g., Ronald Reagan or Martin Luther King), major historical events (e.g., September 11th), or renowned sports figures (e.g., Muhammad Ali). *Confabulatory (incorrect)* responses occur with severe amnestic disorders, come quickly, and patients have no insight into the fact that they are totally confused.

- **Step Five: Testing for emotional and higher cognitive functions**

    These components of the mental status exam are listed in Table 2.1 and are usually not anatomically localizable and not essential to test in all cases. They are primarily of value for identifying complex cognitive and neuropsychiatric disorders.

CRANIAL NERVES

CN 1   Olfactory nerve

Testing for olfactory nerve function is rarely needed and is usually omitted.

CN 2   Optic nerve

1. **Fundus**

    Check for papilledema, optic disk pallor or atrophy, retinal hemorrhages or exudates, spontaneous venous pulsations, and hypertensive microvascular changes (arteriovenous [AV] nicking and copper wiring) (Fig. 2.2).

2. **Visual fields**

    Stand facing the patient, instruct him or her to look at your nose, and have the patient count fingers in all four quadrants (Fig. 2.3). Test each eye separately. Check lateralized blink to threat if the patient is inattentive.

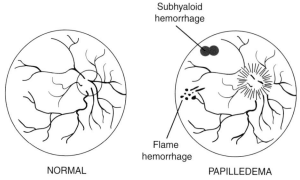

FIG. 2.2 Common abnormalities found on examination of the optic fundus. Papilledema is characterized by optic disk congestion and the loss of distinct vessels crossing the blurred disk margin.

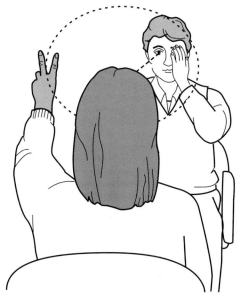

FIG. 2.3 Technique for visual field testing.

3. **Visual acuity**

Test acuity with eyeglasses, one eye at a time, using a pocket Snellen chart or "near card"

4. **Color vision**

This is usually tested only by an ophthalmologist. Color desaturation occurs with optic nerve disorders.

CN 3, 4, 6 Oculomotor, Trochlear, and Abducens nerves

1. **Eyelids**

Check for *ptosis,* which is defined as a drooping eyelid that does not clear the upper margin of the pupil. Ptosis occurs with oculomotor nerve (CN 3) injury or with *Horner syndrome* (ptosis, miosis, facial anhidrosis), which results from injury to central or peripheral sympathetic nerve pathways.

2. **Pupils**

Check for shape, symmetry, reactivity to light, and accommodation. *Anisocoria* (pupillary asymmetry) can result from *miosis* (an abnormally small pupil) or *mydriasis* (an abnormally large pupil), and in some cases, examination in both light and dark conditions is necessary to determine which pupil is abnormal.

An *afferent pupillary defect* (APD), or Marcus Gunn pupil, results from a lesion of the optic nerve (e.g., optic neuritis in multiple sclerosis). It is elicited using the swinging flashlight test: as the light swings from one eye to the other at 3-second intervals, the abnormal pupil will *dilate* rather than constrict when the light shines on it.

3. **Extraocular movements**

Ask the patient to fixate on and follow your finger in all directions of gaze. Unilateral impairment of ocular motility usually results from an isolated cranial nerve deficit. Along with checking for limitations of eye movement, look for abnormalities of *fixation* (square wave jerks, nystagmus, opsoclonus), *smooth pursuit* (saccadic pursuit), and *saccadic eye movements* (hypometric saccades, ocular dysmetria). Test saccades by asking the patient to rapidly switch fixation from one hand to the other.

Opticokinetic nystagmus (OKN) is a normal physiologic nystagmus that occurs when the patient is asked to fixate on a series of moving visual stimuli (e.g., striped OKN tape). Asymmetric loss of OKN results from frontal or parietal lobe lesions on the side to which the tape is moving.

CN 5 Trigeminal nerve

Sensory function of V1, V2, and V3 is evaluated by testing for deficits to light touch, pinprick, and temperature on the

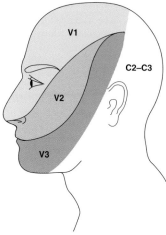

FIG. 2.4 Sensory distribution of the trigeminal nerve.

forehead, cheek, and chin, respectively (Fig. 2.4). Motor function can be tested by checking for asymmetry of lateral jaw movements. Lateral pterygoid muscle weakness results in ipsilateral deviation on jaw opening and weakness of lateral movement to the opposite side.

The *corneal reflex* (mediated by V1) is elicited by lightly touching the cornea with a cotton wisp, which results in contraction of the orbicularis oculi (CN 7). It usually needs to be tested only in comatose patients, or if focal brain stem or cranial nerve pathology (e.g., an acoustic neuroma) is suspected.

CN 7   Facial nerve

A *widened palpebral fissure* and *flattened nasolabial fold* are indicative of facial weakness. Ask the patient to grin and raise the eyebrows, and check the strength of eye and lip closure against active resistance. Upper motor neuron facial weakness tends to spare the contralateral forehead because it has bilateral upper motor neuron innervation, whereas the lower portion of the face does not.

Taste usually requires testing only when there is evidence of facial weakness. Dip a wet cotton swab in sugar or salt and apply it to the tip and side of the tongue with the tongue kept protruded. Absence of taste confirms a peripheral CN 7 lesion proximal to the junction of the chorda tympani.

CN 8 Vestibulocochlear nerve

Auditory deficits can be screened for by testing appreciation of *finger rub* in each ear. If unilateral hearing loss is present, sensorineural and conduction deafness can be differentiated using a 512-Hz tuning fork:

- *Weber test* is performed by striking the tuning fork and placing it against the middle of the forehead. Ask the patient if the tone is equal in both ears. Diminution in the affected ear indicates sensorineural hearing loss. A louder tone in the affected ear results from *conduction deafness* (disease of the ossicles in the middle ear). In conduction deafness, a pure tone transmitted through the skull is appreciated in the affected ear, whereas the tone sounds softer in the normal ear because of competing ambient noise transmitted via the tympanic membrane and ossicles.
- *The Rinne test* is performed to confirm the presence of conduction deafness in the affected ear. Strike the tuning fork, place it on the mastoid process, and ask the patient when the tone can no longer be heard. Then place it over the external auditory meatus. Normally, the patient will hear the tone again; if not, conduction deafness is present.

CN 9, 10 Glossopharyngeal and Vagus nerves

Ask the patient to say "ah," check for symmetry and adequacy of soft palate elevation, and listen for hoarseness or nasal speech (all motor functions of CN 10). The gag reflex, tested by lightly touching the posterior oropharynx with a cotton swab (CN 9 sensory, CN 10 motor), is often absent or depressed in older patients. *Dysphagia* and risk for aspiration are best screened for by asking the patient to swallow a small quantity of water (3 ounces); coughing indicates aspiration and inability to protect the airway.

CN 11 Spinal accessory nerve

Have the patient flex and turn the head to each side against resistance (tests the sternocleidomastoid muscle). Contraction of the left sternocleidomastoid muscle turns the head to the right and vice versa. Have the patient shrug the shoulders against resistance to test the trapezius muscle.

CN 12 Hypoglossal nerve

Have the patient stick out the tongue and push it into each cheek. Unilateral CN 12 dysfunction results in deviation of the tongue to the weak side on protrusion and in inability to push the tongue into the opposite cheek.

MOTOR

1. **Inspection**

   Look for *muscle wasting* (atrophy), *fasciculations,* and *adventitious movements.* Preferential spontaneous movement of the limbs on one side suggests paresis of the unused limbs. If the patient is comatose, check for a preferential localizing response to sternal rub.

   Tremor should be evaluated at rest (rest tremor), with sustained posture (postural tremor), and with active movement (action or intention tremor).

2. **Tone**

   Have the patient relax; check muscle tone by passively moving the elbows, wrists, and knees.

   a. **Hypotonia** occurs with acute paralysis, lower motor neuron disease, ipsilateral cerebellar lesions, and chorea.

   b. **Hypertonia** comes in three varieties:

      (1) **Spasticity** develops as a consequence of upper motor neuron lesions. It is generally characterized by a sudden increase in tone (a "catch") as the limb is passively flexed or extended. The clasp-knife phenomenon is a particular form of spasticity sometimes encountered in the legs; muscle tone is greatest at the beginning of movement and slowly decreases until there is a sudden loss of resistance.

      (2) **Rigidity** occurs with disease of the basal ganglia. Increased resistance is present throughout the full range of motion. *Cogwheel rigidity,* characterized by a regular ratchet-like loss of resistance, is especially characteristic of parkinsonism. Cogwheel rigidity at the wrist can often be accentuated if the patient is asked to repeatedly open and close the opposite hand.

      (3) **Gegenhalten** (holding against), or paratonia, occurs with dementia and frontal lobe syndromes. It is characterized by a variably and inconsistently increased tone that alternates with relaxation.

3. **Screening tests for hemiparesis**

   In many instances, cerebral lesions lead to subtle hemiparesis with normal strength against resistance. Check the following to screen for subtle indications of hemiparesis (Fig. 2.5):

   a. **Pronator drift**

      Have the patient hold both arms forward, palms up, with eyes closed. Check for pronation and downward drift.

   b. **Rapid finger taps**

      Check thumb and forefinger taps in each hand separately. Although often considered a sign of cerebellar dysfunction, slowing of fine rapid finger movements also occurs with corticospinal tract lesions.

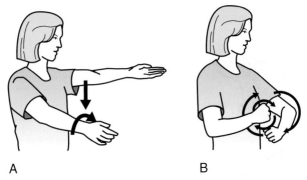

FIG. 2.5 Screening procedures for mild hemiparesis. (A) Pronator drift. The weaker right arm drifts downward and pronates. (B) Arm-rolling test. The stronger left arm tends to "orbit" the weaker right arm.

BOX 2.2	Muscle Strength Grading Scale
0	No muscle contraction detected
1	A barely detectable flicker or trace of contraction
2	Movement occurs only in the plane of gravity
3	Active movement against gravity but not against resistance
4	Active movement against resistance but less than normal strength (may be graded as 4+, 4, or 4−)
5	Normal strength

    c. **Arm-rolling test**

        Have the patient make fists and rotate the forearms around each other. With hemiparesis, the normal arm will tend to orbit the weaker arm.

4. **Power**

    Detailed testing of strength against active resistance in multiple individual muscle groups is usually unnecessary unless a peripheral cause of weakness is suspected. *For screening purposes, testing of strength at the shoulders, wrists, hips, and ankles will often suffice.* Be aware that estimates of lower extremity strength in bedridden patients are often unreliable and that walking is the best way to screen for leg weakness.

    By convention, muscle strength is graded as shown in Box 2.2.

COORDINATION

Disease of the cerebellar hemispheres leads to limb ataxia, whereas midline cerebellar lesions lead to gait ataxia. The following tests can be used to detect incoordination and ataxia.

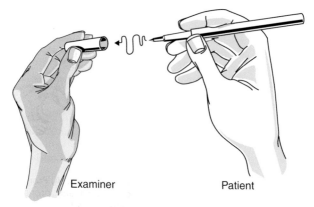

FIG. 2.6 Screening procedure for subtle dysmetria. Hold a pen cap, and look for an intention tremor as the patient tries to guide the pen into the cap.

1. **Finger-to-nose test**

   Have the patient alternately touch a fingertip to his or her nose and your finger. Check for intention tremor (irregular chaotic movements as the target is approached) and past pointing (often easier to elicit when the eyes are closed). Subtle dysmetria can be detected by holding the cap of a pen and having the patient slowly place the pen into the cap (Fig. 2.6).

2. **Rapid rhythmic alternating movements**

   Have the patient touch each of the fingers to the thumb in rapid succession, turn the hand over and back (pronation-supination) as fast as possible, and touch the toe and the heel to the floor in rapid succession. With cerebellar disease, these movements are slow and awkward *(dysdiadochokinesis)*.

3. **Heel-to-shin test**

   Have the patient slide the heel up and down the front of the shin. Limb ataxia results in a side-to-side "tremor" as the test is performed.

REFLEXES

1. **Deep tendon reflexes**

   Striking the muscle tendon with a reflex hammer normally leads to a reflex muscle contraction mediated by the lower motor neuron reflex arc. *Hyperreflexia* results from upper motor neuron lesions as a result of release from normal descending inhibition, whereas *hyporeflexia* results from lesions of the lower motor neuron. The principal deep tendon reflexes and their corresponding spinal roots are listed in .Table 2.3. Severe hyperreflexia results in *clonus,* which is repeated rhythmic contraction elicited by striking a tendon or dorsiflexing the ankle (see Table 2.3).

By convention, deep tendon reflexes are graded on a scale of 0 to 5 (Box 2.3).

2. **Plantar reflex**

Firmly stroke the sole of the patient's foot with the handle end of your reflex hammer, beginning at the heel and following up the lateral margin and across the ball of the foot to the base of the big toe. Flexion of the big toe at the metatarsophalangeal joint is the normal response; extension *(Babinski sign)* occurs with upper motor neuron lesions. If the patient is sensitive, lightly stroking the lateral heel alone is often enough to elicit a normal response.

3. Cutaneous reflexes

These reflexes do not require routine testing, but their testing is useful when a spinal cord or a cauda equina lesion is suspected. They are frequently absent in otherwise normal elderly or obese individuals. The presence of these reflexes implies

TABLE 2.3	Deep Tendon Reflexes
Reflex	**Segments**
Jaw jerk	Trigeminal nerve (CN 5)
Biceps reflex	C5 and C6
Brachioradialis reflex	C5 and C6
Triceps reflex	C7 and C8
Finger flexion (Hoffman) reflex	C8 and T1
Knee reflex	L2, L3, and L4
Ankle reflex	S1

BOX 2.3	Tendon Reflex Grading Scale
0	Absent
1	Diminished
2	Normal
3	Increased (may spread to adjacent muscles)
4	Unsustained clonus (a few beats)
5	Sustained clonus

normal function of the spinal cord and corresponding sensory and motor nerves at the level tested.

a. **Abdominal reflexes**

Use a key, wooden stick, or reflex hammer handle to lightly stroke from the lateral to the medial section of the abdomen above (T8-T9) and below (T11-T12) the umbilicus. The normal response is local contraction of the ipsilateral rectus abdominis muscle.

b. **Cremasteric reflex**

Striking the medial thigh (L1-L2) results in ipsilateral retraction of the scrotum (S1).

c. **Bulbocavernosus reflex and anal wink**

Squeezing the head of the penis (S2-S3) or stroking the perianal skin (S3-S4) results in reflex contraction of the external anal sphincter (S3-S4).

4. **Frontal release signs**

These primitive reflexes are typically seen with dementia or frontal lobe disease, but they may also occur in normal individuals.

a. **Snout, suck, and root reflexes**

These reflexes are elicited by lightly tapping the upper lip or the side of the mouth.

b. **Palmomental reflex**

Lightly stroking the palm results in ipsilateral contraction of the mentalis muscle. A unilateral palmomental contraction implies contralateral frontal lobe disease.

c. **Grasp reflex**

Placing two fingers in the palm results in involuntary grasping.

d. **Glabellar reflex**

Obligatory blinking occurs each time the glabellar area between the eyes is tapped.

SENSORY

Sensory testing, because of its subjectivity, is the most difficult and least reliable part of the neurologic examination. In patients with depressed level of consciousness or severe inattention, sensory testing usually provides little useful information and should be omitted. In most cases, testing for signs of sensory loss is unnecessary unless the patient has symptoms of sensory loss. **The key to a successful and efficient sensory examination is to know what you're looking for.** Sensory loss typically occurs in specific patterns, which you should try to rule in or rule out (Box 2.4).

A few simple rules can help make the sensory examination easier and are noted in Box 2.5.

BOX 2.4	Patterns of Sensory Loss

- Hemisensory loss (cortical lesions)
- Stocking-glove sensory loss (neuropathy)
- Spinal level and Brown-Séquard syndrome (spinal cord lesions)
- Dermatomal sensory loss (nerve root lesions)
- Peripheral nerve sensory loss (mononeuropathy)
- Saddle anesthesia (lesion in cauda equina or conus medullaris)

BOX 2.5	Rules for Sensory Examination

1. *Do not ask leading questions.*
   When testing for hemisensory loss, ask "Does this feel the same on both sides?" If you ask "Which side feels sharper?," you are likely to get inconsistent (and insignificant) lateralizing responses.
2. *When mapping a region of sensory loss, move from the affected into the normal region.*
   Patients are better able to detect when a pinprick turns sharp than when it becomes dull.
3. *Beware of fatigue.*
   Cooperation in the sensory examination takes concentration, and patients may become fatigued. Rather than taking a thorough, top-to-bottom approach, start your sensory examination by getting right to the point.

1. **Primary sensory modalities**

   Sensation is mediated by two pathways: the dorsal columns, which mediate vibration and joint position; and the spinothalamic tracts, which mediate pain and temperature. Touch is mediated by both sensory pathways and is usually the last modality to be affected.

   a. **Light touch**

      Test by lightly touching with fingertips or cotton wool. *Allodynia* refers to pain in response to a normally nonpainful stimulus (e.g., light touch).

   b. **Pinprick**

      Use a clean safety pin. *Hyperalgesia* refers to an exaggerated painful sensation; *hyperpathia* refers to an abnormal painful sensation (e.g., burning, tingling).

   c. **Temperature**

      Test with the handle of a reflex hammer or tuning fork submerged under cold tap water.

   d. **Vibration**

      Apply a 128-Hz tuning fork to the toes, medial malleolus, patella, fingers, wrist, and elbow, and ask when the sensation stops. In the elderly, vibration is commonly absent or reduced in the feet.

e. **Joint position (proprioception)**

Grasp the sides of the digit and ask the patient to identify small (5–10 degrees), random, up or down movements. Remember that even with complete proprioceptive loss, 50% of responses will be correct!

2. **Cortical sensory modalities**

If the primary sensory modalities are intact, disturbances of these modalities imply dysfunction of the contralateral parietal lobe. *The main utility of cortical sensory testing is for the detection of subtle hemisensory neglect.*

a. **Double simultaneous stimulation (face–hand test)**

Have the patient close the eyes; quickly touch one cheek and the contralateral hand at the same time. *Extinction* refers to consistent neglect of the hand stimulus on one side and implies a lesion of the contralateral parietal lobe. *Caudal neglect* refers to the tendency to consistently neglect the hand stimulus on either side; it occurs with dementia and frontal lobe disease.

b. **Graphesthesia**

Have the patient close the eyes and identify a number traced on the palm.

c. **Stereognosis**

Ask the patient to close the eyes and identify a key, coin, paperclip, or similar object placed in the palm.

GAIT AND STATION

Disturbances of gait can result from dysfunction in one of many neurologic subsystems, including the motor cortex, corticospinal tracts, basal ganglia, cerebellum, vestibular system, peripheral nerves, muscles, and visual and proprioceptive afferent tracts (Table 2.4). **Hence, gait testing is an excellent screening procedure, and many practitioners make it the first part of the neurologic examination.**

Specific components of gait analysis include *posture, width of stance, length of stride, arm swing,* and *balance.* Specific types of gait disturbance are listed in Table 2.4. Test the following:

1. **Natural gait**
2. **Tandem gait**

Have the patient walk a straight line, touching toe to heel.

3. **Toe walking**
4. **Heel walking**
5. **Sitting to standing**

TABLE 2.4	Some Abnormalities of Gait

Gait	Features
Hemiparetic	Patient drags or circumducts the affected leg (moves stiffly in a circular motion outward and forward) and has a reduced ipsilateral arm swing
Ataxic	Patient has a wide-based stance with a veering and staggering gait; patient may consistently fall to the same side as the affected cerebellum
Parkinsonian	Patient has a stooped posture, takes small steps (festination), hesitates and freezes, and turns "en bloc"
Steppage	Patient lifts the knee high off the ground because of inability to dorsiflex at the ankle; patient has foot slap (results from peripheral neuropathy)
Waddling	Patient's pelvis drops on non–weight-bearing side with each step (results from myopathy with hip girdle weakness)
Scissor	Patient's gait is stiff, with short steps that cross forward on each other (results from spastic paraparesis)
Apraxic	Patient's gait is slow and unsteady; patient has trouble initiating steps, and the feet barely elevate off the floor (i.e., "magnetic gait") (results from hydrocephalus or frontal lobe disease)
Hysterical	Patient has a bizarre, wild, careening gait but never falls; patient shows excellent balance

To assess proximal leg strength, have the patient stand up from a chair with the arms folded.

6. **Romberg test**

Have the patient stand with eyes open and feet together. If the patient cannot do so, suspect a severe cerebellar or vestibular disturbance. *If substantial instability or falling occurs only after the patient closes the eyes, then the Romberg test is positive.* A positive test indicates either *proprioceptive* (i.e., neuropathy or dorsal column disease) or *vestibular* dysfunction.

7. **Pull test**

Stand behind the patient and pull back on the shoulders. Normally, the patient should be able to regain balance after one step. Falling or retropulsion (many backward steps) suggests *impaired postural reflexes,* which occurs with Parkinsonism.

Diagnostic Studies

A thorough history and examination should enable you to localize the disease process and generate a differential diagnosis. Confirmation of the diagnosis will usually require neurodiagnostic testing. When any of the tests described here is performed, it is essential to know what you are looking for and to understand the sensitivity (likelihood of a true positive result if the disease is present) and specificity (likelihood of a true negative result if the disease is absent) of each test for diagnosing the disease in question. Risks, benefits, and cost must also be considered.

LUMBAR PUNCTURE

Examination of the cerebrospinal fluid (CSF) by lumbar puncture (LP) is essential for diagnosing meningitis and subarachnoid hemorrhage when computed tomography (CT) is negative. It also can be helpful in evaluating peripheral neuropathy, carcinomatous meningitis, pseudotumor cerebri, multiple sclerosis (MS), and a variety of other inflammatory disorders.

- **Technique of LP**

  Proper positioning is the key to success (Fig. 3.1). Position the patient's back at the edge of the bed, with the head flexed and the legs curled up in the fetal position. Place a pillow under the head; it may be helpful to place another pillow between the legs. *Ensure that the shoulders and hips are parallel to each other and perpendicular to the bed* (i.e., not tilted forward). Locate the interspace between L4 and L5, which lies at the intercristal line (across the tops of the iliac crests), and insert the needle one level above, between L3 and L4. After sterilizing the area and locally injecting 2% lidocaine, insert a 20-gauge or 22-gauge needle, parallel to the bed and tilted slightly cephalad. As you enter the subarachnoid space, you will feel a slight "pop." Measure the opening pressure and collect the CSF.

- **Examination of the CSF**

  This examination should always include a cell count (2 mL), protein and glucose analysis (2 mL), a Gram stain and culture

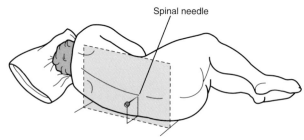

FIG. 3.1 Positioning for lumbar puncture. A pillow should be placed beneath the head. Hips and shoulders should be parallel to each other and perpendicular to the bed. The spinal needle should be parallel to the bed.

TABLE 3.1	Cerebrospinal Fluid Tests

- Cell count
- Protein and glucose levels
- Gram stain and culture
- VDRL test
- India ink test (for *Cryptococcus neoformans*)
- Wet smear (for fungi and amebae)
- Stain and culture for AFB (for tuberculosis)
- Cryptococcal antigen titers
- pH and lactate levels (abnormal in MELAS)
- Oligoclonal bands (abnormal in multiple sclerosis)
- IgG index (intrathecal IgG production)
- IgG and IgM viral antibody studies
- Latex agglutination bacterial antigen tests (for pneumococcus, meningococcus, and *Haemophilus influenzae*)
- Viral isolation studies
- Cytology (requires fixation in formalin)
- Lyme disease antibody titers (compare with serum titers) and Western blot
- Polymerase chain reaction for Lyme disease, tuberculosis, and causes of viral encephalitis
- 13-9-9 protein and RT-QuIC (elevated in Creutzfeldt-Jakob disease)

AFB, Acid-fast bacteria; *Ig,* immunoglobulin; *MELAS,* mitochondrial encephalomyopathy, lactic acidosis, and stroke; *RT-QuIC,* real-time quaking-induced conversion; *VDRL,* Venereal Disease Research Laboratory.

(2 mL), and a CSF Venereal Disease Research Laboratory (VDRL) test (1 mL). Additional CSF tests are listed in Table 3.1. If red blood cells (RBCs) are encountered, check for xanthochromia, which is a yellowish tinge that differentiates true subarachnoid hemorrhage (>12 hours old) from a

traumatic tap. To evaluate the significance of white blood cells (WBCs) in a traumatic tap, recall that the normal ratio of WBCs to RBCs in peripheral blood is 1:700.

- **Complications of LP**

    The most frequent complication (in approximately 5% of patients) of LP is *spinal headache,* which results from persistent leakage of CSF from the entry site, leading to low intracranial pressure (ICP) and traction on the pain-sensitive intracranial dura when the patient is upright. The risk is minimized by using a thin (22-gauge) pencil-tipped spinal needle with a side hole (Sprotte or Gertie Marx), as opposed to a conventional bevel-tipped end hole (Quincke) spinal needle. Other complications are rare and occur only in patients with predisposing conditions: (1) *meningitis* can result if the needle is passed through infected tissue (e.g., cellulitis) before penetrating the dura; (2) *epidural hematoma* with compression of the cauda equina can result in patients with coagulopathy; (3) *tentorial herniation* can result in patients who have space-occupying lesions or severe basilar meningitis; and (4) *complete spinal block* and cord compression can result in patients who have a partial spinal block. These predisposing conditions are relative (not absolute) contraindications to LP, and the risk/benefit ratio of performing or not performing the procedure must be considered in each case.

Computed Tomography

CT provides "slice" images of the brain by sending axial X-ray beams through the head. The amount of radiation involved is essentially harmless. Tissues are differentiated by the degree to which they attenuate the X-ray beams:

Low attenuation (appears black)	Air (darkest) Fat Water
Medium attenuation (appears gray)	Edematous or infarcted brain Normal brain Subacute hemorrhage (3–14 days old)
High attenuation (appears white)	Acute hemorrhage Intravenous contrast material Bone or metal (brightest)

- **Intravenous contrast**

    When injected, contrast material is normally confined to the cerebral vessels. Hence, *contrast enhancement detects the presence of a disrupted blood–brain barrier.* Contrast is useful in patients with suspected neoplasm, abscess, vascular malformation, or new-onset seizures.

- **CT perfusion imaging**

    Single or multislice CT perfusion scans are obtained after an intravenous (IV) contrast bolus is injected via an 18-gauge IV. The images must be reconstructed using computerized software. Color-coded maps of cerebral blood flow, cerebral blood volume, and mean transit time can be obtained. The main utility of CT perfusion imaging is to demonstrate a region of non-infarcted hypoperfused brain in patients with acute ischemic stroke or subarachnoid hemorrhage.

- **CT angiography**

    After an IV contrast bolus and computerized image reconstruction, these three-dimensional images can provide good to excellent resolution of the cervical and large proximal intracranial arteries (Fig. 3.2). The main utility of CT angiography is for the diagnosis of extracranial carotid stenosis, proximal intracranial stenoses or occlusions, and saccular intracranial aneurysms. Beware that resolution of the distal vasculature for detecting more subtle lesions such as vasculitic beading, a mycotic aneurysm, or a dural arteriovenous fistula is limited.

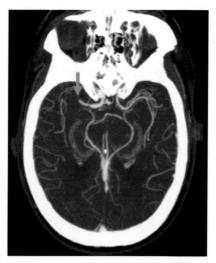

FIG. 3.2 Computed tomography angiogram corresponding to a right middle cerebral artery occlusion

Magnetic Resonance Imaging

Magnetic resonance imaging (MRI) provides greater resolution and detail than does CT but takes longer to perform. MRI is superior to CT for evaluating the brain stem and posterior fossa and is superior to myelography for identifying intramedullary spinal cord lesions. Because it uses a powerful magnetic field, there is no exposure to radiation. However, MRI is contraindicated in patients with implanted ferromagnetic objects such as pacemakers, orthopedic pins, and older aneurysm clips.

- **T1 images**

  T1 images (TE [echo time] < 50 ms, TR [repetition time] < 100 ms) are best for showing *anatomy*. CSF and bone appear black, normal brain appears gray, and fat and subacute blood (>48 hours old) appears white. Most pathologic processes (e.g., infarction, tumor) are associated with increased water content and hence appear darker than normal brain. *Fat suppression T1 images* are useful for identifying intramural thrombus (appears white) in cases of cervicocranial arterial dissection.

- **T2 and fluid attenuation inversion recovery (FLAIR) images**

  T2 (TE >80 ms, TR >2000 ms) and FLAIR images are best for showing *pathology*. Most pathologic processes (e.g., infarction, tumor) lead to bright high-signal (white) changes, which reflect increased tissue water content. FLAIR is somewhat more sensitive than T2 in general; the CSF appears dark on FLAIR but bright on T2. Blood on T2 varies in signal intensity according to the age of the hemorrhage, as depicted in Table 3.2.

- **Diffusion-weighted imaging**

  Diffusion-weighted imaging (DWI) is useful for detecting *hyperacute ischemia* in patients with acute stroke. Cerebral

TABLE 3.2	Evolution of Appearance of Hemorrhage on Magnetic Resonance Imaging		
Feature	**T1 Image**	**T2 Image**	**Metabolic Change**
Blood			
4–6 hours	No change	○	Intact RBC with oxyhemoglobin
7–72 hours	No change	●	Intact RBC with deoxyhemoglobin
4–7 days	○	●	Intact RBC with methemoglobin
1–4 weeks	○	○	Free methemoglobin
Months	●	●	Hemosiderin with macrophages
Edema	●	○	Increased water content

●, Low signal, appears dark; ○, high signal, appears bright; *RBC*, red blood cell.

ischemia produces an immediate reduction in the diffusion coefficient of water, resulting in high-intensity (white or bright) signal changes on these images within minutes. Over several hours, DWI lesions become associated with high-intensity lesions seen on T2 and FLAIR as the ischemic tissue progresses to infarction. "T2 shine-through" refers to the tendency for high-intensity T2 lesions to produce increased signal on DWI, falsely indicating reduced diffusion.

- **Apparent diffusion coefficient (ADC) maps**

    Compared with DWI, ADC maps are a purer image of restricted diffusion caused by ischemia and cytotoxic edema. ADC maps are mathematically calculated (hence they have lower sharpness and resolution) to have T2 shine-through effects removed. *Restricted diffusion caused by ischemia appears black or dark on ADC.* A bright region on DWI corresponding with a bright region on ADC is consistent with vasogenic edema.

- **Proton density images**

    Proton density images are partway between T1 and T2 images in signal density. Their main utility is for differentiating periventricular pathology (e.g., white matter demyelination) from CSF.

- **Short tau inversion recovery (STIR) sequences**

    STIR sequences allow summation of T1 and T2 signals and dropout of fat. They are useful for evaluating mesial temporal sclerosis in patients with epilepsy.

- **Flow voids**

    Flow voids appear black on both T1 and T2 images, and they represent high-velocity blood flow (e.g., normal cerebral vessels or arteriovenous malformation [AVM]).

- **Magnetic resonance angiography (MRA)**

    MRA produces images of the extracranial and intracranial cerebral circulation with the brain and skull "subtracted out." The resolution is adequate for the evaluation of large-scale lesions (e.g., internal carotid artery [ICA] stenosis and large aneurysms) but is inferior to standard angiography for evaluating smaller lesions (e.g., beading, distal spasm). *Time-resolved contrast-enhanced MRA* offers improved resolution over conventional MRA, particularly for evaluating high-grade stenosis of the cervical arteries.

- **MR venography**

    MR venography provides subtraction images of the major venous sinuses. It can be useful for diagnosing dural sinus thrombosis but is less sensitive than angiography for detecting cortical vein thrombosis.

Myelography

Myelography consists of injecting radiopaque dye into the spinal canal via either a lumbar or a suboccipital approach. After the patient is tilted, X-rays and axial CT slices allow visualization of the spinal subarachnoid space and can reveal extradural compressive lesions, ruptured intervertebral disks, and vascular malformations on the surface of the cord. In recent years, this test has been largely supplanted by MRI; however, myelography can still be useful if MRI is equivocal, and it remains essential for ruling out cord compression if MRI is not available. Complications are generally the same as those associated with LP.

Doppler Ultrasonography

- **Carotid duplex Doppler ultrasonography**

    This imaging technique can provide an accurate and noninvasive estimate of the degree of stenosis of the extracranial internal carotid arteries. B-mode ultrasonography gives a graphic image of the arterial wall and can detect plaques, whereas pulsed Doppler ultrasonography analyzes velocity and turbulence related to stenosis. Results are generally classified as (1) normal, (2) <40% stenosis, (3) 40% to 60% stenosis, (4) 60% to 80% stenosis, (5) 80% to 99% stenosis, and (6) occlusion. If carotid Doppler scans suggest occlusion, then confirmation with angiography is required because high-grade stenosis cannot be ruled out in all cases. Positioning of the transducer over the posterior neck can also differentiate normal, high-resistance, and absent flow in the proximal vertebral arteries.

- **Transcranial Doppler (TCD) ultrasonography**

    This technique measures the velocity of blood flow in the intracranial proximal cerebral arteries (ICA siphon, middle cerebral artery [MCA], anterior cerebral artery [ACA], posterior cerebral artery [PCA], ophthalmic, basilar, and vertebral). The main parameters obtained by TCD ultrasonography are blood flow velocity and pulsatility. TCD ultrasonography can be useful for the following:

    1. Diagnosing intracranial stenosis or occlusion
    2. Evaluating the hemodynamic significance of carotid stenosis or occlusion (look for blunted poststenotic flow in the MCA and reversed collateral flow in the ACA or ophthalmic artery)
    3. Assessing vasospasm in patients with subarachnoid hemorrhage (high-velocity flow)
    4. Screening for AVMs (high-velocity flow, very low pulsatility)

5. Identifying severely increased ICP (low-velocity flow, high pulsatility)
6. Diagnosing brain death (systolic spikes with absent diastolic flow)

Angiography

Cerebral angiography provides high-resolution images of the extracranial and intracranial cerebral vasculature (Fig. 3.3). Angiography has also become an increasingly important therapeutic modality for the treatment of stroke. The procedure is performed by threading a small catheter into the cerebral vessels via the femoral artery. Angiography is useful for identifying the following:

1. Occluded or stenotic vessels
2. Arterial dissections
3. Aneurysms
4. AVMs
5. Vasculitic narrowing ("beading")
6. Dural venous sinus thrombosis

- **Complications of angiography**

   Although infection or bleeding at the puncture site can occur, the most important complication (in 1%–2% of patients) is stroke, which results from emboli generated by the catheter, and which occurs most frequently in older patients with atherosclerotic disease.

Electromyography and Nerve Conduction Studies

Electromyography (EMG) and nerve conduction studies assess the integrity and function of muscle and nerve, respectively, and essentially serve as extensions of the clinical examination.

- **EMG**

   This test can help distinguish neuropathic from myopathic disease, define the precise distribution of muscle involvement, and aid in the diagnosis of specific muscle disorders with unique features (e.g., myotonia). The procedure is performed by inserting a needle electrode into a muscle and analyzing motor unit potentials, both at rest (spontaneous activity) and with varying degrees of muscle contraction. The following parameters are analyzed:

1. **Insertional activity.** Excessive insertional activity is seen in both neuropathic and myopathic disease and hence is nonspecific.
2. **Spontaneous activity.** Normal muscle is electrically silent. Spontaneous muscle fiber contractions (*fibrillation potentials* and *positive sharp waves)* and spontaneous motor unit discharges (*fasciculations)* usually signify muscle denervation.

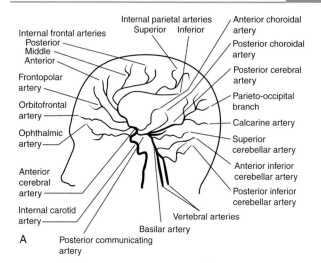

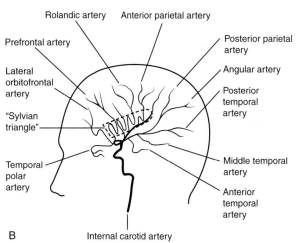

FIG. 3.3 Diagram of a lateral cerebral angiogram. (A) Anterior cerebral and posterior cerebral arteries. (B) Middle cerebral artery.

After an acute nerve injury (e.g., disk herniation and nerve root compression), spontaneous activity usually takes 2 weeks to appear. *Paraspinal muscle denervation* implies nerve root injury as opposed to more distal lesions of the plexus or peripheral nerve. *Myotonia* is a special form of continuous motor unit activity characterized by high-frequency waxing and waning discharges, producing a "dive bomber" sound.

3. **Motor unit potential.** This parameter can differentiate myopathy from denervation. Neuropathic features reflect reinnervation of previously denervated motor units, resulting in *high-amplitude, polyphasic potentials*. Myopathic features reflect loss of muscle fiber mass, resulting in *low-amplitude, polyphasic potentials of short duration*.

4. **Recruitment pattern.** Voluntary muscle contraction leads to progressive recruitment of motor units and to a dense interference pattern that completely obliterates the baseline. In neuropathic disease there are fewer motor units in the affected muscle, resulting in a *reduced* or *discrete recruitment* of motor units. Myopathic disease, with random loss of muscle fibers, leads to *early recruitment* and a *low-amplitude interference pattern*.

5. **Single-fiber EMG (SFEMG).** This technique examines the temporal relationship between firing of single muscle fibers innervated by the same motor neuron. Impaired neuromuscular transmission (e.g., in myasthenia gravis) results in a varying interval, referred to as "jitter."

- **Nerve conduction studies**

  Nerve conduction studies can be performed on motor or sensory nerves. The procedure is performed by applying electrical stimulation to skin sites overlying a peripheral nerve and recording the speed of conduction and amplitude of the "downstream" action potential. The following parameters are analyzed:

  1. **Conduction velocity.** This is generally reduced (<60% of normal) in demyelinating neuropathy. *Conduction block* reflects focal demyelination and is identified when nerve stimulation proximal to the block leads to a compound muscle action potential (CMAP) amplitude that is less than 50% of that obtained by stimulating distal to the block.

  2. **Amplitude.** The amplitude of the CMAP correlates with the number of muscle fibers activated by stimulation of the peripheral nerve. In general, reduced CMAP amplitude with relatively preserved conduction velocity is characteristic of *axonal neuropathy*.

  3. **Late responses.** *F waves* result from antidromic conduction followed by orthodromic conduction in the same nerve. Delayed or absent F waves, in combination with normal peripheral nerve conduction, implies disease of the proximal nerve (e.g., root compression, early Guillain-Barré

syndrome). The *H reflex* is the electrical counterpart of the ankle jerk and can be performed to assess the integrity of the S1 root; the antidromic potential travels down a sensory nerve, synapses in the spinal cord, and then travels orthodromically down a motor nerve.

4. **Repetitive stimulation.** Muscle responses to repetitive stimulation are useful for assessing neuromuscular junction disease. In myasthenia gravis (see Chapter 16), repetitive stimulation at 2 to 3 Hz produces a characteristic *decremental response* (>10% drop in amplitude between the first and the fifth CMAP).

Electroencephalography

Electroencephalography (EEG) provides a multichannel recording of the surface electrical activity of the brain. Background rhythms (Fig. 3.4) are analyzed regarding amplitude and frequency (delta waves, <4 Hz; theta waves, 4–7 Hz; alpha waves, 8–13 Hz; and beta waves, >13 Hz). In the awake, normal adult, a posterior dominant alpha rhythm is detected when the eyes are closed and the patient is in a relaxed state. Sleep results in characteristic sequential changes (progressive slowing, vertex transients, sleep spindles, and K complexes) that reflect highly organized synchronous activity. The primary utility of a conventional 20- to 40-minute EEG examination is for evaluating epileptiform disorders.

Continuous 24-hour EEG (cEEG) over a period of one or more days is rapidly replacing briefer conventional EEG examinations for hospitalized patients because it is vastly more sensitive for detecting nonconvulsive electrographic seizure activity. In the intensive care unit, long-term monitoring with cEEG is mandatory

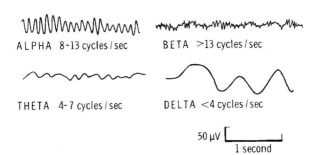

ALPHA 8–13 cycles/sec

BETA >13 cycles/sec

THETA 4–7 cycles/sec

DELTA <4 cycles/sec

50 μV

1 second

FIG. 3.4 Basic electroencephalography rhythms. (From Solomon GE, Kutt H, Plum F. *Clinical Management of Seizures.* 2nd ed. Philadelphia, PA: WB Saunders; 1983.)

for titrating therapy in stuporous or comatose patients with refractory nonconvulsive status epilepticus. Routine surveillance cEEG is also increasingly being used for the general evaluation of comatose states; with 48 hours of monitoring, otherwise undetectable electrographic seizure activity can be detected in 10% to 30% of patients (see Chapter 4).

- **Seizure disorders**

  The main value of EEG in patients with epilepsy is for detecting *interictal epileptiform activity* (isolated spikes and sharp waves). Focal epileptiform activity reflects a single irritative focus and corresponds with partial-onset seizures, whereas paroxysmal spike-and-wave discharges of diffuse origin correspond with generalized-onset seizures (Fig. 3.5). The absence of epileptiform discharges does not rule out a seizure disorder, however, because 20% to 40% of EEG recordings in patients with epilepsy appear normal. Sleep, sleep deprivation, hyperventilation, and photostimulation can be used to elicit epileptiform activity or

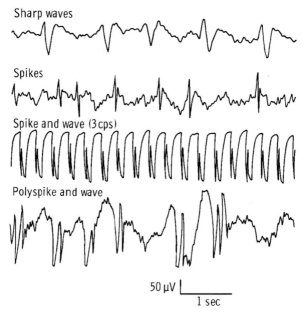

FIG. 3.5 Paroxysmal electroencephalography patterns seen in patients with epilepsy. (From Solomon GE, Kutt H, Plum F. *Clinical Management of Seizures.* 2nd ed. Philadelphia, PA: WB Saunders; 1983.)

absence seizures, and they are collectively referred to as activation procedures. *Electrographic seizures are characterized by the distinct onset, evolution, and offset of rhythmic spikes, sharp waves, or ictal-appearing discharges, lasting at least 10 seconds.* Electrographic seizures typically evolve regarding frequency, amplitude, location, or morphology. cEEG is essential for confirming the diagnosis of *nonconvulsive status epilepticus* (complex-partial or absence status) in patients with prolonged postictal or otherwise unexplained impairment of consciousness.

- **Evaluation of stupor and coma**

  Diffuse background slowing (in the range of theta and delta waves) is an almost universal finding in patients with impaired level of consciousness of any cause. In patients with focal lesions (e.g., stroke or brain tumor), the slowing is usually more pronounced in the ipsilateral hemisphere. In patients with coma of unknown etiology, cEEG may be particularly helpful both for detecting nonconvulsive seizure activity or for showing unique background patterns that can point to a specific diagnosis:

  1. **Periodic epileptiform discharges (PEDs).** These discharges can occur with large destructive lesions of any type or in the aftermath of focal seizure activity. Although PEDS are not generally believed to represent ictal activity per se, in some cases of prolonged nonconvulsive status epilepticus, intermittent or evolving runs of high-frequency PEDs (>2 Hz) may reflect ongoing seizures; otherwise they should not be treated aggressively. PEDs can be further categorized as lateralized (LPEDs), bilateral and independent (BiPEDs), or generalized (GPEDs). When PEDs are identified, it means that the patient is at increased risk for having additional seizures on long-term cEEG.

  2. **Triphasic waves.** These are nonspecific but can occur with high frequency in patients with metabolic encephalopathy (e.g., in hepatic, renal, and pulmonary failure).

  3. **Beta activity.** Combined with diffuse slowing suggests intoxication with barbiturates, benzodiazepines, or other sedative-hypnotic drugs.

  4. **Pseudoperiodic discharges.** Consisting of repeated but irregular bisynchronous bursts of high-amplitude, sharp waves are characteristic of subacute sclerosing panencephalitis (SSPE) and Jakob-Creutzfeldt disease.

  5. **Stimulus-induced rhythmic, periodic, or ictal discharges (SIRPIDs).** These are a phenomenon unique to coma in which noxious stimuli (such as squeezing a fingernail) result

in brief, nonsustained run of high-amplitude rhythmic activity, PEDs, or an ictal-appearing discharge. The cause appears to be hyperexcitable cortex, and they most often occur in postictal coma. SIRPIDs are identified in approximately 10% of comatose patients. Their prognostic significance remains unclear.

- **Prognosis in coma**

  In hypoxic-ischemic coma, prognosis for recovery of consciousness is related to the severity of slowing and attenuation of the background rhythm. A *burst-suppression pattern, diffuse low-amplitude attenuation, lack of reactivity,* and *electrographic seizures* imply a poor prognosis after cardiac arrest and other causes of coma. Keep in mind, however, that prognosis is usually related more to the cause of coma than to the depth of coma. *Alpha coma* and *spindle coma patterns* tend to occur with brain stem coma, are usually associated with lack of reactivity to stimuli, and portend a poor prognosis.

- **Brain death**

  .Electrocerebral silence can be used as a confirmatory test for brain death (see Chapter 19).

Evoked Potentials

Evoked potentials provide a recording of electrical activity in central sensory pathways produced by visual, auditory, or sensory stimulation. Signals are recorded by placing electrodes over the scalp or the spine and using a computer to average and amplify the signal, which results in a characteristic pattern of waveform peaks that have approximate anatomic correlates. There are three types of evoked potential studies:

- **Visual evoked responses (VERs)**

  The visual stimulus is delivered as an alternating checkerboard pattern or a stroboscopic flash; the waveform corresponds with stimulation of the occipital cortex.

- **Brain stem auditory evoked responses (BAERs)**

  Auditory signals are delivered by clicks through earphones. The waveform corresponds with stimulation of CN 8, the cochlear nucleus, pons, and inferior colliculus.

- **Somatosensory evoked potentials (SSEPs)**

  Electrical stimuli are delivered to peripheral nerves. The waveform corresponds with stimulation of the lumbosacral or the brachial plexus, the cervicomedullary dorsal column nuclei, and the sensory cortex (the N20 potential).

  The uses of evoked potentials in clinical practice are as follows:

1. **Multiple sclerosis.** Evoked potentials can be used to support the diagnosis in a patient with a single symptom by identifying

subclinical demyelination at a different anatomic site (e.g., abnormal VERs in a patient with transverse myelitis).

2. **Brain stem lesions.** These can be verified and localized with BAER.
3. **Acoustic neuroma.** BAER can be used to verify CN 8 injury.
4. **Spinal cord injury.** SSEP can be used for prognosis by differentiating complete from partial injury.
5. **Hypoxic-ischemic coma.** Bilateral absence of the N20 cortical potentials by SSEP on day 5 or later implies with a high degree of certainty that consciousness will not be regained.

Muscle and Nerve Biopsy

Muscle and nerve biopsy specimens are extremely fragile, and the procedure should be performed only by an experienced surgeon with adequate neuropathology backup for processing and analysis. The sural nerve and gastrocnemius muscle are often examined together, although biopsy of almost any muscle can be performed. Muscle biopsy is essential for diagnosing causes of myopathy such as polymyositis, genetic biochemical deficiencies, mitochondrial disease, sarcoidosis, critical illness myopathy, and infection (e.g., trichinosis). The causes of neuropathy that can be diagnosed by nerve biopsy are listed in Table 20.4.

Brain Biopsy

Brain biopsy can be performed either as an open procedure, usually of the anterior nondominant temporal lobe, or by using stereotactic needle localization. Although stereotactic biopsy is often necessary for deep lesions, the diagnostic yield is better with the open procedure because more tissue can be obtained. Regardless of the suspected condition, the diagnostic yield of brain biopsy is always maximized when areas of enhancement or signal abnormality on MR are targeted. The main complication is hemorrhage (in approximately 1% of cases). Brain biopsy is of value for diagnosing brain tumors or abscess, central nervous system (CNS) vasculitis, neurosarcoidosis, viral encephalitis, heritable metabolic disorders, and Jakob-Creutzfeldt disease.

Patient-Related Problems: The Common Calls

Acute Seizures and Status Epilepticus

Seizures are abnormal, paroxysmal synchronous discharges of cortical neurons resulting in abrupt neurologic manifestations that depend on the area of the brain involved. Seizures are classified as generalized (Fig. 4.1) when they involve the entire brain, producing an abrupt alteration in consciousness with or without motor manifestations. Focal seizures (see Fig. 4.1) involve a single brain region, causing limited dysfunction, which may include motor manifestations or nonmotor manifestations such as sensory disturbances, behavioral/cognitive changes, automatisms, or abnormal speech. Focal seizures are further subdivided into those with preserved consciousness and those without. Status epilepticus is defined as 5 minutes or more of continuous clinical and/or electrographic seizure activity, or repeated seizures between which the patient fails to return to baseline. Status epilepticus is a neurologic emergency that results when intrinsic mechanisms to terminate seizures fail with associated enhancement of excitatory pathways, culminating in neuronal death, increased mortality, and worsening clinical outcomes.

Seizures can be dramatic and frightening for those who witness the event, inducing panic rather than rational thought, even on a neurology or emergency room service. Effective management (Fig. 4.2) requires rapid yet comprehensive simultaneous assessment and treatment to ensure

1. Provision of supportive care as required;
2. Cessation of ongoing seizures and prevention of further seizures; and
3. Identification and treatment of the underlying cause of the seizures.

The acute management of seizures and status epilepticus is discussed in this chapter. Epilepsy, a chronic condition defined as recurrent, unprovoked seizures is discussed in Chapter 26.

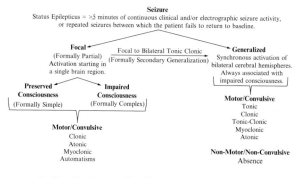

Seizure

Status Epilepticus = ≥5 minutes of continuous clinical and/or electrographic seizure activity, or repeated seizures between which the patient fails to return to baseline.

Focal ←── Focal to Bilateral Tonic Clonic ──→ **Generalized**
(Formally Partial)   (Formally Secondary Generalization)   Synchronous activation of
Activation starting in   bilateral cerebral hemispheres.
a single brain region.   Always associated with
impaired consciousness.

Preserved ←──────→ **Impaired**
Consciousness   **Consciousness**   **Motor/Convulsive**
(Formally Simple)   (Formally Complex)   Tonic
Clonic
Tonic-Clonic
Myoclonic
Motor/Convulsive   Atonic
Clonic
Atonic   **Non-Motor/Non-Convulsive**
Myoclonic   Absence
Automatisms

Non-Motor/Non-Convulsive   Note: Seizures with subtle or no motor manifestations that occur
Sensory   in patients with altered consciousness may only be detected on
Behavior/Cognitive Changes   electroencephalography. These seizures are commonly refered to
Autonomic   as electrographic or non-convulsive seizures.

FIG. 4.1 Seizure classification.

PHONE CALL

Questions

1. **What are the vital signs? Is the airway secured?**
2. **Is the patient still seizing?**
   - If yes, how long has it been going on?
   - If no, has the patient had multiple seizures without return to baseline?

   Status epilepticus is a neurologic emergency defined as ≥5 minutes of continuous seizure or repeated seizures without return to baseline in between. Any patient seizing with no known time of onset should be considered to be in status epilepticus until proven otherwise.

3. **What is the patient's level of consciousness?**

   A patient may have a decreased level of consciousness because of ongoing nonconvulsive status epilepticus, postictal state, as a result of medications given to abort the seizures, or because of the underlying cause of the seizure. One should never assume an altered level of consciousness is caused by a postictal state or medications until nonconvulsive status epilepticus and underlying pathologies are excluded with further investigations, including an electroencephalogram (EEG).

4. **What are the patient's finger stick glucose level and vital signs?**

   Focal and generalized seizures can be caused by hyperglycemia or hypoglycemia, and they may remain refractory to

Status Epilepticus

Seizure lasting ≥ 5min OR ≥ 2 seizures without return to baseline in between

	Supportive Care	Stop & Prevent Seizures See Table 4-3	Identify and Treat Etiology See Tables 4-1, 4-2, & 4-3

Emergent Initial Rx	• Remain calm
	• Crowd control
	• **Protect patient** - clear bed, lateral decubitus, rails up
	• Obtain 2 IVs
	• Apply monitors & obtain vitals
	• Apply O₂
	• Obtain **ABG** if ↓LOC
	• Address ABCs if needed
		• 1ˢᵗ line AED
		  ○ Lorazepam 4 mg (or 0.1mg/kg) IV push, may give additional 4 mg if seizures don't stop.
		  ○ Alternative benzos - see Table 4-3
			• Classify seizure- Figure 1
			• Bedside **glucose**
			  ○ Hypoglycemia Rx: **Thiamine 100mg** + **50mL D50W**
			• **Labs** (review past/obtain new)
			  ○ CBC, electrolytes, Mg, Ca, PO4, Cr, BUN, AST, ALT, ALP, bilirubin +/- AED levels and Toxicology panel

Urgent Control Rx	• **Continue monitoring for complications** of Sz/AED
	  ○ Beware ↓LOC, ↓HR, ↓BP, ↓RR
	  ○ Consider slowing AED infusion administer fluids, insert nasal airway, intubate, etc.
		• 2ⁿᵈ line AED should be given unless the cause is identified and immediately corrected.
		  ○ **Fosphenytoin** 20mg/kg @ 200mg/min (if using Phenytoin max rate 50mg/min)
		  ○ **Valproic Acid** 20-40mg/kg IV @ 3-6mg/kg/min
		  ○ **Levetiracetam** 20mg/kg IV over 15 min
		  ○ **Phenobarbital** 20mg/kg @ 75mg/min
			• Treat immediate reversible causes-see Table 4-4
			• Once able perform preliminary **history** and focused **exam** - Tables 4-5 & 4-7
			• Obtain **continuous EEG** to assess for NCSz

Refractory Rx	• If seizure continues (convulsive or non-convulsive) call **ICU**
	• Patient requires
	  ○ ICU level monitoring
	  ○ Intubation + Mechanical Ventilation
	  ○ +/- IV fluids
	  ○ +/- Vasopressors
		• 3ʳᵈ line AED:
		  ○ **Midazolam** 0.2mg/kg IV load → 0.2-2mg/kg/min infusion
		  ○ **Propofol** 1-2mg/kg IV load → 20-200mcg/kg/min infusion
		  ○ Additional 2ⁿᵈ line agents
			• Once stabilized consider **additional investigations** based on History/Exam
			  ○ Neuroimaging
			  ○ Lumbar Puncture
			  ○ Paraneoplastic panel
			  ○ Vasculitic work-up
			  ○ Toxicology work-up
			• Treat underlying causes accordingly.

Super Refractory Rx	• Continue monitoring for complications of ongoing seizures, AEDs, and underlying etiology	• 4ᵗʰ line AED:
		  ○ **Pentobarbital** 5-20mg/kg IV load @ ≤ 50mg/min → 0.5-5mg/kg infusion
		  ○ Additional 3ʳᵈ line agents
		• **Titrate in additional AEDs** to assist in weaning of infusions.
		• **Other options:** ketamine, inhaled anesthetics, ketogenic diet, steroids, IVIG, PLEX, Surgery, VNS
			• Continue investigations and treatment accordingly.

Ongoing Management: Once seizures controlled ensure seizure precautions maintained (Table 4-7), continue monitoring, complete investigations, continue treatment, titrate AEDs accordingly, and educate regarding seizure safety(Table 4-7).

FIG. 4.2 Management of status epilepticus. *ABG,* arterial blood gas; *AED,* antiepileptic drug; *ALP,* alkaline phosphatase; *ALT,* alanine aminotransferase; *AST,* aspartate aminotransferase; *BP,* blood pressure; *BUN;* blood urea nitrogen; *CBC,* complete blood count; *Cr,* creatinine; *EEG,* electroencephalography; *HR,* hear rate; *ICU,* intensive care unit; *IV,* intravenous; *LOC,* level of consciousness; *NCSz,* nonconvulsive seizure; *RR,* respiratory rate; *Sz,* seizure.

antiepileptic drugs (AEDs) unless the glucose is corrected. Knowing the patient's vital signs (even if no longer seizing) is crucial to assess the urgency of the situation.

5. **Is this the first known seizure for this patient?**

   In patients with known epilepsy, there may be records available detailing their history, including AEDs that have worked/ failed in the past, or allergies and complications from AEDs that should be avoided.

6. **Is the patient on antiepileptic medications?**

AED levels need to be checked for any seizure patient on medication. Noncompliance with medication in patients with epilepsy is the most common cause of status epilepticus. In some cases, AEDs may be epileptogenic at toxic levels.

Orders

1. **Protect patient** from potential harm. Place the patient in the lateral decubitus position to prevent aspiration, clear sharp or hard objects from the bed, put side rails up, and pad side rails.
2. Obtain a full set of **vitals** and place patient on monitors if possible.
3. Ensure that **two working intravenous (IV) lines** present.
4. Ensure that **airway equipment** such as oxygen, suction, oral airway, and Ambu bag are present at bedside.
5. For any seizure lasting ≥2 minutes **Lorazepam 0.1 mg/kg** should be given by IV push. For most patients, a total of 8 mg given in four repeated 2-mg boluses is required. Although the seizures may stop after the initial 2 mg is given, consider a full loading dose to minimize the chance of recurrent seizures during the next 6 to 12 hours.
6. Perform a bedside **finger stick glucose test**. If results are available and confirm hypoglycemia, then **100 mg IV thiamine followed by 50 mL of IV D50W** should be administered.
7. Send **stat labs** including complete blood count, electrolytes, calcium, magnesium, phosphate, creatinine, and a liver panel. If the patient has depressed level of consciousness, then send an arterial blood gas (ABG). Depending on the clinical scenario, a tox panel or AED levels also may need to be sent.

Inform RN

"Will arrive at the bedside in…minutes."

If the patient is still seizing, it must be considered an emergency. Even if the patient has stopped seizing, the patient may remain unstable because of aspiration or depressed level of consciousness, and another seizure may occur within minutes requiring urgent assessment.

ELEVATOR THOUGHTS

What is the differential diagnosis of seizures?

On your way to the bedside, you should generate a list of probable diagnoses based on the initial information you obtained from your telephone conversation, keeping in mind two rules:

- **Rule 1: Not all paroxysmal spells are seizures**. Beware seizure mimics including hypoglycemia, syncope, asterixis, stroke/

transient ischemic attack, myoclonus, dystonia, tremor, narcolepsy, complicated migraine, panic attack, transient global amnesia, hyperventilation, paroxysmal nonepileptic spell, or malingering. These mimics require different management than seizure.

- **Rule 2: A seizure is a symptom, not a disease**. One must always determine the underlying cause of the seizure. Generate a differential diagnosis using the mnemonic **VITAMIN CD** (Tables 4.1 and 4.2).

MAJOR THREAT TO LIFE

- **Inability to protect airway** with potential for **aspiration** of gastric contents, **upper airway obstruction,** and resulting **hypoxemic/hypercarbic respiratory failure.**
- **Head injury resulting from convulsions.**
- **Lactic acidosis, hyperthermia, rhabdomyolysis, cerebral edema, or hypotension** from a prolonged seizure may produce permanent brain injury.

BEDSIDE

Quick-Look Test

1. *Is the patient still seizing?*

   Most seizures will have stopped by the time you arrive at the bedside. If there is still seizure activity when you arrive, then you are almost certainly dealing with status epilepticus, and the seizure must be stopped immediately.

2. *If the patient has stopped seizing, assess the patient's level of consciousness.*

   Is the patient awake and alert? A period of reduced consciousness or agitation may follow a generalized seizure. Focal deficits such as a hemiparesis may also be apparent. Remember, a patient may have a decreased level of consciousness because of ongoing nonconvulsive status epilepticus, postictal state, as a result of medications given to abort the seizure, or because of the underlying cause of the seizure.

3. *Is there any sign of respiratory distress?*

   Is there significant tachypnea, labored respirations, desaturation, or oropharyngeal obstruction? Is there profound hypercarbia or hypoxemia on the previously sent ABG (if not already sent, consider sending a stat ABG if the patient is obtunded). Call for help immediately for potential intubation if there is any concern.

TABLE 4.1 Diseases Causing Seizures

Category		Diseases
V	Vascular	Intracranial hemorrhage, ischemic infarction (acute or chronic[a]), venous sinus thrombosis, posterior reversible encephalopathy syndrome, subarachnoid hemorrhage, vascular malformation, amyloid angiopathy
I	Infection	CNS Infections: meningitis/encephalitis (bacterial, viral, fungal), or abscess (bacterial, fungal, or parasitic) Systemic infections: pneumonia, urinary tract infection, bacteremia, etc.; can lower a patient's seizure threshold and should be considered
T	Trauma	Acute or chronic traumatic brain injury with or without subdural/epidural hematomas, contusions, or traumatic subarachnoid hemorrhage
A	Autoimmune	Autoimmune encephalitis (e.g., NMDA), primary or secondary CNS vasculitis (e.g., systemic lupus erythematosus), multiple sclerosis, acute disseminated encephalomyelitis, and other inflammatory demyelinating conditions
M	Metabolic/ toxic	Hypoglycemia or hyperglycemia, hyponatremia or hypernatremia, hypocalcemia or hypercalcemia, hypomagnesemia, hyperthyroidism, uremia, and hyperammonemia Table 4.2 lists common illicit drugs and medications that can cause seizures
I	Idiopathic	Idiopathic epilepsy
N	Neoplastic	Brain metastasis, primary CNS tumors, paraneoplastic encephalitis
C	Congenital	Congenital brain malformations, inborn errors of metabolism
D	Degenerative	Certain types of dementia both rapidly progressive (e.g., Creutzfeldt-Jakob disease) and slowly progressive (e.g., Alzheimer's disease) can cause seizures although rarely

[a]Chronic ischemic cerebrovascular disease is the most common cause of new-onset seizures in adults.

CNS, Central nervous system; *NMDA*, N-methyl-D-aspartate.

TABLE 4.2	Medications That May Cause Seizures	
Categories	**Classes**	**Drugs**
Antimicrobials	Quinolones	Ciprofloxacin, levofloxacin, moxifloxacin
	Carbapenems	Imipenem, meropenem
	Cephalosporins	Cefepime, cefixime, ceftazidime, cefuroxime, cephalexin
	Penicillins	Penicillin, ampicillin, synthetic penicillins
	Other	Metronidazole, isoniazid (T), zidovudine, pyrimethamine
Antidepressants	SNRI	Bupropion, venlafaxine, duloxetine
	SSRI (T)	Fluoxetine, escitalopram
	TCA (T)	Amitriptyline, nortriptyline, imipramine, clomipramine, maprotiline
	Other	Lithium (T)
Antipsychotics	Typical	Haloperidol, chlorpromazine, thioridazine, trifluoperazine, perphenazine
	Atypical	Sertraline, risperidone, quetiapine, loxapine, clozapine
Analgesics	Opioids	Fentanyl, meperidine, oxycodone, propoxyphene, pentazocine
	NSAIDs	Indomethacin, ketorolac
Anesthetics	Local (T)	Lidocaine, bupivacaine, procaine,
	Inhalational	Enflurane
Cytotoxics	Calcineurin inhibitors	Tacrolimus, cyclosporine
	Alkylating agents	Cyclophosphamide, chlorambucil, cisplatin
	Antimetabolite	Methotrexate, mycophenolate
	Other	Vincristine, doxorubicin
Sedatives (W)	Benzodiazepines	Lorazepam, temazepam, clonazepam, etc. Flumazenil, a benzodiazepine antagonist, can also cause seizures
	Other	Zolpidem, zaleplon, sodium oxybate, alcohol
Sympathomimetics	—	Ephedrine, cocaine, amphetamines
Others[a]	—	Insulin (via hypoglycemia), antihistamines, anticholinergics, cholinergics, certain bronchodilators and antihypertensives

[a]The list of potential seizure-inducing medications is extensive, and should there be any concern of drug-induced seizures, further review by a pharmacy is suggested in addition to stopping all unnecessary medications.

Common culprits in bold. *NSAIDs*, Nonsteroidal antiinflammatory drugs; *SNRI*, serotonin-norepinephrine reuptake inhibitor; *SSRI*, selective serotonin reuptake inhibitor; *T*, seizures occur with toxicity; *TCA*, tricyclic antidepressant; *W*, seizures occur with withdrawal.

MANAGEMENT

Effective management (see Fig. 4.2) of seizures and status epilepticus requires rapid yet comprehensive simultaneous assessment and treatment to ensure:

1. Cessation of ongoing seizures and prevention of further seizures;
2. Identification and treatment of the underlying cause of the seizures; and
3. Provision of supportive care as required.

Although much of what is presented in the following section is in list format, it is important to remember that most steps should occur in parallel as they are completed by members of the health care team under the guidance of the physician.

Emergent Initial Therapy

1. **Keep calm.** It is likely that others in the room are reacting with fear or panic. Controlling the room is essential for streamlining management. Ask family members to leave the room. Assure them you will speak with them as soon as the situation is under control. You may need to remind the other health care workers in the room to quiet down and provide explicit instructions for management.
2. **Protect the patient.** Have one or two people maintain the patient in a lateral decubitus position. Clear sharp or hard objects from bed, put side rails up, and pad side rails.
3. **Administer oxygen,** particularly if the patient is older or has a history of cardiac disease.
4. **Ensure two working IVs.** If the patient has no IV access, have one or two people hold the forearm while the most experienced person available inserts two IV lines and draws blood. Avoid the antecubital area because convulsions may cause flexion of the arm and block off the IV site.
5. Check **vitals and the finger stick glucose** level.
   - Hypoglycemia is corrected with **glucose (50 mL of D50W)** by slow, direct injection. If there is any history or suspicion of alcoholism, administer **thiamine 100 mg by slow, direct injection over 3 to 5 minutes** prior to the D50W. The administration of thiamine will prevent susceptible patients from developing Wernicke encephalopathy. If hypoglycemia is the cause of the seizure, then the seizure should stop, and the patient should wake up soon after the glucose administration.
   - Hyperglycemia treatment should commence with 10 units of IV insulin and then be titrated according to the follow-up glucose level.

6. If the seizure just started, **watch and wait for 2 minutes.** A majority of seizures will stop spontaneously within a short time. There is no immediate risk to the patient, provided the risks of aspiration and physical injury have been addressed. During the waiting period, do the following:
   - Ask for **lorazepam 8 mg** in a 10-mL syringe. This may need to be administered if the seizure does not stop spontaneously (see below).
   - **Elicit further history** not obtained in the initial phone call. Ask for the chart to be brought to the bedside. Is this a first-ever seizure? Is the patient on AEDs? What is the patient's admitting diagnosis? Is the patient diabetic? Is the patient immunocompromised? Has the patient been febrile in the last 24 hours? What other medications is the patient taking?
   - **Observe and classify the seizure type** (see Fig. 4.1). Most seizures manifest as one of two types: *convulsive* and *non-convulsive*. Generalized convulsive seizures are characterized by bilateral tonic-clonic activity and altered level of consciousness. Much more challenging to detect are "non-convulsive" seizures, which present primarily as a paroxysmal alteration in level of consciousness, with or without subtle motor manifestations such as eyelid blinking, facial twitching, head turning, or motor automatisms.

7. **If the seizure has not remitted in 2 minutes:**
   - If glucose levels are normal or after glucose has been given, administer **lorazepam 4 mg (0.1 mg/kg) by IV push** (Table 4.3). An Ambu bag with face mask should be at the bedside because benzodiazepines can cause respiratory depression and sedation.
   - Alternatives to IV lorazepam included in Table 4.3:
     - **Midazolam 10 mg intramuscularly (IM) or 0.2 mg/kg IV or sublingually.**
     - **Diazepam 5 to 10 mg IV push or 20 mg per rectum (PR).**
     - Lorazepam 0.1 mg/kg IM if no IV access is available. Intranasal formulas are also available.
   - Order the following **blood tests** to search for correctable underlying causes: complete blood count, electrolytes, magnesium, calcium, phosphate, glucose, creatinine, urea, liver panel, ammonia, EtOH level, toxicology screen, and AED levels (if applicable). See Table 4.4 for details regarding the treatment of specific reversible causes of seizures.

Urgent Control Therapy

1. After a full dose of benzodiazepine has been given regardless of if the seizures have stopped or not, a **second antiepileptic medication** should be administered unless the cause of the seizure

TABLE 4.3   Drugs Used for the Treatment of Status Epilepticus

Medication	Dose	Side Effects	Considerations
Emergent Initial Therapy			
Lorazepam	Load: 4 mg (0.1 mg/kg) may give additional to total of 8 mg IV IM (IM if no IV)	Respiratory depression Sedation	Ensure airway equipment nearby
Midazolam	10 mg IM or 0.2 mg/kg IV/SL		
Diazepam	5–10 mg IV or 20 mg PR		
Urgent Control Therapy			
Fosphenytoin or phenytoin	Load: 15–20 mg/kg IV @ 200 mg/min (fosphenytoin) or 50 mg/min (phenytoin) Additional 10 mg/kg if still seizing after initial load	Arrhythmias Hypotension Hepatotoxicity Pancytopenia Steven-Johnson syndrome Purple glove syndrome	Monitor ECG continuously for bradycardia, prolonged QTc, etc. BP should be checked regularly Slow infusion if hypotension or arrhythmia occur.
Valproic acid	Load: 20–40 mg/kg IV @ 3–6 mg/kg/min Additional 20 mg/kg if still seizing after initial load	Hepatotoxicity Hyperammonemia Pancreatitis Thrombocytopenia Hypofibrinogenemia	Ideal medication in patients with do not intubate status as nonsedating and rarely causes hypotension Preferred in GBM patients
Levetiracetam	Load: 20 mg/kg IV over 15 min	Psychosis Agitation	Minimal drug interactions Dose adjustment required with reduced CrCl and RRT

TABLE 4.3   Drugs Used for the Treatment of Status Epilepticus—cont'd

Medication	Dose	Side Effects	Considerations
Phenobarbital	Load: 15–20 mg/kg IV @ 75 mg/min	Sedation Respiratory depression Hypotension	Requires close observation because of side effect profile
Refractory Status Epilepticus Therapy			
Midazolam	Load: 0.2 mg/kg IV q5min until seizures stop Infusion: 0.2–2 mg/kg/min IV	Sedation Respiratory depression Hypotension	Requires ICU monitoring, intubation ± vasopressors Titrated to EEG for seizure cessation or burst suppression
Propofol	Load: 1–2 mg/kg IV Infusion: 20–200 µg/kg/min IV	Sedation Respiratory depression Hypotension Bradycardia Propofol infusion syndrome	
Super Refractory Status Epilepticus Therapy			
Pentobarbital	Load: 5–20 mg/kg IV @ ≤50 mg/min Infusion: 0.5–5 mg/kg/h IV	Sedation Respiratory depression Hypotension Ileus Immunosuppression	Requires ICU monitoring, intubation ± vasopressors Titrated to EEG for burst suppression
Ketamine	Load: 0.5–4.5 mg/kg Infusion: up to 5 mg/kg/h	Sedation Hypertension Neurotoxicity	Add to ongoing midazolam infusion

BP, Blood pressure; *CrCl,* creatinine clearance; *ECG,* electrocardiogram; *EEG,* electroencephalogram; *GBM,* glioblastoma multiforme; *ICU,* intensive care unit; *IM,* intramuscularly; *IV,* intravenous; *PR,* per rectum; *RRT,* renal replacement therapy; *SL,* saline lock.

TABLE 4.4 Acute Treatment of Reversible Causes of Seizures

Condition	Treatment
Acute stroke	Consideration of tPa ($\leq$4.5 h) and endovascular clot retrieval ($\leq$6 h)
ICH/SAH/PRES	Lower SBP $\leq$ 140–160 Labetalol 10 mg IV q10 min maximum 300 mg/24 h. Hold if HR < 60 Hydralazine 5–10 mg IV q15–30min Enalaprilat 1.25 mg IV q6h
Infection	Empiric antibiotics targeting suspected infection Ceftriaxone 2 g IV q12h Vancomycin 1–1.5 g q12h Empiric encephalitis coverage Acyclovir 10 mg/kg IV q8h
Autoimmune/ inflammatory	Solumedrol 1 g IV daily × 3–5 days Further immunosuppressive medications will depend on underlying etiology (autoimmune/paraneoplastic encephalitis, vasculitis, demyelinating condition)
Hypoglycemia	Thiamine 100 mg IV followed by D50W 50 mL IV Hold insulin and hypoglycemic medications
Hyperglycemia	Insulin 10 units IV. Titrate further doses according to glucose level Assess for and treat diabetic ketoacidosis/hyperglycemia hyperosmolar state
Hyponatremia	3% NaCl 50–100 cc IV boluses (only given if hyponatremia associated with seizures/coma) Identify and treat underlying cause
Hypomagnesemia	$MgSO_4$ 2 g IV over 5 min (only given if extreme hypomagnesemia is causing seizures) Identify and treat underlying cause
Hypocalcemia	10 mL (1 g) CaCl/Ca gluconate IV over 5 min Identify and treat underlying cause
Hypercalcemia	Aggressive hydration combined with Lasix followed by renal replacement therapy Identify and treat underlying cause
Hypophosphatemia	Sodium phosphate 0.32–0.64 mmol/kg IV @ $\leq$7 mmol/h (only given if extreme hypophosphatemia causing seizures)
Toxicity/overdose	Speak with poison control center regarding antidote/supportive care

HR, Heart rate; *ICH,* intracerebral hemorrhage; *IV,* intravenous; *PRES,* posterior reversible encephalopathy syndrome; *SAH,* subarachnoid hemorrhage; *SBP,* systolic blood pressure; *tPa,* tissue plasminogen activator.

has been definitely corrected. The Established Status Epilepticus Treatment Trial (ESETT) is currently underway to help define the best second-line agent. If the patient is a known epileptic on a known AED-available IV, then a load of that medication can be given; otherwise the most commonly used medications include (see Table 4.3):

- **Fosphenytoin or Phenytoin** are the most commonly used.
  - Loading dose: **20 mg/kg IV at rate of 150 mg/min (fosphenytoin) and 50 mg/min (phenytoin).** Fosphenytoin can also be given IM. If the patient is known to be on phenytoin already and is suspected of having subtherapeutic levels or if they continue seizing after an initial load, then a bolus dose of 10 mg/kg may be given.
  - Adverse effects: both medications can cause cardiac arrhythmias, prolongation of the QT interval, and hypotension. Hepatotoxicity, pancytopenia, Steven-Johnson syndrome, and purple glove syndrome are other potential side effects.
  - Considerations: The electrocardiogram (ECG) should be monitored continuously, and the blood pressure should be checked periodically during the infusion. The rate of administration should be slowed if ECG changes or hypotension occurs. Beware numerous drug interactions.
- **Valproic acid**
  - Loading dose: **20 to 40 mg/kg IV at a rate of 3 to 6 mg/kg/min** followed by an additional 20 mg/kg if remain seizing 10 minutes after initial load.
  - Adverse effects: hepatotoxicity, hyperammonemic encephalopathy, pancreatitis, thrombocytopenia and qualitative platelet dysfunction, and hypofibrinogenemia.
  - Considerations: nonsedating and rarely causes hypotension, making it an ideal medication for patients with do-not-intubate status. May be the preferred agent in patients with glioblastoma multiforme.
- **Levetiracetam**
  - Loading dose: **20 mg/kg IV over 15 minutes**
  - Adverse effects: psychosis, agitation.
  - Considerations: Minimal drug interactions. Requires dose adjustment in patients with poor renal function or on renal replacement therapy.
- **Phenobarbital**
  - Dose: **20 mg/kg IV** at maximal rate of 75 mg/min.
  - Adverse effects: sedation, respiratory depression, hypotension.

2. Approximately 70% of prolonged convulsive seizures will be brought under control with a combination of lorazepam and

fosphenytoin. The likelihood of success with this therapy is directly correlated to the interval between seizure onset and initiation of treatment. When AEDs are initiated within 30 minutes of seizure onset, 80% of patients respond, but if the patient has been seizing for greater than 2 hours prior to treatment, the success rate falls to 40%.

3. **Consider nonconvulsive status epilepticus:** By this time the convulsive activity may diminish/stop and the patient may remain unresponsive regardless of if the seizure has stopped or not. A patient may have a decreased level of consciousness because of ongoing nonconvulsive status epilepticus, postictal state, as a result of medications given to abort the seizures, or because of the underlying cause of the seizure. **Patients who fail to awaken (i.e., follow commands) after convulsive status epilepticus has been terminated require continuous EEG (cEEG) to detect ongoing nonconvulsive seizure activity.** cEEG will detect additional electrographic seizure activity in 30% to 50% of these patients and ongoing nonconvulsive status epilepticus in approximately 15%. Left unchecked, these seizures can lead to a state of prolonged unconsciousness and secondary brain injury.

Treatment of Refractory Status Epilepticus

Patients who continue to experience clinical or electrographic seizures after receiving adequate doses of benzodiazepine and a second AED are considered to be in refractory status epilepticus. These patients have a mortality of 25% to 60% depending on the study, and they **require intensive care unit admission** for aggressive management including intubation, continuous monitoring (including cEEG), and administration of continuous infusions of sedatives with optimization of other AEDs.

The most common error in the management of status epilepticus is under treatment. Patients need to be treated rapidly and aggressively until the seizures have been stopped.

1. The therapeutic options that are reasonable at this stage include (see Table 4.3):
   - **Midazolam.** This short-acting benzodiazepine is the favored agent because it is relatively safe, easy to titrate, and has a rapid onset/offset.
     - Dose: **0.2 mg/kg IV bolus q5min** until seizures stop followed by **0.2 to 2 mg/kg/h IV infusion** titrated via cEEG
     - Adverse effects: respiratory depression, hypotension, sedation.
   - **Propofol**
     - Dose: **1 to 2 mg/kg IV** load followed by **20 to 200 µg/kg/min IV infusion** titrated via cEEG

- Adverse effects: respiratory depression, hypotension, bradycardia sedation, propofol infusion syndrome (rhabdomyolysis, metabolic acidosis, renal failure, and cardiovascular collapse).
- **Additional AED loads**: in some circumstances (e.g., patients who cannot or should not be intubated) additional loads of AEDs can be tried. Valproic acid is typically favored in this setting if not already given.

Treatment of Super Refractory Status Epilepticus

If there is **no response to full doses of a benzodiazepine and two additional AEDs, patients are considered to be in super refractory status epilepticus.**

1. At this point definitive therapy in the form of total barbiturate anesthesia or ketamine infusion is often required (see Table 4.3).
   - **Pentobarbital**
     - Dose: **5 to 20 mg/kg IV at a rate ≤50 mg/min followed by 0.5 to 5 mg/kg IV infusion** titrated to burst suppression on cEEG.
     - Side effects: hypotension, sedation, respiratory depression, ileus, immunosuppression.
     - Considerations: vasopressors are generally required for hypotension.
   - **Ketamine**
     - Dose: 0.5–4.5 mg/kg loadi followed by 1–5 mg/kg/hr
     - Side effects: sedation, hypertension, neurotoxicity
     - Considerations: add on to ongoing midazolam infusion, maintain high normal masgnesium levels for maximum effect.
2. Electrographic **seizure control (or EEG showing suppression burst) is typically maintained for 24 to 48 hours** followed by a gradual withdrawal of the continuous infusion of the medications discussed previously. To allow for transition from continuous infusions of sedatives, additional maintenance AEDs are titrated accordingly.
3. **Alternative therapies** for status epilepticus, include ketamine, inhaled anesthetics, corticosteroids, IV immunoglobulins, plasma exchange, hypothermia, vagus nerve stimulation, and surgical management. These are selected based on the underlying cause and have variable success.

Ongoing Management

When managing seizures or status epilepticus, the priority is to abort the seizures as quickly as possible while providing supportive care. However, in parallel with the previously mentioned efforts, and certainly after the seizures have ceased, one must **consider and address**

the underlying cause of the seizures. Although the vast majority of seizures may be brought under control with anticonvulsant therapy, continued control may be impossible until the underlying cause is identified and treated. The underlying cause may also directly contribute to morbidity and mortality unless appropriately addressed. To identify the underlying cause one should:

1. Perform a **selective history and chart review**
   - **Characterize the spell** to ensure the event was a seizure and not a mimic (Table 4.5). This is done via talking with the patient and/or witnesses in a chronological manner as follows:
     - **Preevent phase:** An aura may be present at the onset of a focal seizure. Epileptic auras are most commonly olfactory, gustatory, or other visceral sensations that

TABLE 4.5	Differentiating Between Seizures and Mimics		
	History		
	Preevent	**Event**	**Other**
Seizure	Various auras possible: Psychiatric Olfactory Gustatory Visual Visceral sensation	Stereotypical events Motor activity: focal or generalized. If generalized, ensure synchronous Altered LOC Focal features: head or eye deviation, automatisms, tonic posturing May have tongue biting, urinary/fecal incontinence, cyanosis Confusion Agitation Post-ictal Todd's paralysis	ROS: may reveal preceding systemic symptoms suggesting clue to underling etiology Preceding sleep deprivation may lower seizure threshold Past medical history: febrile seizure, head trauma, stroke, encephalitis, brain tumor Medications: see Table 4.2 Social history: alcohol, drug use
Migraine	Various auras Visual Sensory	Severe headache Associated phonophobia, photophobia, nausea/vomiting	Past medical history: migraines Family history: migraines

TABLE 4.5	Differentiating Between Seizures and Mimics—cont'd		
	History		
	Preevent	**Event**	**Other**
Syncope	Prolonged standing Lightheadedness Diaphoresis Chest pain Palpitations Tunnel vision Shortness of Breath	Flaccid Pallor Eyes closed Urinary incontinence possible Note: Convulsive syncope may mimic seizures Resolution with recumbency Minimal postevent confusion	ROS: may reveal preceding cardiac symptoms Past medical history: cardiac disease Medications: new antihypertensives
PNES	Stressful circumstances Emotional outburst/upset	Nonstereotyped Bilateral movements but preserved consciousness Nonsynchronous bilateral movements Head shaking Pelvic thrusting Immediately back to normal	Past medical history: epilepsy (many PNES patients also have epilepsy), psychiatric comorbidities
TGA	No warning	Hours of amnesia with all other neurologic function preserved	Nil
TIA	No warning	≤1 h of negative neurologic symptoms localizing to a vascular territory. No alteration in consciousness Full resolution	Past medical history: stroke risk factors Social history: smoker

LOC, Level of consciousness; *PNES*, paroxysmal nonepileptic spell; *ROS*, review of systems; *TGA*, transient global amnesia; *TIA*, transient ischemic attack.

precede motor or sensory activity. Whereas syncope may be preceded by dizziness, diaphoresis, turning pale, blurry vision, chest pains, palpitations, or shortness of breath. What the patient was doing immediately prior to the event may also be helpful (e.g., a patient who just stood up and then became lightheaded with a loss of consciousness is more likely to have fainted rather than seized.)

- **Event:** Try to identify any focal onset of the seizure. A seizure that begins focally can aid in the localization of the underlying pathology. Were there head and eye deviation at the beginning? Were automatisms noted? Was there motor activity that began in one part of the body prior to generalizing? If generalized motor activity occurred was it rhythmic and synchronous? Did the patient lose consciousness, become incontinent, or bite their tongue or mouth? Seizure mimics will have very different semiologies (see Table 4.5). Try to quantify the duration of the event.
- **Postevent phase:** After the event was the patient somnolent, confused, agitated, or immediately back to normal? Were any focal deficits transiently noted after the event including weakness (Todd paralysis) or aphasia?
- Further history and chart review should inquire about:
  - Potential underlying etiologies
  - Review of systems may reveal preceding symptoms such as headaches, fever, neck stiffness, sleep deprivation, cardiac symptoms, and so forth, that may give clues to the underlying etiology.
  - Review of past medical history/past surgical history could reveal underlying medical problems that could cause seizures, e.g., previous strokes, traumatic brain injury, known malignancy (lung, breast, and colon are the most common malignancies to metastasize to the brain), HIV or other immunodeficiencies that predispose to opportunistic infections, hepatic or renal disease, and so forth. Previous cardiac conditions may be suggestive of syncope.
  - Medications should be reviewed for potential epileptogenic medications, and compliance with AEDs. Recent addition or changes to blood pressure medications may be suggestive of syncope.
  - Social history should be reviewed for illicit drug and alcohol use.
  - Recent laboratory results may give clues to the underlying etiology.

- Relevant social history
  - In addition to inquiring about drug and alcohol use, one should also inquire about the patient's current occupation, hobbies, and modes of transportation, as this becomes relevant for discussing seizure safety and driving/job restrictions.

2. Perform a **selective physical examination**
   - Physical examination (Table 4.6) of a patient with seizures will vary depending on the clinical scenario and how involved the patient can be in the examination. Patients who have a single seizure and return to baseline can engage in a full neurologic examination, whereas patients requiring intubation and sedation to control seizures can only have a limited neurologic examination. Regardless, a full systemic physical examination should be performed. The examination is conducted to assess for clues to the etiology of the seizure. It is important to pay particular attention to unilateral focal neurologic deficits that could indicate a structural lesion.

3. **Perform and review investigations**
   - Having accumulated information for the history, physical examination, and preliminary investigations, a working differential diagnosis should be generated. As always, in an

TABLE 4.6	Focused Physical Examination for Seizures
Examination	**Interpretation of Findings**
Vital Signs	
Temperature	Fever may suggest infection, although fever can also be seen after prolonged seizures
Heart rate	Sinus tachycardia may be seen post seizures, but persistent sinus tachycardia or arrhythmias may be suggestive of syncope, a cardioembolic event, or underlying infection or toxidrome
Blood pressure	Hypertensive encephalopathy can present with seizures
O_2 saturation	Oxygen desaturations may be indicative of aspiration
Respiratory rate	Tachypnea can be seen postictal, but persistent tachypnea may be suggestive of an underlying infection, metabolic disturbance, or toxidrome
Neurologic	
Level of consciousness	A period of lethargy, stupor, or inattentiveness may follow a generalized seizure; if awake have patient count backward from 20 to 1 as a screening for attentiveness

TABLE 4.6	Focused Physical Examination for Seizures—cont'd
Examination	**Interpretation of Findings**
Language exam	Abnormalities in fluency/naming/repetition/comprehension in an attentive patient may indicate a focal lesion affecting the dominant hemisphere
Cranial nerves	Persistent gaze deviation, hippus, or subtle eyelid/face twitching may suggest ongoing seizure activity; bilateral visual deficits suggest PRES; other deficits would help localize a focal lesion
Motor and reflexes	Hemiparesis may be obvious or subtle; hemiparesis may be transient because of Todd paralysis or persistent; either way it is suggestive of a focal lesion
	Reflex asymmetry or unilateral Babinski sign may be indicative of a focal lesion
Sensory exam	Hemibody numbness or extinction/neglect to sensory stimuli may help localize a focal lesion
Head and Neck	
Assess for trauma	Acute or chronic head trauma may indicate a cause of the seizure or be a result of the seizure; patients who experience seizures may also bite their tongue, lips, or buccal mucosa
Fundoscopy	Papilledema suggests high intracranial pressures
Neck mobility	Meningismus suggests an underlying meningitis/meningoencephalitis
Respiratory	
Auscultate lungs	Focal bronchial breath sounds or rhonchi suggests aspiration
Cardiac	
Auscultate heart	New cardiac murmurs may be suggestive of a cardioembolic source (if fever present consider infective endocarditis)
GI and GU	
Observation	Incontinence
MSK and Skin	
Observation	Cafe au lait spots, port-wine stains, etc., suggest underlying neurocutaneous disorders; hematomas, lacerations, or fractures may result as a consequence of seizures

GI, gastrointestinal; GU, genitourinary; MSK, musculoskeletal; PRES, posterior reversible encephalopathy syndrome; RR, respiratory rate; T, temperature; UE, upper extremities.

acute situation, the differential diagnosis should include the most dangerous diagnosis as well as the most likely. Further investigations should proceed from the differential diagnosis:

- If not already performed, an **EEG** should be obtained if the diagnosis of seizure is at all uncertain. The finding of interictal epileptiform activity implies an increased risk of seizures and need for maintenance therapy with antiepileptics. If the patient remains obtunded, then an EEG should be obtained to assess for potential ongoing nonconvulsive seizures.

- If the examination reveals a focal deficit, if the onset of the seizure appeared to be focal, or if the patient has new-onset seizures, then a **computed tomography (CT) scan** should be obtained. Depending on the clinical scenario, a magnetic resonance imaging (MRI) and vessel imaging via magnetic resonance angiography (MRA)/magnetic resonance venography (MRV) or computed tomography angiography (CTA) may also be indicated. Keep in mind that an acute infarction may not be visualized on a noncontrast CT scan for 6 hours.

- If an infection is suspected because of the preceding symptoms, fever, meningismus, or leukocytosis, then an infectious workup should be completed trying to identify the most likely source. This may include a **lumbar puncture**, blood and urine cultures, viral serologies, and chest X-ray.

- **AED levels** should be ordered for the next morning for any known AEDs that the patient had been prescribed, and for all AEDs administered during the acute management.

- If clinical history suggests drug use or a toxidrome is suspected (Table 4.7), then a toxicology panel should be sent if not already done so.

- If a metabolic cause was identified on the original assessment and treatment was given to correct abnormal laboratory results, then further investigations including repeat testing of the abnormal values may be indicated.

- Further investigations may include autoimmune/paraneoplastic antibody panels and rheumatologic/vasculitis antibody panels, depending on the clinical scenario.

- If no underlying cause for seizures is determined, then idiopathic epilepsy may be the diagnosis. An EEG can be helpful in differentiating specific epileptic syndromes.

- The identified underlying etiology should, if possible, be addressed (see Table 4.4). AEDs should be titrated as

TABLE 4.7	Seizure Precautions and Seizure Safety

Seizure Precautions	Seizure Safety
Bed: should be at the lowest position **Side rails:** should be up and padded **Ambulate:** to bathroom only with supervision **Vital signs:** only axillary temperatures should be measured **Supervision:** when using sharp objects	**Driving:** patients must be seizure free for a set time prior to driving (jurisdiction specific). **Occupational:** patients working in transportation, or jobs with moving equipment/open flames/chemicals/at heights may need to consider a leave of absence, modified duties, or change of career **Leisure:** isolated sports, cycling, swimming/diving/snorkeling may need to be modified **Home:** avoid baths, do not lock bathroom door, turn down hot water heater, cook with back burners, limit EtOH, avoid sleep deprivation, avoid heights, avoid power tools, etc. **Women:** those of childbearing age require contraception to avoid teratogenicity of AEDs

AED, Antiepileptic drug; *EtOH,* ethanol.

needed. Note, however, that a single first seizure that has stopped often does not need to be treated with AEDs. Antiepileptic therapy should be reserved for patients who have more than one seizure or who have risk factors that make another seizure more likely (see Chapter 26 for more details). Patients who remain hospitalized should be placed on **seizure precautions** (Table 4.7) to ensure their safety should they have another event. Patients who are discharged should be educated about **seizure safety and restrictions** (see Table 4.7).

Stupor and Coma

Stupor and coma refer, respectively, to moderate and severe depression of the level of consciousness. The acute onset of stupor or coma is a medical emergency. A wide variety of metabolic and structural disorders can produce this state. Management should focus on stabilizing the patient, establishing a diagnosis, and treating the underlying cause.

PHONE CALL

Questions

1. **What are the vital signs?**
2. **Is the airway protected?**

    Stuporous and comatose patients are at high risk for *aspiration* because of impaired cough and gag reflexes, and *hypoxia,* which results from diminished respiratory drive. Endotracheal intubation is the most effective method for securing the airway and ensuring adequate oxygenation.

3. **Is there any history of trauma, drug use, or toxin exposure?**

    Obtain a quick description of recent events and preexisting medical or neurologic conditions. Check the Emergency Medical Service run sheet.

4. **Is someone available to provide further history?**

    Relatives, friends, ambulance personnel, or anyone else who has had recent contact with the patient should be identified and instructed to wait for further questioning.

Orders

1. **Call the anesthesiology service for intubation if the patient is deeply comatose or exhibiting signs of respiratory compromise.**

    In stuporous or comatose patients with normal respirations, begin 100% oxygen via bag mask ventilation until hypoxemia is ruled out with pulse oximetry.

2. **Order an intravenous line.**
3. **Order pulse oximetry.**

4. **Order a finger-stick glucose measurement.**

   This should always be checked immediately because hypoglycemia is a rapidly treatable cause of stupor or coma that can coexist with other diagnoses (e.g., sepsis, cardiac arrest, or trauma).

5. **Order diagnostic blood tests.**
   - Serum chemistries (glucose, electrolytes, blood urea nitrogen [BUN], creatinine)
   - Complete blood count (CBC)
   - Arterial blood gas
   - Calcium, magnesium
   - Prothrombin time (PT)/partial thromboplastic time (PTT)

6. **If the etiology of stupor or coma is unclear,** order toxicology screen, thyroid function tests, liver function tests, serum cortisol, and ammonia level.

7. **Insert a Foley catheter.**

8. **Order urinalysis, electrocardiogram (ECG), and chest X-ray.**

9. **Give emergency treatment.** These measures are often given in the field, or whenever the cause of stupor or coma is unclear.
   - **Thiamine 100 mg IV**

     Thiamine reverses stupor or coma resulting from acute thiamine deficiency (Wernicke encephalopathy). It must be given *before* dextrose because hyperglycemia can lead to consumption of thiamine and acute worsening of Wernicke encephalopathy.
   - **50% dextrose 50 mL (1 ampule) IV**
   - **Naloxone (Narcan) 0.4 to 0.8 mg IV**

     Naloxone reverses coma caused by opiate intoxication. Up to 10 mg may be required to reverse severe intoxication.
   - **Flumazenil (Romazicon) 0.2 to 1.0 mg IV**

     Flumazenil reverses stupor or coma caused by benzodiazepine intoxication. Up to 3 mg may be required. Do not give flumazenil if seizures have occurred because flumazenil may precipitate further seizures.

ELEVATOR THOUGHTS

What causes stupor or coma?

Stupor and coma result from diseases affecting either both of the cerebral hemispheres or the brain stem. As a rule, *unilateral hemispheric lesions* do not produce stupor or coma unless there is mass effect sufficient to raise the intracranial pressure (ICP), or compress either the contralateral hemisphere or the brain stem. *Focal brain stem or bilateral thalamic lesions* produce coma by disrupting the reticular activating system. *Metabolic and ictal disorders* impair consciousness by disrupting normal brain metabolism and electrical function. The causes of stupor and coma (Table 5.1) can be broadly grouped into four categories:

1. **Structural intracranial disorders**

   In most cases, these disorders are diagnosed by positive brain imaging (computed tomography [CT] or magnetic resonance imaging [MRI]) or by lumbar puncture (LP) in the case of meningitis or encephalitis.

TABLE 5.1	Causes of Stupor and Coma

1. Structural intracranial disorders
   a. Trauma
      (1) Epidural, subdural, intracerebral, or subarachnoid hemorrhage
      (2) Diffuse axonal injury
      (3) Concussion
   b. Cerebrovascular events
      (1) Intracerebral or subarachnoid hemorrhage
      (2) Hemispheric or brain stem infarction
      (3) Dural sinus thrombosis
      (4) Posterior reversible encephalopathy syndrome
   c. Infection
      (1) Meningitis
      (2) Encephalitis
      (3) Abscess
   d. Inflammatory disorders
      (1) Autoimmune vasculitis or cerebritis
      (2) Demyelinating disease (e.g., multiple sclerosis)
   e. Neoplasm
   f. Hydrocephalus
2. Toxic or metabolic disorders
   a. Global hypoxia-ischemia
   b. Electrolyte or acid-base disorders
      (1) pH disturbances
      (2) Hypernatremia or hyponatremia
      (3) Hyperglycemia or hypoglycemia
      (4) Hypercalcemia or hypocalcemia
   c. Drug intoxication or withdrawal
   d. Temperature disorder (hyperthermia or hypothermia)
   e. Organ system dysfunction
      (1) Liver (hepatic encephalopathy)
      (2) Kidney (uremia)
      (3) Thyroid (myxedema, thyrotoxicosis)
      (4) Adrenal (hyperadrenalism or hypoadrenalism)
      (5) Multisystem organ failure
   f. Seizure and postictal states
   g. Thiamine or vitamin B_{12} deficiency
3. Psychogenic unresponsiveness

2. **Toxic or metabolic disorders**

   Abnormal blood tests usually, but not always, confirm these disorders. Drug intoxication, sepsis, renal failure, hypoxia, hypoglycemia, and multisystem systemic organ failure are common causes of toxic-metabolic encephalopathy.

3. **Ictal or postictal states**

   Emergency continuous electroencephalopathy (EEG) monitoring is crucial for diagnosing active, ongoing electrographic seizure activity or epileptiform activity such as spikes or periodic epileptiform discharges (PEDs) that occur in the aftermath of seizures.

4. **Psychogenic unresponsiveness**

   Technically a behavioral disorder, psychogenic unresponsiveness is a mimic of coma because normal brain function is maintained. These states are defined by their reversibility.

MAJOR THREAT TO LIFE

Three common and treatable causes of coma can rapidly lead to death:

- **Herniation and brain stem compression**

  Space-occupying mass lesions that produce stupor or coma are a neurosurgical emergency (Fig. 5.1).

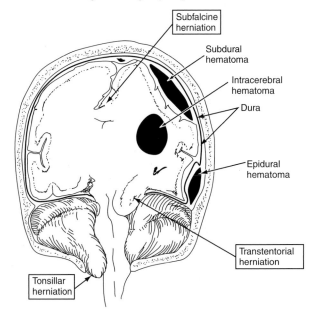

FIG. 5.1 Types of brain herniation that can occur in patients with compartmentalized intracranial pressure.

- **Increased ICP**

  Increased ICP can lead to impaired cerebral perfusion and global hypoxic-ischemic injury (see Chapter 13).
- **Meningitis or encephalitis**

  Death from bacterial meningitis or herpes encephalitis can be prevented with early treatment (see Chapter 22).

BEDSIDE

Selective History

The cause of coma can frequently be determined by the history. Ask family, friends, ambulance personnel, or others who have had recent contact with the patient about the following:

1. *Recent events*

   When was the patient last seen? How was the patient discovered? Were there any preceding neurologic complaints? Was there any recent trauma or toxin exposure?
2. *Medical history*
3. *Psychiatric history*
4. *Medications*
5. *Use of drugs or alcohol*

Selective Physical Examination

With or without history, clues to the etiology of coma can be elicited from the physical examination.

General Physical Examination

Vital signs	*Severe hypertension* suggests a structural CNS lesion caused by stroke, increased ICP, or hypertensive encephalopathy
Skin	Look for external signs of trauma, needle marks, rashes, cherry redness (suggests carbon monoxide poisoning), or jaundice
Breath	Alcohol, acetone, or fetor hepaticus (from liver failure) can lead to a pungent or "fruity" smell
Head	The skull should be inspected for fractures, hematomas, and lacerations
ENT	*CSF otorrhea or rhinorrhea* results from skull fracture with disruption of the dura (a positive dextrose stick test, indicating a high level of glucose, differentiates CSF from mucus)
	Hemotympanum is also highly suggestive of skull fracture
	Tongue biting suggests an unwitnessed seizure

Neck (do not manipulate the neck if there is suspicion of cervical spine fracture)	Stiffness suggests meningitis or subarachnoid hemorrhage

CNS, Central nervous system; *CSF,* cerebrospinal fluid; *ENT,* ear, nose, and throat; *ICP,* intracranial pressure.

Neurologic Examination

The goals of the neurologic examination are (1) to determine the depth of coma and (2) to localize the process leading to coma.

1. **General appearance**

    Open eyelids and a slack jaw indicate deep coma. Head and gaze deviation suggest a large ipsilateral hemispheric lesion. Observe for *myoclonus* (which suggests a metabolic process), *rhythmic muscle twitching* (which is indicative of seizure activity), or *tetany* (spontaneous, prolonged muscle spasms).

2. **Level of consciousness**

    Many inexact terms are used to describe depressed level of consciousness (e.g., somnolent, clouded, drowsy, obtunded). Because of the lack of precision associated with these terms, it is much more useful to document **the response of the patient to a specific stimulus;** for example, "opens eyes temporarily and responds with brief phrases to repeated questioning," or "moans and localizes to sternal rub." *Remember that the defining feature of coma is the lack of ability to follow simple one-step commands.*

    Responses to verbal and noxious stimuli can be used to generate a **Glasgow Coma Scale score** (Table 5.2), which is a reproducible and widely used method for quantifying level of consciousness. For the sake of simplicity, we advocate describing nonalert patients as *lethargic, stuporous,* or *comatose.*

    a. **Lethargy**

        Lethargy resembles sleepiness, except that the patient is incapable of becoming fully alert. These patients are conversant but inattentive and slow to respond. They are unable to adequately perform simple concentration tasks, such as counting from 20 to 1 or reciting the months in reverse.

    b. **Stupor**

        Stupor is defined by a state in which the best motor or verbal response requires a painful stimulus. There is little or no response to verbal commands. Painful stimulation results in brief responses to questions, exclamations

TABLE 5.2	Glasgow Coma Scale	
Parameter	**Patient Response**	**Score**
Eye-opening	Spontaneous	4
	To voice	3
	To pain	2
	None	1
Best motor response	Obeys commands	6
	Localizes to pain	5
	Withdraws to pain	4
	Flexor posturing	3
	Extensor posturing	2
	None	1
Best verbal response	Conversant and oriented	5
	Conversant and disoriented	4
	Uses occasional words	3
	Makes incomprehensible sounds	2
	None	1

For charting, Glasgow Coma Scale (GCS) scores should be documented in the chart by subscore and not added into a total score. For instance, e2 m5 v2 indicates a person who opens eyes to pain, localizes but does not follow, and grunts and groans to painful stimuli without speaking words.

("ouch"), or moaning. The patient may obey commands temporarily when aroused by noxious stimuli but more often only localizes to pain.

c. **Coma**

Coma is defined by the absence of verbal or complex motor responses to any stimulus. Coma patients are unable to follow or imitate verbal commands, are not conversant, and do not nod to questions. *A Glasgow Coma Scale score of 8 or lower is frequently used to define coma.*

3. **Respirations**

Abnormal respiratory patterns (Fig. 5.2) occur frequently with coma and can aid in localization. Respirations in intubated patients can be observed by briefly disconnecting the endotracheal tube from the ventilator.

a. **Patterns without localizing value**

(1) **Depressed respirations** can occur with severe coma of any cause but especially with intoxication.

(2) **Cheyne-Stokes respiration is** characterized by alternating periods of hyperventilation and apnea. It usually occurs with bihemispheric lesions or metabolic **en-cephalopathy.** Slow-cycling Cheyne-Stokes respirations are considered to represent a "stable" breathing

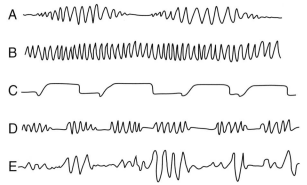

FIG. 5.2 Abnormal respiratory patterns associated with coma. Tracings represent chest wall excursion; upward deflections represent inspiration. *A,* Cheyne-Stokes respiration. *B,* Central neurogenic hyperventilation. *C,* Apneustic breathing. *D,* Cluster breathing. *E,* Ataxic breathing.

pattern that does not imply impending respiratory arrest. Rapid-cycling Cheyne-Stokes respirations may be more ominous.

(3) **Hyperventilation** in comatose patients is most often caused by systemic disease. Hyperventilation associated with metabolic acidosis can result from lactic acidosis, ketoacidosis, uremia, or organic acid poisoning. An association with respiratory alkalosis can result from hypoxia or hepatic encephalopathy. **Central neurogenic hyperventilation** is sometimes associated with central nervous system (CNS) lymphoma or brain stem damage from tentorial herniation.

b. **Patterns with localizing value**

(1) **Apneustic breathing** is characterized by a prolonged inspiratory phase (the inspiratory cramp) **followed** by apnea. It implies pontine damage.

(2) **Cluster breathing** consists of brief cycles of shallow hyperventilation with periods of **apnea.** It has less of a crescendo-decrescendo quality than Cheyne-Stokes respiration and is often a sign of pontine or cerebellar damage.

(3) **Ataxic (Biot) breathing,** which is an irregular, chaotic breathing pattern, implies **damage** to the medullary respiratory centers and is usually seen in association with posterior fossa lesions. Progression to apnea occurs frequently.

4. **Visual fields**

Visual fields should be tested with threatening movements, which normally evoke a blink. Asymmetry of this response implies hemianopia.

5. **Fundoscopy**

Papilledema occurs after prolonged (>12 hours) elevation of ICP, and only rarely does it develop acutely. Thus the absence of papilledema does not rule out increased ICP. *Spontaneous venous pulsations* are difficult to identify, but their presence implies normal ICP. *Subhyaloid hemorrhages* appear as globules of blood on the retinal surface and are commonly associated with subarachnoid hemorrhage.

6. **Pupils**

The shape, size, and reactivity to light of the pupils should be noted.

a. **Symmetry and normal reactivity to light** implies structural integrity of the midbrain. Reactive **pupils** in conjunction with absent corneal and oculocephalic responses are highly suggestive of metabolic coma.

b. **A unilateral dilated and fixed pupil** usually occurs with cranial nerve (CN) 3 **compression** in the setting of ipsilateral uncal transtentorial herniation. Ptosis and exodeviation of the eye are also seen. On CT there is usually midline shift and effacement of the ambient cistern (lateral to the midbrain) caused by encroachment of the medial temporal lobe. A "false localizing" third nerve palsy, with the mass lesion contralateral to the affected eye, can also sometimes occur. An acutely "blown" pupil represents an immediate threat to life and requires urgent intervention to reduce ICP.

c. **Midposition (2- to 5-mm) fixed or irregular pupils** imply a bilateral focal midbrain lesion, or progression of herniation to the level of the midbrain.

d. **Pinpoint reactive pupils** occur with pontine damage. Opiates and cholinergic intoxication (e.g., with pilocarpine) also produce small reactive pupils.

e. **Bilateral fixed and dilated pupils** can reflect central herniation; global hypoxia-ischemia; or **poisoning** with barbiturates, scopolamine, atropine, or glutethimide.

7. **Ocular movements**

Horizontal conjugate gaze is mediated by the *frontal eye fields* and the *pontine gaze centers*. The frontal eye fields, when activated, drive gaze to the opposite side. The pontine gaze centers, when activated, drive gaze to the same side. Vertical conjugate gaze is mediated by centers in the *midbrain tegmentum and lower diencephalon*. In unresponsive patients, conjugate eye movements can be actively elicited by testing the

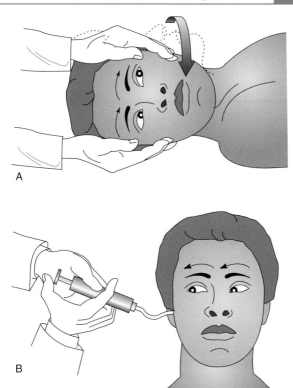

FIG. 5.3 (A) "Doll's eye" maneuver (oculocephalic reflex). With an intact brain stem (cranial nerves 3 through 8), the eyes move opposite to the direction of head turning. (B) Cold caloric test (oculovestibular reflex). With an intact brain stem, injecting cold water in the auditory canal results in tonic conjugate eye deviation toward the cold ear.

oculocephalic and oculovestibular reflexes (Fig. 5.3). Both reflexes are mediated by stimulating the semicircular canals, with CN 8 input to the vestibular nuclei and bilateral connections to the third, fourth, and sixth nuclei. *Thus intact eye movements indicate brain stem integrity from the level of CN 3 to CN 8 (midbrain and pons).*

a. **The position of the eyes at rest** should be noted.
    (1) **Gaze deviation away from the hemiparesis** results from hemispheric lesions contralateral to the hemiparesis.

(2) **Gaze deviation toward the hemiparesis** can result from the following:
   (a) Pontine lesions contralateral to the hemiparesis
   (b) "Wrong-way gaze" from thalamic lesions contralateral to the hemiparesis
   (c) Seizure activity in the hemisphere contralateral to the hemiparesis
(3) **Forced downward eye deviation** results from lesions of the midbrain tectum. Association with impaired pupillary reactivity and refractory nystagmus is known as *Parinaud syndrome*.
(4) **Slow roving eye movements** may be conjugate or dysconjugate and are indicative of bilateral hemispheric dysfunction with intact brain stem function. They are typically associated with intact and active oculocephalic reflexes.
(5) **Ocular bobbing** consists of fast downward "bobbing" with slow return to the primary position. It results from bilateral damage to the pontine horizontal gaze centers and is typically seen in locked-in syndrome.
(6) **Saccadic (fast) eye movements are not seen in coma and imply psychogenic unresponsiveness.**

b. Check for a **visual orienting response** and **ocular tracking**. These cortically mediated eye movements (Table 5.3) often recover *before* patients begin to follow verbal commands as they emerge from coma.

Stand at the bedside and state in a loud voice, "Hey Mr. Jones, look at me!" A visual orienting response is when the patient opens their eyes and looks in your general direction. If they orient, move your face around the bedside. If they track your face, then ask the patient to look at your moving finger.

c. **The oculocephalic (doll's eye) reflex** should be noted.

This reflex is elicited by briskly turning the head side to side. In alert patients, supranuclear cortical inputs to the oculomotor nuclei control eye movement, and the response

TABLE 5.3	**Hierarchy of Cortically Mediated Eye Movements**

1. Smooth pursuit of a moving finger
2. Broken pursuit of a moving finger
3. Tracks face, not finger
4. Visually orients to examiner with no tracking
5. No visual orienting response

Tracking implies more integrative cortical function and higher level of consciousness. Cortically mediated eye movements often begin to recover before the patient emerging from coma can follow verbal commands.

cannot be elicited. *An intact response consists of full conjugate eye movement opposite to the direction of head movement.*

A full and easy-to-elicit reflex ("ball-bearing eyes") implies bilateral cerebral hemisphere dysfunction and structural integrity of the brain stem, as seen with metabolic coma.

d. **The oculovestibular (cold caloric) reflex** should be tested.
This reflex is a more potent method for eliciting conjugate eye movements. The head is tilted 30 degrees above horizontal, and the ear is lavaged with 30 to 60 mL of ice water using butterfly tubing attached to a syringe. *A normal response consists of tonic eye deviation toward the cold ear and fast nystagmus away from the cold ear (mediated by the frontal lobe contralateral to the direction of the fast component).*

(1) **Tonic phase bilaterally intact, with absent fast responses** suggests coma from bihemispheric dysfunction.

(2) **Conjugate gaze paresis** can result from unilateral hemispheric or pontine lesions.

(3) **Asymmetric eye weakness** implies a brain stem lesion. CN 3 paresis, CN 6 paresis, and internuclear ophthalmoplegia are the most commonly identified abnormalities.

(4) **Absent oculovestibular responses** are seen with deep coma of any cause and imply severe depression of brain stem function.

8. **Corneal reflex**
Stroking the cornea with sterile gauze or cotton normally results in bilateral eye closure. Water drops do not consistently create the same amount of stimulation. The afferent limb of the reflex is mediated by CN 5 and the efferent limb by CN 7.

9. **Gag reflex**
In intubated patients, this reflex can be tested by gently manipulating the endotracheal tube.

10. **Motor responses**
Motor responses are the single best indicator of the depth and severity of coma.

a. **Spontaneous movements** should be observed for symmetry and purpose. Preferential movement on one side indicates weakness of the unused limbs.

b. **Limb tone** should be tested for symmetry.
Axial tone is tested by turning the head side to side. Tone in the upper extremities is tested by passive motion at the elbow and wrist. Lower extremity tone is tested by a quick lifting motion under the thigh; if the heel elevates off the bed, then tone is abnormally increased. *Bilaterally increased lower extremity tone is an important sign of herniation. Generalized increased tone is also characteristic of ictal and postictal states.*

   c. **Induced movements** should be tested systematically by observing responses to stimuli of increasing intensity, in the following order:

     (1) **Verbal command.** Ask the patient to raise one arm and show two fingers and the thumbs-up sign. Sticking out the tongue and wiggling toes are reasonable alternatives. *Eye opening and hand squeezing often occur as automatic, reflexive, nonvolitional responses and always imply verbal comprehension and preservation of consciousness.*

     (2) **Sternal rub.** Apply gentle pressure with fingertips. Placing a sheet over the face is an even milder midline stimulus; an attempt to pull the sheet is evidence of conscious behavior. Proceed to deep knuckle pressure on the sternum if there is no response to milder stimuli.

      (a) **Fending off responses** consists of precise hand movements and active attempts to push away or remove the stimulus

      (b) **Gross localizing responses** are slower and less accurate. They occur with deepening coma or with nondominant hemispheric lesions, causing impaired spatial discrimination.

     (3) **Nailbed pressure.** Use the handle of the reflex hammer and gradually increase the pressure on the nailbed, in each extremity.

      (a) **Withdrawal** is mediated by the motor cortex. The movements are sudden, nonstereotyped, and variable in intensity.

      (b) **Flexor (decorticate) posturing** (Fig. 5.4) results from damage to the corticospinal tracts at the level of the *deep hemisphere or upper midbrain.* The full response consists of flexion with adduction of the arms and extension of the legs.

      (c) **Extensor (decerebrate) posturing** (see Fig. 5.4) consists of extension, adduction, and internal rotation of the arms and extension of the legs. It results from corticospinal tract damage at the level of the *pons or upper medulla.*

11. **Sensory responses**

    Asymmetry of response to noxious stimulation suggests a lateralizing sensory deficit.

12. Reflexes

   a. **Deep tendon reflexes**

     Asymmetry indicates a lateralizing motor deficit caused by a structural lesion.

   b. **Plantar reflexes**

     Bilateral Babinski responses can occur with structural or metabolic coma.

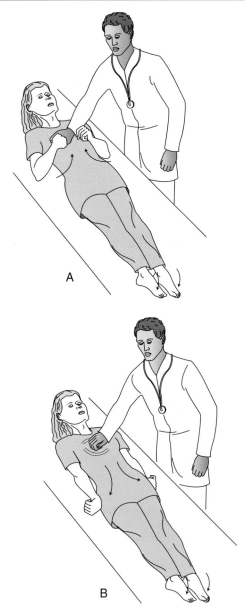

FIG. 5.4 (A) Decorticate (flexor) posturing. (B) Decerebrate (extensor) posturing.

Diagnosis

Once the history and neurologic examination are completed, a differential diagnosis should be generated. Most patients in stupor or coma can be placed into one of three categories on the basis of neurologic findings:

1. **Nonfocal examination with brain stem intact**

    This category is characterized by reactive pupils, full eye movements, and symmetric motor responses and suggests a toxic-metabolic etiology, hypoxic-ischemic encephalopathy, CNS infection, or hydrocephalus.

2. **Focal hemispheric signs**

    These signs are characterized by contralateral hemiparesis and gaze paresis and suggest a structural CNS lesion such as stroke, subdural hematoma, and neoplasm. If CT or MRI are normal, then the most likely cause is a prolonged postictal state with Todd paralysis resulting from metabolic depletion of the seizure focus.

3. **Focal brain stem signs**

    These signs are characterized by abnormal pupil reactivity, cranial nerve signs, and motor posturing and suggest a brain stem lesion or a space-occupying lesion associated with herniation.

Because it is important to quickly rule out life-threatening conditions in patients with coma, diagnostic testing should generally proceed in the following order in all patients until a diagnosis is established:

1. **Noncontrast head CT and CT angiography**

    The CT angiogram is essential for ruling out basilar artery occlusion, which is a highly treatable time-sensitive medical emergency. Look at bone windows if there is a history or suspicion of trauma.

2. **Brain MRI with and without gadolinium**

    MRI is much more sensitive than CT for revealing acute ischemia (i.e., brain stem stroke), demyelination (i.e., acute disseminated encephalomyelitis), or vasogenic edema and microbleeds (i.e., posterior reversible encephalopathy syndrome). Gadolinium IV contrast should be given if a tumor or an abscess is suspected.

3. **LP**

    LP should be performed to rule out meningitis, encephalitis, or subarachnoid hemorrhage if the diagnosis is not established by CT or MRI. *Never postpone empiric treatment for meningitis or encephalitis if there is a delay in obtaining the cerebrospinal fluid (CSF).*

4. **Continuous EEG monitoring**

    An EEG may be necessary to rule out *nonconvulsive status epilepticus,* a postictal state, or metabolic coma if the diagnosis is not established by CT and LP.

Pseudocoma States

These **pseudocoma states** are important to be aware of when considering the cause of coma.

- **Psychogenic unresponsiveness**

    Psychogenic coma occurs in patients who are physiologically awake but unresponsive. Clues to the diagnosis include negativistic behavior (active resistance to eye-opening or passive limb movement), avoidance behavior (the hand avoids the face when dropped from above the head), intact saccadic eye movements, nystagmus on cold caloric testing, and abrupt recovery of alertness in response to painful stimuli.

- **Locked-in syndrome**

    Locked-in syndrome refers to bilateral pontine damage (usually from infarction or hemorrhage) that renders the patient awake but completely paralyzed except for vertical eye movements. *Ocular bobbing* is a common finding. Evidence of consciousness comes from their ability to look up and down to verbal command.

- **Minimally conscious state and akinetic mutism**

    Akinetic mutism refers to states of extreme psychomotor slowing (i.e., severe abulia) resulting from extensive thalamic or frontal lobe damage. These patients appear awake and unresponsive, demonstrate minimal spontaneity, and exhibit only limited verbal or motor responses after extremely long delays. Minimally conscious state (MCS) is a more modern term for the same syndrome that occurs as a transition state between coma and recovery of consciousness.

MANAGEMENT

Emergency Treatments for Patients in Coma

1. **Space-occupying lesions** require prompt neurosurgical evaluation because emergent decompression may be lifesaving.
2. **Increased ICP,** if suspected, should be treated immediately. Stepwise treatment includes:
    a. Head elevation.
    b. Intubation and hyperventilation.
    c. Sedation if severe agitation is present (**midazolam 1 to 2 mg IV** is an effective, short-acting agent).
    d. Bolus osmotherapy with **20% mannitol 1.0 to 1.5 g/kg via rapid IV infusion.** If the patient is hypotensive, a suitable alternative is **0.5 to 2.0 mL/kg of 23.4% hypertonic saline** infused via a central venous line.

        These therapies can be used to "buy time" before definitive neurosurgical intervention.

e. **Dexamethasone 10 mg IV every 6 hours** also may be of benefit for reducing edema associated with tumor or abscess. After these emergency treatments, an ICP monitor should be inserted to further guide management (see Chapter 13).

3. **Encephalitis** from herpes virus infection, if suspected, should be treated empirically with **acyclovir 10 mg/kg IV every 8 hours.** Further diagnostic testing should proceed as outlined in Chapter 22.

4. **Bacterial meningitis,** if suspected, should be treated empirically. Pretreat with **dexamethasone 6 mg IV** before starting **ceftriaxone 2 g IV every 12 hours** and **vancomycin 1 g IV every 12 hours** pending CSF culture results.

5. **Status epilepticus** is a common cause of coma. Clues to the diagnosis of nonconvulsive status may include obvious or subtle "runs" of facial or extremity twitching and directional gaze deviation or nystagmus, but in many cases the seizures may be purely electrographic with no motor manifestations. If ongoing status epilepticus is suspected, order emergency continuous EEG monitoring and begin first-line benzodiazepine therapy. Start with **lorazepam 0.1 mg/kg IV** in repeated 2-mg doses. Second-line agents include **fosphenytoin 20 mg/kg** or **levetiracetam 3 to 4 g IV**. Failing those interventions, third-line therapy in intubated patients starts with midazolam 0.2 mg/kg as an IV loading dose, followed my midazolam infusion 0.2 mg/kg/h. For more details refer to Chapter 4.

6. **Cardiac arrest** resulting in diffuse hypoxic-ischemic brain injury can be cooling the body to 33°C to 36°C for 24 hours, which is a procedure known as **therapeutic temperature modulation** (TTM) (Table 5.4). Advanced feedback-controlled technology to cool the patient rapidly and precisely, in the form of an adhesive surface cooling system or endovascular heat exchange catheter, is typically required. After cooling, the patient can be gradually rewarmed to 37°C at a rate of 0.20°C to 0.33°C per hour. An example of a critical care checklist for TTM is shown in Table 5.5.

General Care of the Comatose Patient

1. **Airway protection**
   Adequate oxygenation and ventilation and prevention of aspiration are the goals. Most patients will require endotracheal intubation and frequent orotracheal suctioning. *Nonintubated stuporous* patients *should always be designated as nothing per mouth (NPO).*

2. **IV hydration**
   Use *only isotonic fluids* (e.g., normal saline) in patients with cerebral edema or increased ICP.

TABLE 5.4	Checklist for Therapeutic Temperature Modulation After Cardiac Arrest

Induction of Hypothermia
- Immediate initiation of cooling to target core body temperature of 33°C to 36°C
- Central temperature monitoring with bladder or esophageal probe
- One-time paralytic dose with rocuronium 1 mg/kg IV for expediting cooling
- Maintain temperature for 24 h after initiation of hypothermia

Shivering
- Goal is to prevent grossly visible shivering in extremities
- Acetaminophen 650 q4h standing
- Buspirone 30 mg po q8 standing
- Bair Hugger set at 43°C for skin counterwarming
- Meperidine 25 mg IV q6h prn shivering
- If shivering is refractory, start magnesium infusion at 0.5–1 g/h with goal magnesium of 3–4 mEq/L
- If shivering is still refractory, can add fentanyl, propofol, or dexmedetomidine drip (must be intubated)
- If shivering remains refractory to sedation, start neuromuscular blockade (must be on sedation) with rocuronium 0.01 mg/kg/min

Seizures and Myoclonus
- Continuous EEG for 48 h to identify seizures
- Treat seizures aggressively with lorazepam, phenytoin, levetiracetam, and midazolam (see text for dosing)
- Treat myoclonus first line with valproic acid 500–2000 mg IV q6h

Rewarming to Normothermia
- Rewarm at 0.20°C–0.33°C per hour to a goal of 37°C
- Maintain normothermia at 37°C with cooling device after rewarming to prevent rebound fever
- Shivering is common during rewarming and should be treated aggressively

Other Monitoring
- Cardiac, pulse oximetry, and capnography monitoring
- Potassium should be monitored and repleted to a goal of K = 3.0 mEq/L, as over repletion can result in hyperkalemia during rewarming
- Insulin drip for blood glucose 120–180 mg/dL (insulin resistance is common with cooling)
- Send serum neuron specific enolase (NSE) daily for five days

EEG, Electroencephalogram; *IV*, intravenous; *mEq*, milliequivalent; *NSE*, neuron-specific enolase; *po*, by mouth; *prn*, as needed; *q*, every.

Adapted from Reynolds A, Agarwal S. Hypoxic-ischemic encephalopathy. In Louis ED, Mayer SA, Rowland LP, eds. *Merritt's Textbook of Neurology.* 13th ed. New York: Wolters Kluwer Publishers, 2016:292

TABLE 5.5	Findings That Imply Poor Prognosis after Cardiac Arrest

Modality	Adverse Prognostic Finding
Neurologic examination off sedation	• Absent corneal or pupillary response • No motor response to pain • Myoclonic status epilepticus
Trend on 48 h of continuous EEG	• Isoelectric or burst suppression background • Lack of reactivity to stimuli • Status epilepticus
Neuron-specific enolase level	• Peak level >80 µg/L (usually at 24 h)
Brain MRI with DWI	• DWI ischemic lesion burden >10% of brain volume
Somatosensory evoked potentials	• Bilaterally absent cortical N20 responses

DWI, Diffusion weighted imaging; *EEG,* electroencephalography; *MRI,* magnetic resonance imaging.

Poor prognosis in this context is defined as failure to recover consciousness, e.g., transition into a persistent vegetative state.

3. **Nutrition**

Administer enteral feeds via a small-bore nasoduodenal tube. Nasogastric tubes impair the integrity of the upper and lower esophageal sphincters and increase the risk of gastro-esophageal reflux and aspiration.

4. **Skin**

Order that the patient be turned every 1 to 2 hours to prevent pressure sores. An inflatable or foam mattress and protective heel pads may also be beneficial.

5. **Eyes**

Prevent corneal abrasion by taping the eyelids shut or by applying a lubricant.

6. **Bowel care**

Constipation can be avoided by giving a stool softener (docusate sodium 100 mg three times a day). Intubation and steroids may predispose to gastric stress ulceration, and this should be prevented by giving an H_2 blocker (ranitidine 50 mg IV every 8 hours).

7. **Bladder care**

Indwelling urinary catheters are a common source of infection and should be used judiciously. Use intermittent catheterization every 6 hours when possible.

8. **Joint mobility**

Order daily passive range-of-motion exercises to prevent contractures.

9. **Deep vein thrombosis (DVT) prophylaxis**

Immobility is a major risk factor for DVT and subsequent pulmonary embolism. Order heparin 5000 units subcutaneously (SC) every 12 hours or enoxaparin 40 mg SC once a day. External pneumatic compression stockings should also be used.

PROGNOSIS AND OUTCOME

The prognosis for recovery from coma depends more on the cause, rather than on the depth, of coma. Coma from drug intoxication and metabolic causes carries the best prognosis, patients with coma from traumatic head injury fare better than those with coma from other structural causes, and coma from global hypoxia-ischemia carries the least favorable prognosis.

A variety of tests can be used to determine prognosis as early as 3 days after cardiac arrest. There five main modalities for evaluating the severity of brain injury in patients with hypoxic-ischemic encephalopathy (see Table 5.5). Be aware that overall prognosis is improving. In the posthypothermia era examples of recovery have now been reported with every single one of the adverse findings listed in the table. For years it was taken on faith that many of these findings meant absolutely no chance of recovery of consciousness.

Persistent vegetative state (PVS), also referred to as unresponsive wakefulness syndrome (UWS), refers to a state of "eyes-open unresponsiveness" that is applied to patients in coma for 30 days or more. These patients regain normal sleep–wake cycles and display primitive responses to stimuli, such as chewing, sucking, and grasping, but demonstrate no evidence of conscious awareness. Prognostication is important because this information may influence decisions to withhold life-sustaining measures such as cardiopulmonary resuscitation (CPR) or intensive care unit (ICU) care.

Recovery of consciousness from coma or PVS is generally defined as return of the ability to convincingly and consistently follow commands. By this criterion, 15% of adult patients with nontraumatic injury and 50% of patients with traumatic injury who are still in a vegetative state after 1 month will recover consciousness by 12 months. **Amantadine hydrochloride 100 mg three times a day** has been shown to accelerate the pace of functional recovery among patients in PVS or MCS after severe traumatic brain injury.

Minimally conscious state (MCS) is when patients have regained the capacity to follow commands but not much else in terms of motor or verbal function. MCS patients are bedbound and display little in the way of higher cognitive functions. Fortunately, MCS is most often a transition state as patients emerge from coma or PVS toward a better level of recovery. Recovery of consciousness after 12 months in a PVS is exceedingly rare.

Acute Stroke

Stroke should be suspected whenever a patient presents with the characteristic sudden onset of focal neurologic signs such as hemiparesis, hemisensory loss, hemianopia, aphasia, or ataxia (Table 6.1). Time is of the essence for treating stroke because reperfusion therapy always works better when given as early as possible. It has been estimated that every 15-minute reduction in onset-to-treatment time translates into a meaningful reduction in the risk of long-term disability at 3 months.

Because of the importance of early intervention in acute stroke, the emphasis of emergency room (ER) management should not be on identifying subtle, unusual, or interesting neurologic signs but on the following five priorities. When a STROKE CODE is called, tasks are ideally performed in parallel by four different personnel immediately on patient arrival (e.g., the emergency department [ED] attending, resident, nurse, and stroke neurologist):

1. **Assess level of consciousness and ensure adequate airway, breathing, and circulation.**
2. **Obtain the history with precise attention to the specific time of onset (or discovery) of symptoms, along with a list of current medications.**
3. **Establish large-bore (preferably 18-gauge) intravenous (IV) access, and obtain admission labs.**
4. **Perform a National Institutes of Health Stroke Scale (NIHSS) examination.**
5. **Obtain head noncontrast computed tomography (NCCT) and CT angiogram imaging as soon as possible.**

It should be kept in mind that mortality is reduced and the likelihood of a good recovery is increased when stroke patients are cared for in a dedicated stroke unit. If your patient is unusually complex or critically ill, consideration should be given to transferring the patient to the nearest comprehensive stroke center once he or she has been stabilized.

This chapter focuses on the emergency management of stroke. Additional information regarding hospital care and long-term management can be found in Chapter 24.

TABLE 6.1	Presentations of Acute Stroke

- Abrupt onset of facial or limb weakness (usually hemiparesis)
- Sensory loss in one or more extremities
- Sudden change in mental status (confusion, delirium, lethargy, stupor, or coma)
- Aphasia (incoherent speech, lack of speech output, or difficulty understanding speech)
- Dysarthria (slurred speech)
- Loss of vision (hemianopic or monocular) or diplopia
- Ataxia (truncal or limb)
- Vertigo, nausea and vomiting, or headache

PHONE CALL

Questions

1. **What were the presenting symptoms?**
2. **Exactly when did the symptoms begin? If the symptoms were unwitnessed, what was the *time last known well* and *time of discovery*?**
3. **Have the symptoms worsened, fluctuated, or improved since onset?**
4. **What are the vital signs?**
5. **Does the patient have a history of hypertension, diabetes, or cardiac disease?**
6. **Is the patient taking any antiplatelet agents or anticoagulants?**
It is particularly important to perform an urgent CT scan on patients taking anticoagulants to rule out intracerebral hemorrhage (ICH), because early treatment reversal agents can be lifesaving.

Orders

1. Establish an IV line with **0.9% normal saline (NS) at 1 mL/kg/h.** Hypotonic fluids such as D5W and half-normal saline aggravate cerebral edema.
2. Place a pulse oximeter and apply oxygen if there is respiratory distress or if the oxygen saturation is <95%.
3. Make sure the patient gets nothing by mouth (is made NPO).
4. Place a portable cardiac monitor.
5. Order a stat noncontrast head CT scan and a CT angiogram (Box 6.1; Fig. 6.1)
6. Order and draw the following diagnostic blood tests, but *do not delay imaging or treatment waiting for lab test results.*
   - Complete blood count (CBC) and platelet count
   - Serum chemistries (glucose, electrolytes, blood urea nitrogen [BUN], creatinine)
   - Prothrombin time (PT)(international normalized ratio [INR])/partial thromboplastin time (PTT)
   - Cardiac troponin level

BOX 6.1	Emergency Computed Tomography Angiography and Perfusion Imaging for Acute Stroke

Increasingly, major stroke centers are routinely incorporating *CTA* into their acute stroke algorithms with the goal of detecting a treatable LVO (see Fig. 6.1). Early detection of LVO is crucial because this is the trigger for proceeding with MT. Stroke centers are increasingly using a *CTA for All* policy, in which a CTA is performed at the same time as the initial noncontrast CT for all stroke codes within 24 hours of last known well, regardless of the baseline NIHSS score.

When an LVO is detected but the patient is presenting between 6 and 24 hours from last known well, *CTP* imaging is then performed to help identify good candidates for thrombectomy. Automated image analysis software calculates the volume (in milliliters) of core infarction (CBF < 30% of normal), ischemic penumbra (mismatch volume, T_{max} > 6.0 seconds) and mismatch ratio (mismatch/core volume).

In these protocols routine documentation of a normal serum creatinine level is waived because of the urgency of the situation and the low risk of serious contrast-induced nephropathy (<1%). Demonstration of a treatable LVO then triggers an interventional "secondary page" that mobilizes the interventional team with the goal of beating a 60-minute "picture-to-puncture" time interval.

CBF, Cerebral blood flow; *CTA,* computed tomography angiography; *CTP,* computed tomography perfusion; *LVO,* large-vessel occlusion; *MT,* mechanical thrombectomy; *NIHSS,* National Institutes of Health Stroke Scale score.

ELEVATOR THOUGHTS

What are the causes of stroke?
1. **Infarction: causes 80% of all strokes**
   a. Embolic
      (1) Cardiogenic embolism
          (a) Atrial fibrillation or other arrhythmia
          (b) Left ventricular mural thrombus
          (c) Mitral or aortic valve disease
          (d) Endocarditis (infectious or noninfectious)
      (2) Embolic stroke of unknown source (ESUS)
      (3) Paradoxical embolism (patent foramen ovale)
      (4) Aortic arch embolism
   b. Atherothrombotic (large-vessel or medium-vessel disease)
      (1) Extracranial disease
          (a) Internal carotid artery (ICA)
          (b) Vertebral artery
      (2) Intracranial disease
          (a) ICA
          (b) Middle cerebral artery (MCA)
          (c) Basilar artery

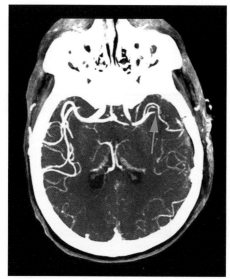

FIG. 6.1 Computed tomographic angiogram demonstrating occlusion of the M1 segment of the left middle cerebral artery *(blue arrow)*. Filling of the anterior temporal branches is evident just proximal to the site of occlusion. Posteriorly, there is markedly reduced filling of the sylvian branches of the middle cerebral artery compared with the contralateral side. (Image provided courtesy Dr. Michael Lev, Massachusetts General Hospital, Boston, Massachusetts).

   c. Lacunar (small penetrating artery occlusion)
   d. Other or unknown
2. **ICH: causes 15% of all strokes**
   a. Hypertensive
   b. Amyloid angiopathy
   c. Arteriovenous malformation (AVM)
3. **Subarachnoid hemorrhage (SAH): causes 5% of all strokes**
   a. Aneurysmal (80%)
   b. Nonaneurysmal (20%)
4. **Miscellaneous causes (can lead to infarction or hemorrhage)**
   a. Dural sinus thrombosis
   b. Carotid or vertebral artery dissection
   c. Central nervous system (CNS) vasculitis
   d. Moyamoya disease (progressive intracranial large artery occlusion)
   e. Migraine
   f. Hypercoagulable state

g. Drug abuse (cocaine or other sympathomimetics)
h. Hematologic disorders (sickle cell anemia, polycythemia, or leukemia)
i. Mitochondrial encephalopathy, lactic acidosis, and stroke (MELAS)
j. Atrial myxoma

MAJOR THREAT TO LIFE

- **Transtentorial herniation**
  Occurs primarily in the following presentations:
  1. Massive hemispheric infarction or hemorrhage
  2. Intraventricular extension of ICH or SAH
- **Cerebellar infarction or hemorrhage**
  All patients with large cerebellar lesions require neurosurgical evaluation because emergent decompression can be lifesaving.
- **Aspiration**
  Aspiration pneumonia is a common cause of death in stroke patients. All patients should be considered to have impaired swallowing until proven otherwise.
- **Myocardial infarction (MI)**
  Acute MI complicates approximately 3% of acute ischemic strokes.

BEDSIDE

Quick-Look Test

What is the patient's level of consciousness?
  The urgency of the situation can be assessed immediately by evaluating the level of consciousness. Patients in stupor or coma are at the highest risk for further deterioration and are most likely to benefit from urgent intervention.

Airway and Vital Signs

Is the patient in respiratory distress?
  If the patient's breathing appears labored, check arterial blood gas levels and start oxygen. **Patients with severe dyspnea or depressed level of consciousness (stupor or coma) should be intubated prior to CT scanning.** Failure to control the airway in either setting can lead to massive aspiration or to respiratory arrest.

What is the blood pressure (BP)?
  Hypertension occurs frequently after stroke as a nonspecific response to cerebral injury. In ischemic stroke, this response may be advantageous because increased cerebral perfusion pressure improves blood flow in regions of marginally perfused brain (the ischemic penumbra) that have lost the capacity to

autoregulate. As a result, *overly aggressive BP reduction in acute ischemic stroke patients can lead to worsened ischemia and neurologic deterioration.* For this reason, only severe hypertension should be treated prior to CT scanning unless there is a nonneurologic indication (Box 6.2).

If the patient meets one of the criteria listed in Box 6.1 and needs urgent BP control, start with **IV nicardipine 5 mg/h (1 mg/10 mL)** and adjust the rate to attain the desired BP target (see Box 6.1), up to a maximum of 15 mg/h. If a second agent is need to control BP, or if rate control is required to maintain heart rate (HR) < 100 beats/min, push **20 mg of IV labetalol** over 2 minutes; then repeat 40, 60, and finally 80 mg at 10-minute intervals until the desired BP is attained, up to a total dose of 200 mg.

Low BP in acute stroke is unusual. Hypotension that is severe enough to precipitate cerebral infarction is rare but can occur in patients with severe carotid artery or intracranial artery stenosis.

What is the HR?

Rapid atrial fibrillation is frequent in acute ischemic stroke and may require treatment with IV labetalol as previously mentioned. Alternatives include **diltiazem 20 to 25 mg** or **verapamil 5 to 15 mg IV push**.

BOX 6.2	Guidelines for Emergency Department Treatment of Hypertension in Acute Stroke

Prior to Computed Tomography Scanning:
Treat hypertension if a nonneurologic hypertensive emergency exists:
1. Acute myocardial ischemia
2. Cardiogenic pulmonary edema
3. Malignant hypertension (retinopathy)
4. Hypertensive nephropathy or encephalopathy
5. Aortic dissection

Also treat hypertension if the BP is highly elevated:
1. SBP > 220 mm Hg
2. DBP > 120 mm Hg
   Otherwise, systolic BPs of 160 to 220 mm Hg should *not* be treated prior to CT scanning.

After Computed Tomography Scanning:
1. If intracerebral hemorrhage is identified, reduce the systolic BP to 140 to 160 mm Hg
2. If the decision is made to give tPA, reduce SBP to ≤180 mm Hg and diastolic BP to ≤105 mm Hg.

BP, Blood pressure; *CT,* computed tomography; *DBP,* diastolic blood pressure; *SBP,* systolic blood pressure; *tPA,* tissue plasminogen activator.

What is the temperature?

The most common cause of fever at onset after stroke is aspiration pneumonia. If fever is present, give acetaminophen 650 mg by mouth (po), and order a cooling blanket and blood and urine cultures. If respiratory distress is present or the patient looks especially sick, consider administering antibiotics empirically (**amoxicillin/sulbactam [Unasyn] 1.5 g IV every 6 hours** or **clindamycin 600 mg IV every 8 hours**).

Selective History

If possible, obtain an eyewitness to corroborate the patient's account. Be sure to check the following:

1. **Exactly what time did the stroke begin?**

   If the symptoms began within 6 hours and an ischemic stroke is confirmed by CT, IV or intraarterial reperfusion therapy may be possible, and the evaluation should proceed as quickly as possible.

2. **What were the initial symptoms?**

   A maximal deficit at onset in a fully alert patient supports cerebral infarction and suggests embolism in particular. Loss of consciousness, headache, or vomiting supports ICH. Inquire specifically about the following:

   - Headache or neck pain (hemorrhage or dissection)
   - Loss of consciousness
   - Confused or slurred speech
   - Visual disturbances
   - Dizziness or vertigo (brain stem ischemia)
   - Weakness or clumsiness
   - Numbness or paresthesias
   - Gait instability

3. **Were there any antecedent attacks consistent with transient ischemic attack (TIA)?**

4. **Was any seizure activity observed?**

5. **What is the patient's medical history?**

6. **Has the patient used drugs or alcohol recently?**

   Cocaine can precipitate infarction or hemorrhage.

7. **What medications is the patient taking?**

Selective Physical Examination
General Physical Examination

Neck: Auscultate for carotid bruits. Neck stiffness suggests subarachnoid hemorrhage.

Lungs: Check for aspiration pneumonia or congestive heart failure.

Heart: Murmurs suggest valvular heart disease and a possible source of embolism.

Neurologic Examination

Because time is of the essence, the initial neurologic examination needs to be systematic and efficient. The goal is to simply localize and characterize the severity of the deficit. An experienced examiner can accomplish this in 10 minutes; a more detailed examination should be performed later. Focusing your examination on these elements will allow you to calculate an *NIH Stroke Scale* score (see www.mdcalc.com/nih-stroke-scale-score-nihss).

- **Mental status**
    1. **Level of consciousness and attentiveness**
    2. **Orientation.** Ask the patient what month it is and how old they are.
    3. **Aphasia.** Check the fluency of spontaneous speech, naming, repetition, and paraphasic errors (word or syllable substitutions). Ask the patient to open and close his or her eyes and grip and release his or her strong hand. Then ask the patient to read some simple sentences and name objects (Fig. 6.2).
    4. **Hemispatial neglect.** Forced head and gaze deviation implies a large hemispheric lesion.
- **Cranial nerves**
    1. **Visual fields.** Ask the patient to count fingers in all four quadrants. Check the patient's blink to threat if the patient is inattentive.
    2. **Pupils.** Assymetry suggests brain stem ischemia.
    3. **Extraocular movements.** Check horizontal eye movements, looking for a conjugate gaze paresis.
    4. **Face.** A widened palpebral fissure and flattened nasolabial fold are indicative of facial weakness.
    5. **Palate and tongue.** Check for symmetry and adequacy of the gag reflex.
- **Motor**
    1. **Spontaneous movements.** Preferential movement of the limbs on one side indicates paresis of the unused limbs. If the patient is unresponsive, check for a preferential localizing response to sternal rub.
    2. **Limb tone.** Increased tone occurs with deep lesions in the internal capsule or brain stem.
    3. **Arm (pronator) and leg drift.** If the patient is unable to follow commands, then passively elevate the arms and legs and check whether one falls preferentially.
    4. **Power.** Check strength against active resistance at the shoulders, wrists, hips, and ankles.
- Reflexes
    1. **Deep tendon reflexes**
    2. **Plantar reflexes**

Proceed with the following elements of the neurologic examination only if the patient's level of consciousness allows:

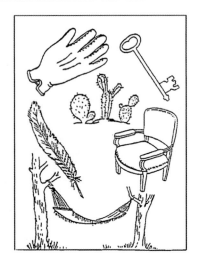

A

You know how.
Down to earth
I got home from work
Near the table in the dining room
They heard him speak on the radio
    last night

B

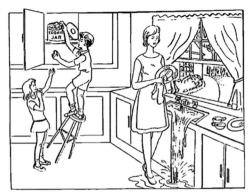

C

FIG. 6.2 Images used to test for aphasia. (A) Objects to name. (B) Sentences to read. (C) A picture to describe.

- **Sensory**
  1. **Pinprick or pinch test** identifies a lateralized deficit.
- **Coordination**
  1. **Finger-to-nose test** identifies intention tremor and past pointing.
  2. **Gait and station.** Check for reduced arm swing on the paretic side. A wide base is indicative of truncal ataxia.

MANAGEMENT

Acute Management

Once the history and examination are completed, you should be able to localize the lesion clinically. **The main differential diagnoses are infarction and hemorrhage, which can be accurately diagnosed only by CT or magnetic resonance (MR).** Hence, all further management decisions (thrombolysis, BP management, or further workup) will depend on the results of brain imaging.

Hemorrhage

Radiographic Assessment

Blood is readily identified by the presence of a high-density (bright) signal (Fig. 6.3). If ICH is present, be sure to check for the following radiographic findings:

- *SAH* (see Fig. 6.3B) in association with intraparenchymal hemorrhage suggests a ruptured aneurysm and requires angiography.
- *Intraventricular hemorrhage* (see Fig. 6.3C) in association with ventricular enlargement requires neurosurgical evaluation for possible emergent ventriculostomy.
- *Fluid/fluid levels* within a hematoma (Fig. 6.3D) result from separation of red blood cells and plasma and are indicative of a coagulopathy.
- *Edema and mass effect* usually lead to delayed neurologic deterioration when associated with a large hemorrhage (>30 mL). An abnormally large or an irregular amount of edema associated with hemorrhage suggests (1) hemorrhagic infarction, (2) bleeding associated with neoplasm, or (3) venous infarction from dural sinus thrombosis.

Checklist for Acute Management of Intracerebral Hemorrhage

1. **Rule out coagulopathy**
   Confirm that the PT/INR and PTT are normal.
   - If the PT is elevated or the patient is actively taking warfarin or another form of oral vitamin K antagonist anticoagulant therapy, give **a four-factor prothrombin complex concentrate (4F-PCC; Kcentra, CSL Behring, King of Prussia,**

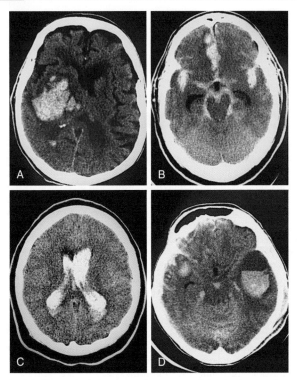

FIG. 6.3 Computed tomography scans of brain hemorrhage. (A) Intracerebral hemorrhage. (B) Subarachnoid hemorrhage. (C) Intraventricular hemorrhage. (D) Acute hemorrhage with fluid/fluid level, indicative of a clotting disturbance.

Pennsylvania) **25 U/kg or 50 U/kg IV push (give the higher dose if the INR is >6.0).** Then give **vitamin K 10 mg by IV push, and repeat as needed daily for the next 3 days** until the INR is normalized to <1.4.

- To reverse unfractionated or low-molecular-weight heparin (LMWH) give **protamine sulfate 10 to 50 mg by slow IV push** (1 mg reverses approximately 100 U of heparin or LMWH; give enough to reverse all of the heparin received within the last 2 hours).
- Reverse dabigatran or other direct thrombin inhibitors with **idarucizumab (Praxbind) 5 g IV.**

- Reverse factor Xa inhibitors (edoxaban, rivaroxaban, apixaban) with **andexanet alpha (Andexxa)**. The low-dose regimen is **400 mg as a bolus followed by 4 mg/min for 120 minutes**. The high-dose regime is **800 mg as a bolus followed by 8 mg/min for 120 minutes**. Give the high dose if the patient last took >10 mg of rivaroxaban, or >5 mg of apixaban, within the last 8 hours.
- Note that platelet transfusion is not recommended for ICH patients on antiplatelet agents, such as aspirin or clopidogrel, based on a clinical trial suggesting that platelet transfusion worsens outcome. It remains reasonable to give platelets for reversing thrombocytopenia, or for patients on antiplatelet therapy who are about to undergo a neurosurgical procedure.

2. **Control severe hypertension**

In contrast to the approach taken with acute cerebral infarction, a somewhat more aggressive approach to BP control is suggested for patients with acute ICH because high levels may lead to worsening of perilesional edema. Although the optimal management has yet to be established, we advocate reduction of systolic BP to a target between 140 and 160 mm Hg using a **labetalol** or **nicardipine** infusion (see the section Airway and Vital Signs).

3. **Consider emergent hematoma evacuation**

The criteria for emergent evacuation of ICH are controversial. It is generally accepted that cerebellar hemorrhages greater than 3 cm in diameter should be evacuated when there is a depressed level of consciousness with clinical signs and radiographic evidence of posterior fossa mass effect. A randomized controlled trial found no benefit when craniotomy was performed for supratentorial ICH within 72 hours of onset compared with best medical therapy. Despite this, patients classically considered good candidates for emergency surgery, such as younger patients with early deterioration caused by symptomatic mass effect from a large lobar hemorrhage, were excluded from the trial, and in selected cases these patients might still benefit from surgery.

Consideration should also be given to inserting a *ventricular drain* in stuporous or comatose patients with intraventricular hemorrhage and obstructive hydrocephalus, or a *parenchymal* intracranial pressure (ICP) monitor in patients with large, deep hemorrhages who are not candidates for surgery.

4. **Consider angiography**

Angiography can rule out an aneurysm or AVM. This is particularly important when SAH is present, in young nonhypertensive patients when a lobar hemorrhage is present, or in any patient with a primary intraventricular hemorrhage. Angiography is almost always negative in chronically hypertensive patients with a hemorrhage in a classic hypertensive location (putamen, thalamus, pons, or cerebellum).

5. **Osmotherapy**

Consider **mannitol (1.0 to 1.5 g/kg IV)** for deepening coma or if clinical signs of brain stem compression are evident (see Chapter 13 for further details). An alternative is 0.5 to 2.0 mL/kg of 23.4% hypertonic saline if the patient is relatively hypotensive or hypovolemic. *Steroids such as dexamethasone have not been shown to be effective in patients with ICH and should not be used.*

6. **Anticonvulsant therapy**

Seizures at onset are unusual but if present should be treated with **phenytoin** or **fosphenytoin 10 to 20 mg/kg IV or levetiracetam 500 to 2000 mg BID.** Prophylactic treatment with phenytoin or a similar anticonvulsant for 7 days is an option in patients whose condition is critical enough to require intubation, treatment for increased ICP, or surgery.

Additional guidelines for the management of ICH or SAH are included in Chapter 24 and in the section Management II: General Care in this chapter.

Infarction
Radiographic Assessment

- **Noncontrast head CT.** Infarction appears as a lucent (dark) signal on a CT scan but may not be apparent until 12 to 24 hours after onset. Early signs of infarction (Fig. 6.4) are important to recognize and include (1) loss of definition of the gray-white junction, (2) mild sulcal effacement, and (3) subtle, hazy

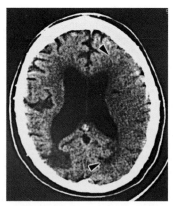

FIG. 6.4 Early cerebral infarction, with loss of gray-white definition and sulcal effacement. (*Arrowheads* indicate anterior and posterior borders of the territory of the middle cerebral artery.)

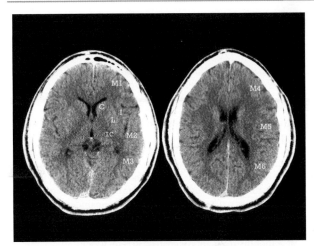

FIG. 6.5 Alberta Stroke Program Early CT Scale (ASPECTS) score. Anatomic regions evaluated in the ASPECTS score. A score of 10 indicates no evidence of early ischemic change, from which one point is subtracted for each region of infarction. Patients with scores below 7 are at high risk for hemorrhagic transformation if given intravenous tissue plasminogen activator. *C*, Caudate; *I*, insula; *L*, lentiform nucleus; *IC*, internal capsule; *M*, middle cerebral artery territories 1 through 6. (Reproduced with permission from *Merritt's Textbook of Neurology*. 13th edition. Wolters Kluwer: New York, 2016:124).

lucency. The extent of early infarction can be quantified with the Alberta Stroke Program Early CT Scale (ASPECTS) score, with 10 indicating no early infarction and 0 representing complete infarction of the entire MCA territory (Fig. 6.5)

- **CT Angiography (CTA) and CT Perfusion (CTP).** At many stroke centers, contrast-enhanced *CTA and CTP* are increasingly being used as adjuncts to standard NCCT imaging in the ED. Demonstration of a large-vessel occlusion (LVO) (see Fig. 6.1) can be used to identify candidates for emergent angiography and mechanical thrombectomy (MT) (see next for further discussion).

- **Magnetic Resonance Imaging (MRI).** Diffusion-weighted imaging (DWI) reveals acute ischemic changes within minutes to hours of onset, which is long before infarction is present on CT or MR fluid attenuation inversion recovery (FLAIR) images. Accordingly, MRI with DWI is probably the imaging modality of choice for patients with acute stroke. Gadolinium-enhanced perfusion-weighted imaging can also be used to identify regions of "perfusion-diffusion mismatch," much in the way that CTP is used. However, logistical problems often limit the timely performance of MR, which can delay therapy. MRI is most often used to assess the final extent of injury once all therapeutic intervention during the acute phase has been completed.

Goals of Management

1. **Give thrombolytic therapy with IV tissue plasminogen activator (tPA) if possible**

   IV thrombolysis with **tPA** within 4.5 hours of symptom onset is the only currently approved medical treatment for reversing ischemia in acute stroke. For eligible patients, 0.9 mg/kg of IV tPA is administered up to a maximum dose of 90 mg, with the initial 10% given as an IV push and the remainder infused over 1 hour. IV tPA only rarely results in immediate early neurologic improvement; rather, it increases the chances of a good recovery at 3 months from approximately 30% to 40%.

   - When given between 3 and 4.5 hours after symptom onset the benefit of tPA is less than when given within 3 hours, but it still improves outcome. However, in this time frame patients must be ≤80 years old, have an NIHSS <25, and not have a history of both stroke and diabetes.
   - Note that BP must be controlled to >180/105 mm Hg prior to giving tPA, and for at least 24 hours thereafter to minimize the risk of hemorrhagic conversion.
   - Hyperglycemia is also an important risk factor for hemorrhage after IV tPA and should be controlled with a regular human insulin infusion of 0.5 to 4.0 U/h to maintain the serum glucose to <180 mg/dL for the first 24 hours.
   - tPA carries a 6% risk of symptomatic intracranial bleeding and should not be given if the head CT scan shows subtle early infarct signs involving more than one-third of the MCA territory, as evidenced by an ASPECTS score of <7.
   - Because the risk of hemorrhage increases significantly after 4.5 hours, this time window must be strictly obeyed. Table 6.2 shows a list of potential contraindications to giving tPA within the 4.5 hour time window, and the strength of these contraindications according to the published literature.

2. **Evaluate for the presence of LVO and perform MT if possible**

   An important limitation of tPA is that it fails to recanalize the occluded vessel in 40% of cases. When larger clots occlude the major large intracranial vessels (the proximal MCA, ICA terminus, or basilar artery) recanalization rates are even worse

TABLE 6.2 **Strength of Evidence for Contraindications to Tissue Plasminogen Activator Therapy**

Clinical Scenario	Strength of Contraindication
• CT evidence of hemorrhage	Absolute
• Early infarct signs involving greater than one-third of the MCA territory	Absolute
• Time of symptom onset unknown	Absolute
• History of coagulopathy or anticoagulant use, or documented elevation of INR (>1.7) or aPTT (>1.5 × control)	Relative, strong
• Thrombocytopenia (platelet count < 100,000)	Relative, strong
• SBP > 185 or DBP > 110[a]	Relative, moderate
• Major surgery or serious trauma within preceding 14 days	Relative, moderate
• Glucose < 50 or > 400 mg/dL[a]	Relative, moderate
• Pregnancy	Relative, moderate
• Stroke or serious head trauma within preceding 3 months	Relative, weak
• Seizure at onset of stroke	Relative, weak
• Rapidly improving or minor symptoms (e.g., pure sensory, minimal weakness)	Relative, weak
• Gastrointestinal, urinary tract, or other significant bleeding within preceding 21 days	Relative, weak
• Significant MI within past 4 weeks or symptoms of post-MI pericarditis	Relative, weak
• Arterial puncture at a noncompressible site within preceding 7 days	Relative, weak
• Lumbar puncture within preceding 7 days	Relative, weak

[a]Blood pressure and glucose can be urgently corrected and then tissue plasminogen activator (tPA) can be administered.

This information is intended to serve only as a guideline. Successful and safe use of intravenous tPA has been reported despite the presence of one or more of these complications. Decisions regarding the risks and benefits of tPA should be individualized.

aPTT, Activated partial thromboplastin time; *CT,* computed tomography; *DBP,* diastolic blood pressure; *INR,* international normalized ratio; *MCA,* middle cerebral artery; *MI,* myocardial infarction; *SBP,* systolic blood pressure.

Reproduced with permission from *Merritt's Textbook of Neurology.* 13th ed. Wolters Kluwer: New York, 2016:127.

and outcomes remain poor despite IV tPA administration. Interventional bridging therapy is the strategy of proceeding immediately to endovascular intervention while tPA is infusing. If a persistent LVO is detected, then angiography (Fig. 6.6) and endovascular intervention to extract the clot from the vessel

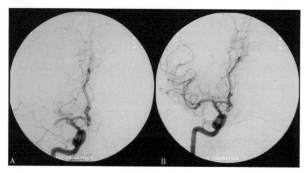

FIG. 6.6 Angiogram (anteroposterior view) demonstrating total occlusion of the right M1 middle cerebral artery segment (A) prior to intraarterial thrombolysis, and complete recanalization (B) after the procedure. (Reproduced with permission from Katzan IL, et al.; Intra-arterial thrombolysis for perioperative stroke after open heart surgery. *Neurology.* 1999;52:1081.)

using a suction or retrievable stent ("stentriever") device can then be attempted (see Chapter 24 for details).

- In 2015, five major randomized trials demonstrated that patients presenting within 6 hours of onset or last known well with LVO documented by CTA benefited substantially from MT. Although there was no consistent reduction in mortality, the ability of the procedure to reduce disability is substantial, with a number needed to treat of 2.6 to reduce disability per patient. The treatment effect is not affected by age >80 or whether or not the patient receives tPA.

- In 2017, two additional studies found that the benefit of MT can be extended to patients presenting within the 6- to 24-hour window from last known well if CTP imaging showed a relatively large penumbra associated with disproportionately small core infarct. As a general rule, CTP should show a ratio of penumbra-to-core of ≥1.8 and a core infarct no larger than 70 mL. As would be expected, patients who meet imaging criteria for thrombectomy in the extended time window tend to have severe deficits (median NIHSS ~16) associated with higher ASPECTS scores (generally >6), indicating a small burden of early infarction. About half of eligible patients treatable in the 6- to 24-hour time window are wake-up strokes, and the others tend to have robust collateral, which extends survival of penumbral tissue. The approximate benefit is an increase in the percentage of patients with minimal deficit at 3 months from 15% to 45%, corresponding to a number needed to treat of about 3.

- Stroke is a team sport. To be successful, rapid evaluation and mobilization of the interventional team requires preparation and interdisciplinary teamwork. Stroke imaging protocols that include CTA and CTP as first-line imaging, without the need for creatinine testing, has been shown to improve LVO detection, increase the MT treatment population, hasten intervention, and improve outcomes after LVO. The outcome benefit primarily affects patients presenting within 6 hours of symptom onset.

3. **Identify the affected vascular territory to determine the mechanism of stroke**

   Identification of the affected vascular territory can provide important information regarding the mechanism of the infarction. The topography of the major arterial territories of the brain is shown in Fig. 6.7. Examples of the three main patterns of infarction, described next, are shown in Fig. 6.8.

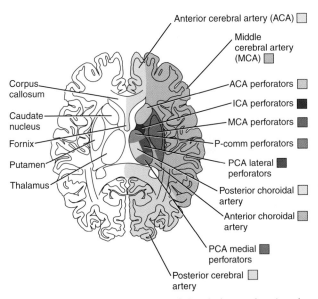

FIG. 6.7 Axial section at the level of the thalamus showing the anatomic distribution of the major cerebral vascular territories. *ICA,* Internal carotid artery; *PCA,* posterior cerebral artery; *P-comm,* Posterior communicating artery. (Redrawn from Tatu L, et al; Arterial territories of the human brain: cerebral hemispheres. *Neurology.* 1998;50:1699–1708.)

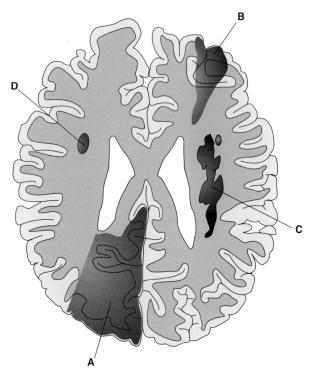

FIG. 6.8 Schematic representation of different topographic patterns of cerebral infarction. (A) Territorial infarction (from posterior cerebral artery occlusion). (B) Watershed border-zone infarction (between the territories of the anterior cerebral artery and the middle cerebral artery). (C) Internal border-zone infarction (deep middle cerebral artery territory). (D) Lacunar infarction (lenticulostriate-penetrating artery occlusion).

- **Territorial infarction** respects the margins of an entire vascular territory or one of its branches. The cause is usually embolism, with infarction occurring in brain regions immediately distal to the site of occlusion.
- **Border-zone infarction** may occur either (1) along the boundaries between different vascular territories (watershed infarction) or (2) in the deepest and least well-collateralized regions of a vascular territory (internal border-zone infarction). In either case, the cause is usually distal hemodynamic

perfusion failure related to a more proximal stenosis or occlusion.

- **Lacunar infarction** appears as a small, deep infarction within the territory of a single, small penetrating artery. The mechanism is usually related to occlusion within the course of the small vessel (microatheroma or lipohyalinosis).

4. **Prevent neurologic deterioration related to an evolving stroke (72-hour window)**

   Once an ischemic stroke is completed, progression occurs in 20% to 40% of hospitalized patients, with the risk highest in the first 24 hours. Clinical deterioration can result from one of three mechanisms:

   - **Extension of ischemic territory.** This may result from either *progressive thrombosis within an occluded vessel* (e.g., progressive brain stem infarction in a patient with basilar artery thrombosis) or *distal perfusion failure related to a more proximal stenosis or occlusion* (e.g., enlargement of internal border-zone infarction in a patient with ICA occlusion).
   - *Approach:* Full anticoagulation with unfractionated heparin may be used to prevent progressive thrombosis, although there is limited evidence of its efficacy, and its use in general is not recommended. Optimization of volume status and blood pressure may be used to mitigate perfusion failure; the best results occur if the patient has a fluctuating deficit or history of crescendo TIAs, which is suggestive of hemodynamic perfusion failure.
   - **Hemorrhagic conversion.** This problem is frequently identified radiographically but seldom results in clinical symptoms. The three main risk factors are increased patient age, large infarct size, and acute hypertension. Risk factors for symptomatic hemorrhagic infarction include age >75, NIHSS score ≥10, hyperglycemia, and extensive early infarct signs.
   - *Approach:* Defer anticoagulation of high-risk patients; treat severe hypertension.
   - **Progressive edema and infarct swelling.** This problem is generally limited to large MCA and cerebellar infarcts. Brain edema generally peaks 3 to 5 days after onset and is rarely a problem within the first 24 hours.
   - *Approach:* Treatment with mannitol or hypertonic saline may be beneficial (see Chapter 13). Avoid hypotonic fluids. *Steroids are not effective.* For patients with significant neurologic worsening (lethargy, pupillary signs, or ipsilateral motor signs) surgical decompression is indicated. *Decompressive hemicraniectomy* increases survival in patients <60 years with malignant MCA syndrome from approximately 25%

to 75%, corresponding to a number needed to treat of just 2 to save a life. Patients aged 60 to 75 also benefit, but the reduction in mortality is somewhat less and there is a relative increase in disability among surgically treated survivors.

5. **Prevent early recurrent stroke (30-day window)**

Approximately 5% of patients hospitalized for ischemic stroke experience a second stroke within 30 days. This risk is highest (greater than 10%) in patients with severe carotid stenosis and cardioembolism and lowest (1%) in patients with lacunar infarction.

Approach: Early treatment (i.e., within the first 30 days) with anticoagulation may reduce the risk of early recurrent stroke in patients with cardioembolism or large-artery stenosis but has not been proven to do so. Carotid endarterectomy or stenting reduces the risk of recurrent stroke in patients presenting with symptomatic high-grade stenosis. Double antiplatelet therapy with aspirin and clopidogrel can reduce the 90-day risk of recurrent stroke to a modest degree in selected patients with stuttering lacunar syndromes.

Secondary Prevention and Hospital Management of Ischemic Stroke

1. **Anticoagulation.** Although the use of **IV heparin** (start at **800 U/h, 20,000 U in 500 mL NS at 20 mL/h**) for acute ischemic stroke is not generally recommended, it may be a reasonable treatment option to prevent progression or recurrence of stroke in the following situations:
   • Stroke in evolution
   • High-grade large-vessel atherostenosis
   • Cardioembolic stroke
   • Arterial dissection
   • Crescendo TIAs
   • Dural sinus thrombosis

   Keep in mind that heparin is relatively contraindicated in patients with large infarcts associated with mass effect or hemorrhagic conversion.

2. **Antiplatelet therapy.** Give **aspirin 81-325 mg poQD** within 48 hours of onset. Aspirin is associated with a very small reduction in mortality and the risk of recurrent ischemic stroke in the first year. In patients with progressive or fluctuating small vessel ischemia ("capsular warning syndrome") and a NIHSS score ≤3, the addition of **clopidogrel 300 mg** on day one, followed by **75 mg** daily for 21 days, is associated with a 3.5% absolute reduction in recurrent stroke at 90 days compared to aspirin alone.

3. **Perform cardiac rhythm monitoring** in all patients on admission for a minimum of 24 to 72 hours to possible paroxysmal atrial fibrillation.

4. **Consider intensive care unit (ICU) observation** in patients with clinical or **radiographic** signs of massive hemispheric or cerebellar infarction, depressed level of consciousness, respiratory distress, or fluctuating deficits or stroke-in-evolution.

5. In selected cases with a *fluctuating deficit and documented large-vessel stenosis or occlusion*, a 30-minute trial of induced hypertension with **phenylephrine 2 to 10 mg/kg/min** targeted to raise the systolic BP by 20% can lead to immediate improvement of the neurologic deficit in approximately one-third of cases. If no improvement is observed after 30 minutes, the infusion should be stopped. Close clinical monitoring of cardiac rhythm and BP is essential.

6. **Obtain a neurosurgical evaluation** for possible decompressive surgery in patients with large cerebellar infarction or complete MCA territory infarction with midline shift and deteriorating level of consciousness.

7. Consider **MRI** including DWI in patients with **posterior** circulation strokes or if the infarction is not well delineated by CT.

8. **Order a noninvasive neurovascular workup.**

   Proper decisions regarding the treatment of cerebral infarction are based on elucidation of the mechanism of the stroke.

   The following tests should be performed in every patient:

   - *Echocardiography* is an important technique for identifying cardiac sources of emboli. In many patients, transthoracic echocardiography is adequate. *Transesophageal echocardiography* provides more detailed views of the left atrium and aortic arch and is a more sensitive test for detecting mural thrombi and valvular vegetations. An *agitated saline study* ("bubble study") is highly sensitive for detecting right-to-left atrial shunts, which are consistent with a patent foramen ovale.

   - *Carotid Doppler ultrasonography, MRA, or CTA* is needed to rule out carotid stenosis that is symptomatic and greater than 70%, which is an indication for carotid endarterectomy.

   The following tests should be performed in selected patients:

   - *Transcranial Doppler ultrasonography* can be used to diagnose occlusion or stenosis of the major intracranial arteries. Abnormal intracranial waveforms and collateral flow patterns can also be used to determine whether a stenosis found in the neck is hemodynamically significant.

- *MR or CTA* can be used to diagnose extracranial or intracranial stenosis or occlusion.
- *Ambulatory electrocardiogram (ECG) monitoring* may be useful for detecting paroxysmal atrial fibrillation in patients with a diagnosis of cryptogenic stroke at discharge, including ESUS. This form of monitoring detects intermittent atrial fibrillation in approximately 15% of patients.

9. **Consider blood testing** to identify unusual causes of stroke, particularly in young patients.
    - *Blood cultures* if endocarditis is suspected
    - *Procoagulant workup:* protein C activity, protein S activity, antithrombin III activity, lupus anticoagulant, anticardiolipin antibodies, factor V Leiden mutation, prothrombin gene mutation. *Note:* These tests should be obtained before anticoagulation is started.
    - *Vasculitis workup:* antinuclear antibody (ANA), rheumatoid factor (RF), rapid plasma reagin (RPR), hepatitis virus serologies, erythrocyte sedimentation rate (ESR), serum protein electrophoresis (SPEP), cryoglobulins, and herpes simplex virus (HSV) serologies
    - *Coagulation profile* to rule out disseminated intravascular coagulation (DIC)
    - *Beta-human chorionic gonadotropin (β-hCG)* testing to rule out pregnancy in young women with stroke

Refer to **Chapter 24** for further discussion of specific ischemic stroke syndromes, evaluation of TIAs, and the secondary prevention of ischemic stroke.

Management II: General Care

Much of the morbidity and mortality associated with stroke is related to nonneurologic complications, which can be minimized by adherence to these guidelines:

1. **Fever**

    Fever exacerbates ischemic brain injury and should be treated aggressively with antipyretics (acetaminophen) or a cooling blanket, if necessary.

2. **Nutrition**

    Stroke patients are at high risk for aspiration. Patients with depressed level of consciousness, brain stem strokes, bilateral strokes, and large hemispheric strokes carry the highest risk. Formal assessment of swallowing ability by a speech pathologist should be completed before patients at risk are fed. Start enteral feeding via a nasoduodenal tube within 24 hours after the stroke if the patient cannot swallow safely.

3. **IV hydration**

    Hypovolemia is common among stroke patients and should be corrected with isotonic crystalloid. Avoiding volume depletion may be particularly important in patients with intra-cardiac thrombi (dehydration has been linked to progressive thrombus formation) or hemodynamic stroke. Hypotonic fluids (e.g., D5W and 0.45% saline) can aggravate cerebral edema and should be avoided.

4. **Glucose**

Hyperglycemia and hypoglycemia can lead to exacerbation of ischemic injury. In critically ill stroke patients it seems prudent to prevent hyperglycemia (glucose level higher than 180 mg/dL) with intensive insulin infusion (0.5–1.0 U/h to maintain glucose levels between 120 and 180 mg/dL).

5. **Pulmonary care**

Chest physical therapy (every 4 hours) should be ordered to prevent atelectasis in immobilized patients.

6. **Head of bed elevation**

Elevate the head of bed 30 degrees to reduce the risk of ventilator-associated pneumonia, improve orientation, and minimize ICP.

7. **Activity**

Patients with stroke should be mobilized and engaged in physical therapy as soon as possible after the first 24 hours. For immobilized patients, order patient turning every 2 hours (to prevent pressure sores) and joint range-of-motion exercises four times a day to prevent contractures. Heel splints to maintain the ankle in dorsiflexion can also prevent shortening of the Achilles tendon. Have the patient taken out of bed to a chair every day as soon as feasible.

8. **Prophylaxis for deep vein thrombosis (DVT)**

Ischemic stroke patients with significant immobility who are not on IV heparin should be treated with enoxaparin 40 mg once daily or heparin 5000 U every 12 hours to prevent formation of DVT. This treatment can be started safely in patients with ICH after 24 hours.

9. **Bladder care**

Indwelling urinary catheters should be used judiciously; order intermittent catheterization every 6 hours when possible.

Spinal Cord Compression

Spinal cord compression is one of the few true neurologic emergencies. The more severe the syndrome, the more acute the injury is likely to have been. Unlike the brain, which may have remarkable functional recovery, the spinal cord, once damaged, rarely recovers function. Patients with cord compression resulting from neoplastic disease of the spine who cannot walk before the onset of treatment will rarely walk again. Diagnosis of spinal cord injury depends on a clear understanding of the anatomy of the cord and the supportive structures.

PHONE CALL

This chapter will be most useful for patients in whom spinal cord compression is known or suspected. The response to such a call should focus on establishing the diagnosis and assessing the acuteness of the injury.

Questions

1. **What is the patient's general condition?**
2. **What are the vital signs? Is the patient in any respiratory distress?**
3. **Does the patient have back pain?**
4. **Is there history of trauma to the neck or back?**
5. **Does the patient have any known cancer or infection?**
6. **Back pain in a cancer patient is considered to result from a vertebral metastasis until it is proved otherwise.**
7. **How long has the problem been going on?**

Orders

If trauma or an unstable spine is suspected, give the following orders:

1. **Immobilize the neck (back)**

    A Philadelphia collar or a backboard should be used to ensure adequate stability (Fig. 7.1). If such equipment is

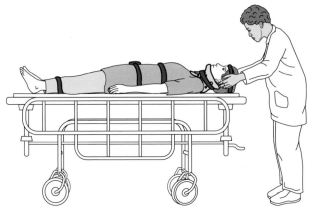

FIG. 7.1 Stabilizing the neck and back with a Philadelphia collar and a backboard.

unavailable immediately, the cervical spine can be immobilized by holding the head firmly in a neutral position, using both hands.

2. **Check vital signs**

   Injury above the C5 level will often acutely compromise respiratory function caused by impairment of diaphragmatic function. Injury of the lower cervical and upper thoracic cord also may cause respiratory failure, although often less acutely. Cervical spinal injury, particularly with complete transection, may result in loss of sympathetic control, causing hypotension and bradycardia. Fever may point to an infectious process.

3. **Obtain imaging**

   In most hospitals, computed tomography (CT) is the initial imaging of choice with consideration of magnetic resonance imaging (MRI) once the patient has been stabilized. If CT is unavailable, X-rays with anteroposterior, lateral, and odontoid views should be done. Even if there is no suspicion of trauma, the pattern of bony abnormality may suggest subluxation, unsuspected pathologic fracture from neoplasm, osteomyelitis, or other infection.

4. **Notify the neurosurgical team or specialized spinal unit, if available**

   Direct trauma to the spinal cord can produce a myelopathy, but it is the secondary effects from bleeding, dislocation, or osseous or articular instability that can be devastating; these secondary effects are preventable if properly identified and addressed.

Inform RN

"Will arrive at the bedside in…minutes."

Spinal cord compression is a medical emergency. Delay may cause irreversible neurologic dysfunction.

ELEVATOR THOUGHTS

What is the differential diagnosis of spinal cord compression?

Physical examination and often radiographic evaluation are needed to confirm a compressive myelopathy. You should be thinking first of the three categories of disease that are the most likely to cause spinal cord compression: trauma, infection, and neoplasm. Four other categories complete the differential diagnosis list.

1. **Trauma**

   Trauma is the most acute form of spinal cord compression. A history of a motor vehicle accident or sports-related accident is commonly elicited. Flexion, extension, compression, or rotation injuries in addition to direct blunt or penetrating trauma may produce a compressive myelopathy. Cervical disks tend to herniate centrally, producing an anterior cord syndrome.

2. **Infection**

   Infections of the spine typically present subacutely, although they can have acute onset of symptoms. They generally present with back pain and fever, and most often occur in the thoracic or lumbar spine. Infections can take the following forms:
   - Epidural abscesses: These are seen commonly in intravenous (IV) drug users and are most often bacterial (e.g., *Staphylococcus aureus*, *Escherichia coli*).
   - Spinal tuberculosis (Pott disease): This occurs in debilitated or immunocompromised patients or in those known to have pulmonary tuberculosis.
   - Vertebral osteomyelitis: This is caused by *Staphylococcus* species, *Streptococcus* species, *E. coli*, or *Brucella* species, which may cause pathologic fractures or produce epidural abscesses.

3. **Neoplasm**

   Metastases are the most common neoplasm seen in bony disease of the spine (Fig. 7.2). The thoracic spine is most often affected because of venous drainage of visceral organs through spinal extradural venous plexuses. Meningiomas may appear as extradural tumors, with a predominance in the thoracic region. Neurofibromas or schwannomas may arise on spinal roots and cause cord compression as they expand. Ependymomas are intrinsic cord tumors that could mimic extraaxial compressive lesions.

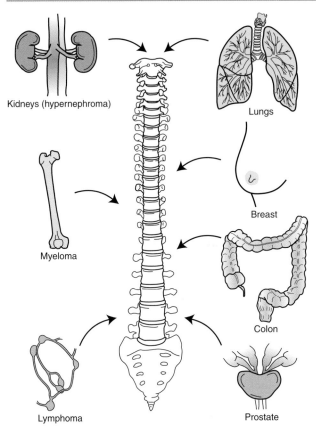

FIG. 7.2 Neoplasms that commonly metastasize to or involve the spine: carcinoma of the lung, breast, colon, and prostate; renal cell carcinoma; myeloma; and lymphoma.

Kidneys (hypernephroma)

Lungs

Myeloma

Breast

Lymphoma

Colon

Prostate

4. **Degenerative disease**

   Cervical disks herniate centrally, in contrast to lumbar disks, which herniate laterally and cause radicular symptoms. Thoracic disk protrusions are rare. An acute cauda equina syndrome may be produced by herniation at L1-L2.

5. **Congenital disease**

   Arnold-Chiari malformation, with or without syringomyelia, may produce cervical myelopathy. Congenital defects of the atlantoaxial joint may predispose to subluxation or dislocation. A *tethered cord* produces a spastic diplegia of the legs.

Relatively minor trauma may bring an occult malformation to clinical prominence.

6. **Inflammatory disease**

Rheumatoid arthritis is the most common disease affecting the stability of the upper cervical spine and may allow atlantoaxial translocations.

7. **Vascular disease**

Spinal cord infarction is rare but may present with acute myelopathy, potentially with back or neck pain. Epidural and subdural hematomas of the spine are also very rare, but they should be considered in patients taking anticoagulant medication. Spinal dural arteriovenous fistulas, arteriovenous malformations, and cavernous malformations of the spine are uncommon.

MAJOR THREAT TO LIFE

- **Respiratory compromise** (cervical lesions) may require immediate intubation. Diaphragm weakness may result in hypoventilation and respiratory acidosis.
- **Autonomic dysregulation may produce hypotension** that does not respond to volume challenge. This phenomenon may be part of spinal shock. The hypotension may respond to vasopressors.

BEDSIDE

Quick-Look Test

1. **What is the general condition of the patient?**

Respiratory distress may necessitate immediate intubation. Look for retraction of the supraclavicular muscles as a sign of accessory respiratory muscle use because of diaphragmatic weakness.

2. **Does the patient look cachectic or ill, suggesting cancer or general debilitation?**

3. **Is there urinary or bowel incontinence, suggesting sacral cord involvement?**

4. **Is there flushing or diaphoresis, suggesting autonomic dysregulation?**

Management

If, after a quick look, the patient appears unstable, notify the surgical team, the anesthesiology service, and/or the neurosurgery service and **address cardiopulmonary dysfunction**. Avoid hypoxia and hypotension. Ensure stability of the neck.

1. **Antiinflammatory treatment**
   a. **Trauma**

      In the past, methylprednisolone has been recommended for treatment of acute spinal cord injury. However, the evidence supporting its use is poor and in fact there is evidence to suggest it is harmful to overall recovery and may even contribute to death. Although this remains a controversial topic, the routine use of methylprednisolone has been removed from the *Guidelines for the Management of Acute Cervical Spine and Spinal Cord Injuries: 2013 Update.*

   b. **Tumor**

      For known or suspected **spinal neoplasm**, administer **dexamethasone 100 mg IV bolus** immediately.

2. **Blood tests**

   In any patient with suspected spinal cord compression, routine blood tests should be performed in preparation for possible surgical decompression: complete blood count (CBC), chemistry panel, coagulation profile, and blood type and hold. Blood and urine toxicology screens may also be helpful in some situations but should not delay initial care and stabilization.

3. **Imaging**

   If the patient is hemodynamically stable and not in respiratory distress, notify the appropriate radiologic personnel. Your patient will require an MRI scan as soon as your examination can provide anatomic localization and a working differential diagnosis. Myelography in combination with CT has nearly uniformly been replaced by MRI. CT may be superior to MRI only in spinal trauma to define subtle bony abnormalities or fractures.

Selective Physical Examination

Do not move the patient with a suspected spine injury until adequate immobilization of the neck or back has been ensured (e.g., with a Philadelphia collar).

The anatomy of the white matter tracts and cell groups in the spinal cord is consistent from patient to patient. Precise localization of the involved level and structure of the cord will, therefore, provide valuable early information about the likely pathogenesis of the injury. An anterior cord syndrome localized to the cervical region, for example, suggests cervical disk herniation. A posterior cord syndrome at the thoracic level suggests bony metastasis. Fig. 7.3 shows a representative cross section of the spinal cord. Table 7.1 outlines the features of the main spinal cord syndromes. Note that at each level, lower motor neuron signs result from cell groups exiting the cord at that level, and upper motor neuron signs are present below the level.

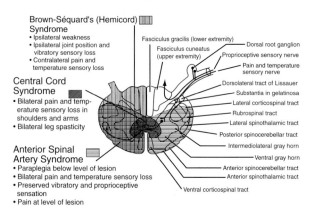

Brown-Séquard's (Hemicord)
Syndrome
• Ipsilateral weakness
• Ipsilateral joint position and vibratory sensory loss
• Contralateral pain and temperature sensory loss

Central Cord Syndrome
• Bilateral pain and temperature sensory loss in shoulders and arms
• Bilateral leg spasticity

Anterior Spinal Artery Syndrome
• Paraplegia below level of lesion
• Bilateral pain and temperature sensory loss
• Preserved vibratory and proprioceptive sensation
• Pain at level of lesion

Fasciculus gracilis (lower extremity)
Fasciculus cuneatus (upper extremity)
Dorsal root ganglion
Proprioceptive sensory nerve
Pain and temperature sensory nerve
Dorsolateral tract of Lissauer
Substantia in gelatinosa
Lateral corticospinal tract
Rubrospinal tract
Lateral spinothalamic tract
Posterior spinocerebellar tract
Intermediolateral gray horn
Ventral gray horn
Anterior spinocerebellar tract
Anterior spinothalamic tract
Ventral corticospinal tract

FIG. 7.3 Cross section of the spinal cord at the cervical level.

TABLE 7.1	Major Spinal Cord Syndromes	
Syndrome	**Common Causes**	**Features**
Hemicord syndrome (Brown-Séquard paralysis)	Penetrating injury Extrinsic compression	Contralateral spinothalamic loss Ipsilateral paresis Ipsilateral dorsal column loss Preserved light touch Note: deficits appear one to two levels below injury
Anterior cord syndrome	Anterior spinal artery infarct "Watershed" (T4-T6) ischemia Acute cervical disk herniation	Bilateral spinothalamic loss Preserved dorsal column sensation Upper motor neuron paralysis below lesion Lower motor neuron paralysis at lesion Sphincter dysfunction
Central cord syndrome	Syringomyelia Hypotensive spinal cord ischemia Spinal trauma (flexion-extension injury) Spinal cord neoplasm Sphincter dysfunction or urinary retention	Lower motor neuron weakness in arms Variable leg weakness and spasticity Severe pain and hyperpathia Spinothalamic loss in arms
Posterior cord syndrome	Trauma Posterior spinal artery infarct	Dorsal column sensory loss Pain and paresthesias in neck, back, or trunk Mild paresis

General Physical Examination

Vital signs: Evaluate as described earlier; look for any signs of autonomic instability.

HEENT: Trauma to the neck should be suspected when there is trauma to the face and body. Battle sign (ecchymosis over the mastoid process), raccoon sign (periorbital ecchymosis), hemotympanum, and cerebrospinal fluid (CSF) otorrhea suggest basilar skull fracture.

Spine: Percuss the spine with a fist or lightly with a tendon hammer. Tenderness to percussion suggests bony disease and will help localize the lesion for the rest of the examination and for a focal radiographic evaluation. Remember that the spinal cord comes down only to L1 in adults, unless there is a tethered cord. Tenderness in the lower lumbar or sacral spine may cause radicular symptoms but does not suggest cord compression.

Musculoskeletal: Look for signs of rheumatoid arthritis, which can be associated with atlantooccipital dislocation.

Neurologic Examination

- **Motor**

    Test strength in the legs and the arms. Symmetric loss of lower extremity power with preserved strength in the arms may be the first clue to thoracic cord involvement. If there is bilateral weakness in both the arms and the legs, suggesting cervical involvement, there should be upper motor neuron signs in the legs. Note that if the spinal injury is acute, muscle tone may be decreased below the level of the injury.

- **Sensory**

    Look for a sensory level. Bilateral weakness with a concordant sensory level is pathognomonic for spinal cord injury. Vibratory sense may be the first to go, particularly with a posterior cord syndrome, but the pinprick test is the most precise and reproducible. Remember, pain and temperature sensory neurons entering the cord ascend ipsilaterally for two to three spinal segments in the dorsolateral tract of Lissauer before crossing just anterior to the central canal to join the contralateral spinothalamic tract located in the lateral cord. Therefore loss of pinprick or temperature sensation at a given level may indicate pathology two to three segments above the level detected on examination. A dermatome chart can be found in Appendix E.

    Perineal sensory loss (saddle anesthesia) suggests injury to the conus medullaris. Patchy sensory loss in the lower extremities with radicular-type pain and bilateral weakness may suggest involvement of the cauda equina, rather than of the spinal cord.

Mark the borders of a sensory disturbance with a pen for comparison with future examinations.

- **Reflexes**

Hyporeflexia is often present at the level of the spinal cord injury, with hyperreflexia below the level of injury. If the injury is acute, then only the upper motor neuron sign may be a Babinski sign. Loss of the "anal wink" (contraction of the anal sphincter in response to pinprick in the perineum) indicates possible conus medullaris involvement.

- **Cranial nerves and mental status examination**

These may be done briefly to rule out involvement of central nervous system (CNS) structures above the spinal cord. A peri-sagittal mass lesion, such as a falx meningioma or a CNS lymphoma, may produce bilateral leg weakness and urinary incontinence, mimicking a thoracic cord lesion. Other mental status signs, such as personality change, lethargy, or disinhibition, may be a clue to CNS pathology. Lower brain stem signs may accompany high cervical cord injury, particularly if there is a congenital deformity of the brain or atlantoaxial joint.

Selective History and Chart Review

1. *Reassess the timing, duration, and course of the symptoms.*

Development over minutes to hours suggests trauma or infarction. Progression over hours to days suggests an infectious etiology. An epidural abscess may be present even in the absence of fever or an elevated white blood cell count. Development of weakness or sensory loss over days to weeks suggests a neoplasm.

2. *Review the presence and character of pain.*

Radicular pain will help localize and confirm extramedullary spinal involvement. Abrupt onset of radicular or diffuse pain, flaccid weakness, sphincter dysfunction, and a thoracic sensory level suggest spinal cord infarction. Bilateral radicular pain in an unusual distribution (e.g., L2 or L3) may indicate a cauda equina syndrome. Rectal pain may be the first sign of a conus medullaris lesion.

3. *Review the chart for history of illicit drug use* (this predisposes to epidural abscess and osteomyelitis), tuberculosis, or cancer.

4. *Check recent laboratory values* to assess for possible infection or chronic disease.

SURGICAL INTERVENTION

Fractures, subluxations, and dislocations require reduction into normal alignment. Cervical traction may succeed in reducing a displacement, but it should be performed only by experienced personnel, usually under radiographic guidance. Open stabilization and fusion operations may be required for unstable, complex fractures or dislocations.

Neurosurgical decompressive laminectomy is the operation of choice for epidural abscess. Investigations should proceed without delay when an epidural abscess is suspected to avoid its progression to irreversible spinal cord injury. Patients who are paraplegic at the start of the operation rarely regain function. For pyogenic osteomyelitis, direct ventral spinal canal decompression is often necessary. A second, reconstructive operation may be required after the infection is brought under control with appropriate antibiotics. Decompressive laminectomy may also be needed for acute myelopathy or cauda equina syndrome resulting from disk herniation in the lumbar region. An anterior approach may be necessary to remove a herniated cervical disk. Finally, in the rare case of epidural or subdural hematoma, decompressive laminectomy is again the treatment of choice.

For **neoplastic spinal cord compression,** a combination of high-dose steroids and radiation should be administered. Surgical decompression is generally reserved for spinal instability, progressive neurologic deterioration from bony collapse, intractable pain, and failure of conservative treatment. Once the pressure has been relieved, further treatment usually requires tissue biopsy. If the surgeons have performed a decompression procedure, open biopsy may be possible. An alternative procedure is CT-guided needle biopsy.

Delirium and Amnesia

The term *delirium* is synonymous with the term *acute confusional state*. Delirium is common in hospitalized patients, particularly in the elderly, and refers to an acute, global disorder of thinking and perception, characterized by impaired consciousness and inattention. Restlessness, agitation, and combativeness may be seen, as well as bizarre behavior and delusions. A call to evaluate delirium may therefore be one for "agitation" or "confusion." Delirium may be distinguished from dementia by the fact that with dementia alone, the sensorium remains clear, despite the occurrence of confusion and disorientation. Furthermore, it should be emphasized that although delirium is often defined as a transient condition, it may take days to weeks to clear, and if delirium is left untreated, the mortality rate may be as high as 25% in elderly inpatients. As with other mental status alterations discussed in this book, delirium is a symptom, not a disease. Successful management depends on accurate diagnosis of the underlying condition.

Amnesia is defined as a pure loss of memory without other cognitive dysfunction. Although memory is affected by delirium, amnesia may occur in isolation, with a clear sensorium. **Retrograde amnesia** refers to loss of memory for events before a specific point in time. **Anterograde amnesia** is the inability to lay down new memory. Memory is often categorized into **immediate recall** (seconds), **short-term memory** (minutes to hours), and **long-term memory** (days to years), with short-term memory being the most vulnerable to pathologic processes, both in acute amnestic states and in dementia syndromes.

The hippocampi and parahippocampal structures, dorsomedial thalamus, and the dorsolateral prefrontal cortex mediate short-term memory function. Long-term, verbal memory is mediated predominantly by the dominant (typically left) hemisphere, and visuospatial memory is mediated by the nondominant (typically right) hemisphere.

Most of this chapter will focus on diagnosis and management of acute confusional state. Two acute amnestic disorders will be discussed in brief here. Dementia as a disorder of memory along with broader cognitive decline will be discussed in depth is Chapter 28.

PHONE CALL

Questions

1. **Is the patient fully awake and alert? In what way is the patient confused? When did the change occur?**

   Clarify the acuteness and nature of the mental status change. It is important to distinguish between acute and chronic changes and also to distinguish delirium from dementia (see Chapter 28) and stupor (see Chapter 5).

2. **What are the vital signs?**

   Fever suggests infection; tachypnea may suggest hypoxia, metabolic acidosis, or hyperglycemia (Kussmaul respiration); and irregular heart rhythm may suggest cardioembolic stroke.

3. **Was there any head injury?**

4. **What is the patient's underlying medical condition?**

   Diseases that are likely to cause metabolic disarray, such as renal or liver disease, endocrinopathies, diarrheal illnesses, or malignancy, may alter electrolytes. HIV infection or AIDS opens a wider array of differential diagnoses.

5. **Is the patient diabetic?**

   Both hypoglycemia and hyperglycemia can cause altered mental status.

6. **Is the patient known to be a user of alcohol, nicotine, or other nonprescription drugs?**

Orders

1. Order a finger stick glucose level.

2. If the patient is tachypneic or drowsy, obtain arterial blood gas measurements. A pulse oximeter may be useful for monitoring oxygen saturation.

3. Provide orientation and reassurance to the patient. Make sure the room is well lit. The treatment of the behavioral and emotional manifestations of delirium, to the extent possible, will make the subsequent etiologic evaluation easier.

4. Restrain the patient with a Posey chest restraint if necessary. Significant agitation or combativeness may put the patient or those nearby at risk for physical injury.

5. If possible, do not medicate. Perform the evaluation first. If sedation is given before a good neurologic examination can be obtained, the opportunity for making a diagnosis may be lost.

Inform RN

"Will arrive at the bedside in…minutes."

ELEVATOR THOUGHTS

What are the causes of delirium?

V (vascular): stroke (infarct or hemorrhage causing a sensory aphasia), subarachnoid hemorrhage, hypertensive encephalopathy, cholesterol emboli syndrome

I (infectious): herpes simplex encephalitis or other viral encephalitis; bacterial, fungal, or rickettsial meningoencephalitis; neurosyphilis; Lyme disease; parasitic abscess (e.g., toxoplasmosis, cysticercosis), bacterial abscess; HIV encephalitis; systemic infection such as urosepsis or pneumonia

T (traumatic): open or closed head trauma, acute or chronic subdural hematoma

A (autoimmune): systemic lupus erythematosus (SLE), multiple sclerosis

M (metabolic/toxic): hypoglycemia or hyperglycemia, hyponatremia, hypercalcemia, hepatic encephalopathy, uremia, porphyria; drug or alcohol ingestion or withdrawal

I (iatrogenic): drug toxicity (particularly in the elderly) such as psychotropic drugs, steroids, digoxin, cimetidine, anticonvulsants, anticholinergics, dopaminergics (see Table 8.1 for common medications with central nervous system [CNS] side effects; Table 8.2 lists medications associated with memory impairment), rare-heavy metal poisoning, pellagra, vitamin B_{12} or folate deficiency, Wilson disease

N (neoplastic): primary brain tumor, metastatic brain disease, paraneoplastic syndrome (limbic encephalitis with small-cell lung cancer)

S (seizure): postictal state, nonconvulsive status epilepticus (rare)

Other (psychiatric): bipolar disorder/mania, psychosis

MAJOR THREAT TO LIFE

- **Expanding mass lesion with impending herniation**

  Although it is rare for a mass lesion to progress to impending herniation without focal neurologic signs, the first changes may be confusion or altered state of consciousness. Progression can be rapid if there is an expanding subdural hematoma or edema from subarachnoid hemorrhage.

- **Bacterial meningitis or encephalitis**

  Bacterial meningitis is a major treatable illness that can be fatal if missed. Other meningitides are likely to be less fulminant yet also can be fatal if left untreated. Herpes simplex encephalitis is the most common sporadic encephalitis. Aside from direct brain damage from infection, encephalitides can produce edema and subsequent herniation.

TABLE 8.1 | **Common Medications That Can Cause Delirium**

Anticholinergics
    Trihexyphenidyl HCl (Artane)
    Benztropine mesylate (Cogentin)
Anticonvulsants
    Levetiracetam (Keppra)
    Phenytoin (Dilantin)
    Valproic acid (Depakene/Depakote)
Antidepressants with serotonergic properties (TCA, SSRI, SNRI)
Antihistamines
    Diphenhydramine (Benadryl)
    Promethazine (Phenergan)
    Cimetidine (Tagamet)
Benzodiazepines
    Diazepam (Valium)
    Temazepam (Restoril)
    Triazolam (Halcion)
Corticosteroids
    Prednisone
    Dexamethasone (Decadron)
Dextromethorphan hydrobromide
Dopaminergic drugs
    L-dopa (Sinemet)
    Pergolide (Permax)
    Bromocriptine (Parlodel)
Digoxin
Disulfiram
Indomethacin
Lithium
Opioids

SNRI, Serotonin/norepinephrine reuptake inhibitor; *SSRI,* selective serotonin reuptake inhibitor; *TCA,* tricyclic antidepressant.

TABLE 8.2 | **Medications That May Be Associated With Memory Impairment**

Anticonvulsants (overdose)	Clioquinol (antifungal)
Antihistamines	Corticosteroids
Antispasmodic urologic agents	Interleukins
Barbiturates	Isoniazid
Benzodiazepines	Methotrexate
Bromides	Tricyclic antidepressants
Chlorpromazine	

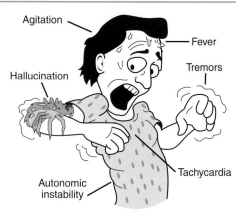

Agitation

Fever

Tremors

Hallucination

Tachycardia

Autonomic
instability

FIG. 8.1 Delirium tremens.

- **Delirium tremens**

Usually occurring more than 48 hours after cessation of alcohol consumption, the autonomic instability of delirium tremens may produce high fevers, tachycardia, and severe fluctuations in blood pressure (Fig. 8.1). The mortality rate is approximately 15%.

BEDSIDE

Quick-Look Test

1. *Does the patient look ill or well?*
2. *Is the patient in respiratory distress?*
3. *What are the vital signs?*

If there is a fever, meningitis must be ruled out; treating meningitis should be strongly considered at the time when diagnosis is first raised, rather than waiting on the workup to be pursued. An irregular heart rhythm may suggest atrial fibrillation. Markedly elevated blood pressure, particularly diastolic blood pressure greater than 120 mm Hg, may produce hypertensive encephalopathy, which is characterized by headache, confusion, and irritability, with lethargy developing over hours to days.

Selective Physical Examination I
General Physical Examination

Breath	The odor of alcohol or fetor hepaticus may suggest the etiology
HEENT	Look for external signs of head or neck trauma scalp lacerations or bruises, Battle sign, raccoon eyes, papilledema

Neck	Nuchal rigidity, Kernig sign, Brudzinski sign
Cardiopulmonary	Tachypnea can indicate hypoxia or metabolic acidosis
	Rales or decreased breath sounds may help diagnose a pneumonia Listen for irregular heart rhythm and for murmurs to suggest valvular heart disease
Abdomen	Percuss the liver; hepatomegaly may be the physical manifestation of hepatic encephalopathy or may direct your management to consideration of alcohol withdrawal; look for ascites.
Extremities	Look for clubbing as a sign of chronic pulmonary disease, peripheral edema as a sign of cardiac or renal failure, and splinter hemorrhages as a sign of emboli; **asterixis** is a sign of metabolic disarray, for example, from renal or hepatic failure.

Neurologic Examination

- **Mental status**
  1. Assess the patient's **alertness:** Is the patient fully awake and alert? Assess the patient's **attentiveness.** Does the patient maintain eye contact? Does he or she glance about the room as if having hallucinations? One simple test of sustained attention is to ask the patient to recite the days of the week backward or to count backward from 20 to 1.
  2. Listen for **fluency** and content of spontaneous spoken language. Abnormalities in including **paraphasias** may suggest an aphasia. Test **comprehension**. Ask the patient to follow progressively complex commands (e.g., "show two fingers," "point to the ceiling and then to the floor," and "tap each shoulder twice with your eyes closed").
  3. Assess **thought content**. Tangential or pressured speech, delusions, flight of ideas, hallucinations, perceptual illusions, and disorientation may be seen with psychiatric disease or acute encephalopathies.
- **Cranial nerves**
  1. **Pupils:** Pinpoint pupils may result from opiate overdose. Widely dilated pupils could be a sign of cholinergic overdose (e.g., organophosphate poisoning). Asymmetric pupils can indicate uncal herniation from intracranial mass effect. Argyll Robertson pupils are seen with CNS syphilis and result from periaqueductal midbrain lesions (see Chapter 22).

2. **Facial asymmetry** in the form of a flattened nasolabial fold or a wider palpebral fissure may be a subtle sign of an intra-parenchymal mass or stroke.
3. Assess swallowing capacity and gag reflex.

- **Motor**

Depending on how cooperative your patient is, you may be able to test strength by confrontation. In an inattentive patient, observe limb movements for asymmetry. Lateralizing weakness suggests an intracranial lesion. Tremor may indicate alcohol withdrawal or intoxication.

- **Sensory**

A detailed sensory examination requires sustained cooperation that an inattentive patient often cannot give. Response to a brief noxious stimulus (e.g., a pinch or pulling hair on the arm) is a quick way to assess gross sensory function. If the limb is paretic, the response may be a facial grimace.

- **Gait**

Ataxia may suggest intoxication.

- **Reflexes**

Babinski response or reflex asymmetry suggests lateralized intracranial pathology.

Selective History and Chart Review

1. **Review medications**

Have any new medications been started recently? Particularly in the elderly, drug toxicity is a common cause of change in mental status. Table 8.1 lists common medications that can cause delirium.

2. **Review medical or psychiatric history**

Known metabolic disorders such as renal or hepatic disease or past episodes of psychosis would be crucial to make a diagnosis.

MANAGEMENT

Control of Delirium

1. **Treatment of agitation**

Treatment of delirium depends on the correct identification of the underlying condition. If agitation or combativeness is likely to interfere with the investigation or if there is a physical threat to the patient or to the staff, the best medications to use are butyrophenones (e.g., haloperidol [Haldol]), benzisoxazoles (e.g., risperidone), dibenzothiazepine derivative (e.g. quetiapine), or benzodiazepines. See Table 8.3 for drugs used to control agitation and delirium.

TABLE 8.3	Drugs Used in the Treatment of Acute Agitation and Delirium

Drug	Starting Dose
Antipsychotics	
Haloperidol (Haldol)	1–2 mg q6h PO/IV
Olanzapine (Zyprexa)	5–10 mg QD BID PO/IM
Quetiapine (Seroquel)	25–50 mg PO
Benzodiazepines	
Lorazepam (Ativan)	0.5–2.0 mg IV/IM/PO
Midazolam (Versed)	1–2 mg IV/PO
Diazepam (Valium)	5–10 mg IV/PO

BID, Twice a day; *IM*, intramuscularly; *IV*, intravenously; *PO*, by mouth; *q*, every; *QD*, daily.

- **Haldol 2 to 10 mg intramuscularly (IM)** may be expected to reach peak serum levels in 20 to 40 minutes. Repeating the dose up to 20 mg may be necessary in severe cases. For mild agitation or in the elderly, atypical antipsychotics are far preferred given lower risk of parkinsonism. Moderate to severe agitation in the elderly can be treated with an initial dose of Haldol 1 to 2 mg, and an additional 2 to 4 mg can be used if violence occurs. If an acute dystonic reaction occurs with Haldol, **diphenhydramine 25 to 50 mg IM** may be given, even though the anticholinergic effect may worsen the delirium.

- Haloperidol should be avoided in alcohol withdrawal, benzodiazepine withdrawal, and hepatic encephalopathy. For acute agitation in these settings, a benzodiazepine such as **lorazepam 1 to 2 mg IMIV** may be given in repeated doses up to every 30 to 60 minutes. Higher doses may be required if tolerance has developed in the setting of chronic alcohol or benzodiazepine abuse.

- Quietipine 25-50 mg PO is usually given qHS for "sundowning," or BID for sustained agitation throughout the day. Compared to haloperidol it causes fewer extrapyramidal side effects, but is slower in onset because it can only be given orally.

  Olazapine 5-10 mg PO is an alternative to Quietipine with a similar efficacy and side effect profile. Both can calm agitation and dysphoria within 30-60 minutes.

- All antipsychotic agents can aggravate QT segment prolongation and can rarely trigger polymorphic ventricular tachycardia (Torsade de Pointes). Patients with preexisiting QTc prolongation (>600 msec), hypokalemia, hypomagnesemia, or hypocalcemia are at risk. IV treatment should be given with cardiac monitoring in susceptible patients.

2. **The following blood tests should be ordered immediately:**
   - Complete blood count (CBC) with differential
   - Electrolyte panel, including stat glucose
   - Full chemistry panel, including liver function tests
   - Urine toxicology screen (if drug intoxication is suspected)
   - Urine and blood cultures (if fever is present)
   - Arterial blood gases
   - Calcium, phosphate
   - Erythrocyte sedimentation rate may be measured, but its specificity is low

3. **A chest X-ray should be obtained if fever or dyspnea is present.**

Treatment of Life-Threatening Disorders

1. **Bacterial meningitis**

   Delirium with fever should be treated as bacterial meningitis until proved otherwise. As a rule, a head computed tomography (CT) scan should be ordered before a lumbar puncture is performed. If there is no papilledema on examination, no coagulopathy, and no focal deficit (including gait ataxia), and a head CT is not readily available, a lumbar puncture may almost always be done without risk of herniation. (See Chapter 3 for a discussion of lumbar puncture.) Cerebrospinal fluid (CSF) should be sent for cell count, protein, and glucose determinations; microbial cultures (bacterial, fungal, mycobacterial); and Venereal Disease Research Laboratory (VDRL) test. It should also be sent for Gram, acid-fast bacillus, and India ink stains. CSF findings in bacterial meningitis are cloudy fluid with 50 to 20,000 white blood cells, predominantly leukocytes, elevated protein level, and decreased glucose level (see Table 21.1). The causative organism may be identified and antibiotic sensitivity may be obtained in more than 80% of the cases. Empirical treatment of bacterial meningitis begins when the diagnosis is first considered, and well before definitive identification of causal organism. Treatment in adults should be **ampicillin 1 g IV every 6 hours** and a third-generation cephalosporin (e.g., **ceftriaxone 2 g IV every 12 hours**). See Chapter 22 for details.

2. **Delirium tremens**

   The autonomic instability of delirium tremens is treated supportively, with acetaminophen (Tylenol) or a cooling blanket for fevers. Continuous cardiac monitoring may be necessary if arrhythmias develop. **Lorazepam 1-2 mg IV/PO or diazepam 5 to 10 mg IV every 6 hours as first line therapy, with** dosing titrated to control the agitation without causing over-sedation and respiratory depression, should be used. Sedation should be titrated to minimize agitation. Tremulousness may be used as a clinical monitor of the effectiveness of the benzodiazepine. An alternative benzodiaezepine with a much longer half life is **chlordiazepoxide (Librium) 25 to 100 mg every 6–12 hours by mouth (PO).** The dose should be tapered as the symptoms subside. **Thiamine 100 mg IV, IM, or PO should** be given daily for 3 days to prevent the development of Wernicke encephalopathy.

3. **Suspected mass lesion**

   If there is bilateral papilledema or a focality on examination, an emergent head CT or magnetic resonance imaging (MRI) scan should be obtained. For mass lesions, refer to the appropriate chapter for treatment of acute stroke (Chapter 6), increased intracranial pressure (Chapter 13), or brain tumor (Chapter 23).

Selective History and Chart Review

Once it is clear that the patient does not have a mass lesion, bacterial meningitis, or delirium tremens, you have time to make a more complete assessment of the situation.

- If family members are available, try to sort out the acuteness of the change. A chronic or fluctuating course in an elderly person may suggest that the apparent delirium is really a component of dementia. Alzheimer's disease and vascular dementia are the most common causes (see Chapter 28). A subacute course over days, with intermittent fevers, suggests a subacute or chronic encephalomeningitis, such as herpes simplex encephalitis, tubercular meningitis, or cryptococcal meningitis.
- Review the chart. What are the patient's medical conditions? What medications is he or she on? Were any medications recently added that are known to have CNS effects (see Table 8.1)? The offending agent should be stopped or substituted. Do the most recent laboratory values suggest metabolic abnormalities? Renal failure and hepatic failure are the most common sources of metabolic encephalopathy (Box 8.1). Is the patient HIV positive? Acute HIV infection may cause a meningoencephalitis. Immunocompromised patients are at risk for a variety of opportunistic infections that can cause encephalopathy, particularly cryptococcal and tuberculous meningitis, toxoplasmosis, and CNS syphilis. Malignancy, most notably small-cell lung carcinoma, can cause a paraneoplastic limbic encephalitis, in addition to altering electrolytes with syndrome of inappropriate antidiuretic hormone

BOX 8.1	Hepatic Encephalopathy

Hepatic encephalopathy usually appears in a patient with liver function already compromised from alcoholic cirrhosis, chronic hepatitis, or malignancy. An increased protein load, such as from a gastrointestinal bleed, causes ammonia to accumulate in the brain. Whether the high level of ammonia itself or the increase in concentration of its metabolites produces the alterations in consciousness is not known. Examination may reveal abdominal ascites, an enlarged (or shrunken) liver, and asterixis, in addition to changes in mental status, namely inattention, disorientation, and confusion. In the later stages, focal signs such as hemiparesis or dysconjugate gaze may appear. Management is directed at reducing the protein load with dietary protein restrictions and **neomycin 2 to 4 g per day PO**, or **rifaximin 200 mg twice a day (BID)**, which reduces the population of ammonia-producing bacteria in the bowel. **Lactulose 15 to 45 mL two to four times per day** to induce diarrhea may also help reduce intestinal bacteria. Ammonia levels should be followed as an indication of the effectiveness of therapy. If acute agitation requires treatment, use benzodiazepines such as **diazepam 5 to 10 mg every 8 hours. Haloperidol should be avoided.** When hepatic encephalopathy is suspected, be sure to obtain a stool guaiac test and a hematocrit.

(SIADH). Several well-described autoimmune limbic encephalitides are known to occur in the absence of malignancy.

Treatment of Other Disorders

1. **Hypoglycemia and hyperglycemia**

   Hypoglycemia may be rapidly corrected with a bolus of **50 mL D50W IV by direct injection.** Do not forget that **thiamine (100 mg PO or IM)** must be given first to prevent possible induction of Wernicke encephalopathy. Maintenance with D5W may be necessary if the hypoglycemia is prolonged. Hyperglycemia (diabetic ketoacidosis) requires administration of insulin, repletion of intravascular volume, and often management of acidosis and potassium. The level of monitoring required is best handled in an intensive care unit (ICU).

2. **Hyponatremia and hypernatremia**

   Management of hyponatremia and hypernatremia usually involves treating the underlying cause (e.g., renal disease, vomiting and diarrhea, hypothalamic or adrenal dysfunction, or SIADH from malignancy or medications). Treatment with IV fluids and electrolytes differs depending on volume status (see Table 21.3). Too rapid a correction of hyponatremia may precipitate central pontine myelinolysis, which is an acute demyelinating syndrome occurring mostly in patients with poor nutritional status, causing quadriplegia, dysarthria, and pseudobulbar palsy.

3. **Hypocalcemia**

Severe hypocalcemia (<7.0 mg/dL) may be treated with **10 to 20 mL (1 to 2 g) of 10% calcium gluconate IV in 100 mL D5W over 30 minutes.** If the patient is hyperphosphatemic, correction with glucose and insulin is required before giving calcium IV. Patients on digoxin should have continuous cardiac monitoring because calcium potentiates digoxin's action.

4. **Uremia with renal failure**

Symptomatic uremia with renal failure causing delirium may necessitate urgent hemodialysis.

5. **Sepsis**

Delirium caused by sepsis should clear spontaneously with appropriate treatment of the infection.

6. **Psychiatric causes**

Psychiatric causes of delirium may generally be treated acutely with haloperidol 1 to 5 mg PO or IM. Atypical antipsychotics should be considered in geriatric patients given lower risk of extrapyramidal symptoms. Psychiatric consultation should be obtained for definitive treatment.

7. **Seizures**

Delirium from a **postictal state** should clear progressively over minutes to hours. An electroencephalography (EEG) should be ordered within the next few days. **Nonconvulsive status epilepticus** is a neurologic emergency that requires EEG for definitive diagnosis. (See Chapter 4 for further discussion of seizure management.)

8. **Nicotine withdrawal**

In rare instances, delirium can occur in heavy smokers caused by nicotine withdrawal. Application of a **transdermal 21-mg nicotine patch** can result in dramatic improvement in some cases.

OTHER AMNESTIC DISORDERS

Transient Global Amnesia

Patients with transient global amnesia (TGA) are middle-aged or older, often with hypertension, prior ischemic episodes, or atherosclerotic heart disease but are otherwise healthy. Typically, they are brought in by a relative or friend because they are "confused." On examination, there are no focal neurologic deficits. Cognitive function and language are intact, except for a profound anterograde amnesia and a retrograde amnesia for the preceding several hours or days. Patients typically appear agitated and will repeat the same question over and over, such as "What am I doing here?" The anterograde amnesia clears gradually after minutes to hours and usually resolves completely within 24 to 48 hours. A residual retrograde amnesia for the hours immediately surrounding the event is often permanent.

- TGA often appears in the setting of an emotional or physical stress. The pathophysiology is unknown; epileptic, migrainous, and vascular mechanisms have been proposed but have not been proved. The differential diagnosis includes unwitnessed head trauma or seizure, drug intoxication, stroke, dissociative states, and neurocognitive disorders associated with thiamine deficiency (including Wernicke encephalopathy and Korsakoff syndrome).
- The EEG is usually negative, but a positive EEG allows treatment with anticonvulsants to be given. MRI should be obtained to evaluate for a seizure-producing lesion; sometimes small unilateral hippocampal signal abnormalities are identified on diffusion-weighted imaging (DWI), particularly when performed 24 to 48 hours after the event.
- The condition is self-limiting and there is no specific treatment, although some physicians have advocated using **aspirin 325 mg per day** for secondary prophylaxis. Addressing underlying neurologic conditions including migraine or pursuing workup for seizures beyond routine EEG can sometimes be helpful. Recurrence occurs in less than one-fourth of the patients.

Thiamine Deficiency Encephalopathies: Wernicke Encephalopathy and Korsakoff Syndrome

Wernicke encephalopathy and the *Korsakoff confabulatory amnestic syndrome* are caused by nutritional thiamine deficiency occurring in chronic alcoholics and other patients with chronic malnutrition (e.g., refugee populations, purposeful starvation related to mood disorders, and chronic ileus, among other risk factors).

- The acute component (Wernicke encephalopathy) is characterized by inattentiveness, lethargy, truncal ataxia, and ocular dysmotility (nystagmus, horizontal with or without a vertical or rotary component and gaze palsy, horizontal or lateral rectus palsy, progressing to complete external ophthalmoplegia). Other signs of nutritional deficiency may be present, such as skin changes or redness of the tongue.
- If left untreated, the condition is fatal in 10% of patients. Treatment is **thiamine 100 mg IV, IM, or PO daily for 3 days,** along with magnesium and multivitamins. If recognized and treated promptly, ataxia, inattentiveness, and ocular dysmotility often resolve.

- Korsakoff syndrome is characterized by moderate to severe anterograde amnesia and patchy long-term memory loss. Unlike patients with TGA, patients with Korsakoff syndrome are not distressed by their amnesia. Confabulation is often present. Even with good nutrition, the amnesia of Korsakoff syndrome rarely resolves. Histopathologic examination shows cell loss and degenerative changes in the dorsomedial thalami, the mamillary bodies, the periaqueductal midbrain, and the Purkinje cell layer of the cerebellar vermis.

Head Injury

The initial assessment of head injury in the emergency room (ER) can be frantic, with resuscitation measures, history taking, and examination occurring simultaneously. An organized approach is essential to ensure that vital components of the evaluation are not omitted. **The immediate goal is to judge the severity of the injury as minimal, moderate, or high.** This aspect of the injury can be quickly assessed at the time of arrival.

PHONE CALL

Questions

1. **What are the vital signs?**

    If the patient is in respiratory distress, the spine should be immobilized (this should have been done already) and endotracheal intubation should be performed.

2. **What were the circumstances and the mode of injury?**

    The force and location of head impact should be determined as precisely as possible.

3. **Did the patient experience loss of consciousness?**

    Concussion refers to the temporary loss of consciousness that occurs at the time of impact. Because patients are amnestic after concussion, only an eyewitness can accurately gauge the duration of loss of consciousness.

4. **Has the patient's neurologic status deteriorated since the time of impact?**

    Progressive decline in level of consciousness after an injury suggests an expanding *subdural or epidural hematoma*.

5. **What is the patient's level of consciousness now?**

    This should be assessed using the Glasgow Coma Scale (see Table 5.2).

6. **Has the patient recently ingested drugs or alcohol?**

   Intoxication can confound assessments of mental status and may lead to withdrawal symptoms.

7. **Is there significant extracranial trauma?**

   The patient should be quickly examined for external signs of trauma to the neck, chest, abdomen, and limbs.

Determination of the Severity of Injury

At this juncture, you should have enough information to classify the injury severity as **minimal, moderate,** or **high.** Subsequent diagnostic testing and management should proceed according to the algorithm in Fig. 9.1.

1. **Minimal-risk group**
   - Glasgow Coma Scale score of 15 (alert, attentive, and oriented) and normal neurologic findings on examination
   - No concussion, or concussion in the absence of moderate-risk group criteria

2. **Moderate-risk group**
   - Glasgow Coma Scale score of 9 to 14 (confused, lethargic, or stuporous) or minor focal neurologic deficit (i.e., nystagmus, facial droop)
   - Concussion if age >60 years, headache, or minor external signs of trauma are present
   - Posttraumatic amnesia
   - Vomiting
   - Seizure
   - Major external trauma (Battle sign, raccoon eyes, etc.)

3. **High-risk group**
   - Glasgow Coma Scale score of 3 to 8 (see Table 5.2)
   - Progressive decline in level of consciousness
   - Major focal neurologic deficit (i.e., hemiparesis, aphasia)
   - Penetrating skull injury or palpably depressed skull fracture

Orders

1. **For *all moderate- and high-risk patients,* order a cervical spine CT scan.**

   All patients with traumatic injury above the level of the clavicles should have cervical spine films to rule out a fracture. Before a cervical collar can be removed, the cervical spine must be cleared completely from C1 to C7.

2. **For all patients with *moderate or severe injury,* give the following orders:**
   a. **Start an intravenous (IV) line with normal (0.9%) saline or Plasma-Lyte solution.**

      Isotonic fluids replace intravascular volume more effectively than do hypotonic fluids, and they do not aggravate cerebral edema.

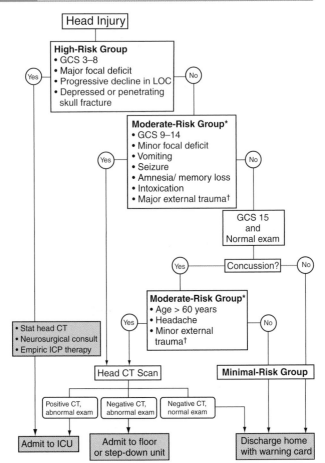

FIG. 9.1 Emergency room diagnostic and treatment algorithm for head injury. (Refer to text for details.) *CT,* Computed tomography; *GCS,* Glasgow Coma Scale score; *ICP,* intracranial pressure; *ICU,* intensive care unit; *LOC,* level of consciousness. *One or more criteria may be present; †above the level of the clavicles.

b. **Order diagnostic blood tests.**
   (1) Hemoglobin and hematocrit
   (2) Complete blood count (CBC) and platelet count
   (3) Serum chemistries (glucose, electrolytes, blood urea nitrogen, creatinine)

    (4) Prothrombin time (PT)/partial thromboplastin time (PTT)

    (5) Toxicology screen and serum alcohol level

    (6) Type and hold

c. **Obtain a head computed tomography (CT) scan with bone windows.**

    Intracranial hemorrhage will be detected in approximately 90% to 100% of high-risk patients, 5% to 10% of moderate-risk patients, and 0% of minimal-risk patients. CT scans should be assessed for the following (Fig. 9.2):

    (1) Epidural and subdural hematoma

    (2) Subarachnoid and intraventricular blood

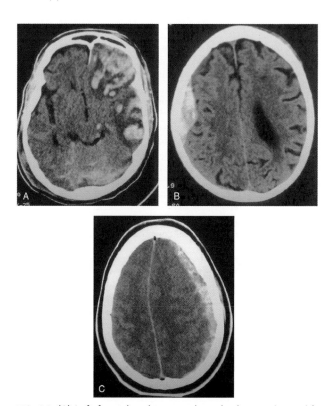

FIG. 9.2 (A) Left frontal and temporal cerebral contusions with surrounding edema. (B) Small right parietal epidural hematoma *(convex shape)*. (C) Thin left subdural hematoma *(crescentic, convex shape)*. (Images courtesy Dr. Robert De La Paz.)

    (3) Parenchymal contusions and hemorrhages
    (4) Cerebral edema
    (5) Effacement of perimesencephalic cisterns
    (6) Midline shift
    (7) Skull fractures, sinus opacification (air-fluid levels), and pneumocephalus

3. **For *comatose patients* (Glasgow Coma Scale score ≤ 8) or in patients with signs of herniation, give the following orders:**

   a. **Elevate head of the bed 30 degrees.**

   b. **Control the airway.**
   Intubate the patient. Place the patient on either volume or pressure control settings to achieve normal minute ventilation between 6 and 8 mL/min with tidal volumes set to 8 to 10 mL/kg (ideal body weight). The goal should be normocapnia (Pco$_2$: 35 to 40 mm Hg). Hypocapnia (Pco$_2$: 25 to 30 mm Hg) should be only be used in setting of brain herniation. Severe hypocapnia (<25 mm Hg) may lead to excessive vasoconstriction and cerebral ischemia and should be avoided.

   c. **Administer either hypertonic saline or mannitol 20%.**
   The typical initial dose for hypertonic saline is a 250-cc IV bolus of 3% saline. High concentrations of saline such as 30 cc of 23.4% require central venous access. Mannitol is dosed between 0.5 and 1.0 g/kg IV bolus. The patient should be reexamined 30 minutes after administration of either agent to assess for signs of improvement. Additional doses should be guided by an intracranial pressure (ICP) monitor (see Chapter 13).

   d. **Insert a Foley catheter.**

   e. **Obtain a neurosurgical consultation.**

ELEVATOR THOUGHTS

What are the most important sequelae of traumatic head injury?

1. **Concussion**
   Concussion refers to temporary loss of consciousness that occurs at the time of impact. It is usually associated with a short period of amnesia. The majority of patients with concussion have normal CT or magnetic resonance imaging (MRI) scans, reflecting the fact that concussion results from physiologic (rather than structural) injury to the brain. *Approximately 5% of patients who have sustained concussion will have an intracranial hemorrhage.*

2. **Epidural hematoma**
   Epidural bleeding usually results from a tear in the middle meningeal artery. Approximately 75% of such cases are

associated with a skull fracture. The classic clinical course (seen in only one-third of patients) proceeds from immediate loss of consciousness (concussion) to a lucid interval, which is followed by a secondary depression of consciousness as the epidural hematoma expands. Epidural blood takes on a bulging convex pattern on the CT scan (see Fig. 9.2) because the collection is limited by firm attachments of the dura to the cranial sutures. Progression to herniation and death can occur rapidly because the bleeding is from an artery.

3. **Subdural hematoma**

   Subdural bleeding usually arises from a venous source, with blood filling the potential space between the dural and arachnoid membranes. CT usually reveals a crescentic collection of blood across the entire hemispheric convexity (see Fig. 9.2). *Elderly and alcoholic patients are particularly prone to subdural bleeding;* in these patients, large hematomas can result from trivial impact or from acceleration/deceleration injuries (e.g., whiplash injury).

4. **Parenchymal contusion and hematoma**

   Cerebral contusions result from "scraping" and "bruising" of the brain as it moves across the inner surface of the skull. The inferior frontal and temporal lobes are the common sites of traumatic contusion (see Fig. 9.2). With lateral forces, contusions can occur just deep to the site of impact (coup lesions) or at the opposite pole as the brain impacts on the inner table of the skull (contrecoup lesions). Contusions frequently evolve into larger lesions over 12 to 24 hours, and, in rare instances, contusions can develop de novo 1 or more days after injury ("spät hematoma").

5. **Diffuse axonal injury (DAI)**

   Persistent coma occurs frequently in patients with severe head injury with normal CT scans and normal ICP. In these cases, coma results from widespread stretching, shearing, and disruption of axons as a result of rotational forces. Bilateral motor posturing, hyperreflexia, and dysautonomia are common and result from injury to the corticospinal tracts and autonomic centers in the brain stem. MRI scans show characteristic "shearing lesions" in the dorsolateral midbrain, posterior corpus callosum, and centrum semiovale (Fig. 9.3). DAI is thought to be the single most important cause of persistent disability in patients with traumatic brain damage.

6. **Skull fracture**

   Skull fractures are important markers of potentially serious intracranial injury, but they rarely cause symptoms themselves. If the scalp is lacerated over the fracture, it is considered an

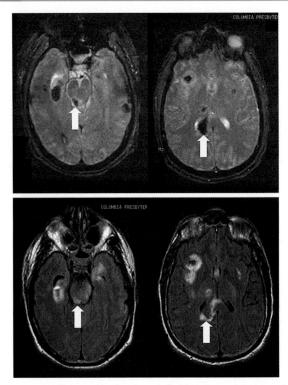

FIG. 9.3 Gradient echo *(top)* and fluid attenuation inversion recovery *(bottom)* magnetic resonance images showing hemorrhagic lesions characteristic of axonal shearing injury involving the right dorsolateral midbrain *(right)* and right posterior splenium *(left)*. Small contusions of the temporal lobes are also present. (Reproduced with permission from Mayer SA. Head Injury. In Rowland LP, ed. *Merritt's Textbook of Neurology.* 11th ed. Baltimore, MD: Lippincott Williams, & Wilkins; 2005:483–485.)

open, or compound, fracture. *Linear fractures* account for 80% of all skull fractures and can usually be managed conservatively. *Basilar skull fractures* occur with more serious trauma and are frequently missed on routine skull X-ray films. These fractures may be associated with cranial nerve injury or cerebrospinal fluid (CSF) leakage from the nose or ear. *Comminuted and depressed fractures* are often associated with contusions of the underlying brain and usually require surgical debridement.

MAJOR THREAT TO LIFE

- Epidural hematoma
- Subdural hematoma
- Increased ICP

BEDSIDE

Quick-Look Test

What is the level of consciousness?

Almost all patients with potentially life-threatening lesions will have depressed level of consciousness (lethargy, stupor, or coma).

Airway and Vital Signs

Is the airway protected? What is the respiratory rate?

Indications for intubation include depressed level of consciousness with inability to protect the airway, respiratory distress (rapid, shallow breathing), or respiratory depression.

What is the heart rate and blood pressure (BP)?

If the patient is *hypotensive,* bleeding into the abdomen, thorax, retroperitoneal space, or tissues surrounding a long-bone fracture should be excluded. *Spinal shock* can occur with cord injury and results from acute loss of sympathetic outflow. *Hypertension* associated with a wide pulse pressure and bradycardia (Cushing reflex) may reflect increased ICP.

Selective Physical Examination
General Physical Examination

Head	The skull should be palpated for fractures, hematomas, and lacerations
	Battle sign (ecchymosis over the mastoid process) and *raccoon sign* (periorbital ecchymosis) suggest, but do not confirm, basilar skull fracture
Ear, nose, and throat	*CSF otorrhea* and *CSF rhinorrhea* result from skull fracture with disruption of the dura
	CSF can be differentiated from mucus by its high glucose content on dipstick testing; bloody CSF can be differentiated from frank blood by a positive *halo test* (a "halo" of CSF forms around the blood when CSF is dropped on a cloth sheet)

	Hemotympanum is also highly suggestive of skull fracture
	Tongue biting suggests an unwitnessed seizure
Neck	Do not manipulate the neck until a cervical fracture has been ruled out
Chest, abdomen, back, pelvis, and extremities	It is essential to rule out important coexisting injuries in patients with head injury The patient should be thoroughly examined, and X-rays, diagnostic peritoneal lavage, and other interventions should be performed prior to CT scanning as clinically indicated

CSF, Cerebrospinal fluid; *CT,* computed tomography.

Neurologic Examination

Rapid neurologic examination of the patient with head injury should focus on the following:

- **Mental status**
  1. **Level of consciousness**

     Level of consciousness is best documented by using the Glasgow Coma Scale (see Table 5.2) and by describing specific stimuli and responses (e.g., "answers with brief confused responses to repeated questioning" or "moans and vocalizes in response to sternal rub").
  2. **Attention and concentration**

     Ask the patient to count from 20 to 1 or recite the months in reverse.
  3. **Orientation**

     Check for orientation to time, place, and situation.
  4. **Memory**

     Document *retrograde amnesia* by asking the patient to recall the last thing he or she remembers prior to the injury. Check for *anterograde amnesia* by asking about the first thing remembered after the injury. Check recall for three objects at 5 minutes.
- Cranial nerves
  1. **Pupils**
  2. **Extraocular movements**

     Nystagmus may be found in alert patients with dizziness or vertigo after concussion. An *exodeviated eye with a large pupil* suggests cranial nerve (CN) 3 compression from uncal herniation.
  3. **Facial nerve**

     The facial nerve is the most commonly injured cranial nerve in patients with closed head injury.

- **Motor**
  1. **Spontaneous movements**

     Preferential movement of the limbs on one side indicates paresis of the unused limbs. If the patient is unresponsive, check for a lateralized localizing response to sternal rub.
  2. **Limb tone**

     Increased tone may reflect an early stage of decortication (flexor posturing) or decerebration (extensor posturing).
  3. **Arm (pronator) drift**

     If the patient is unable to follow commands, passively elevate both arms and check to see whether one falls preferentially.
  4. **Power**

     Check strength against active resistance at the shoulders, wrists, hips, and ankles.
- **Reflexes**
- **Gait**
  1. **Normal gait**
  2. **Tandem (heel-to-toe) gait**

     It is particularly important to check gait in patients with "mild injury" who are treated and released without a CT scan.

MANAGEMENT

Minimal-Risk Group

Patients in this group (see Fig. 9.1) can generally be discharged from the ER **without a head CT scan** as long as the following criteria are met:

- Neurologic examination (especially mental status and gait) is normal.
- Cervical spine is clinically cleared (no pain or tenderness and full range of motion).
- A responsible person is available to observe the patient over 24 hours, with instructions to return the patient to the ER if late symptoms (listed on a head injury warning card) develop.

Moderate-Risk Group

In patients who have suffered concussion, normal findings on neurologic examination and CT scan eliminate the need for hospital admission. These patients can be discharged home for observation, even in the presence of headache, nausea, vomiting, dizziness, or amnesia because the risk of development of a significant intracranial lesion thereafter is minimal. Criteria for hospital admission after head injury are shown in Box 9.1.

| BOX 9.1 | Criteria for Hospital Admission After Head Injury |

- Intracranial blood or fracture identified on head CT scan
- Confusion, agitation, or depressed level of consciousness
- Focal neurologic signs or symptoms
- Alcohol or drug intoxication
- Significant comorbid medical illness
- Lack of a reliable environment for subsequent observation

CT, Computed tomography.

Severe Head Injury

After initial assessment and stabilization, the immediate consideration in the patient with severe head injury is whether there is an indication for emergent neurosurgical intervention. If the decision is made to operate, surgery should proceed immediately because delays can only increase the likelihood of further brain damage during the waiting period.

The medical management of patients with severe injury should be performed in a Neuro-Intensive Care Unit (NICU). Although little can be done about brain damage that occurs on impact, NICU care can play a major role in reducing secondary brain injury from hypoxia, hypotension, or increased ICP.

CHECKLIST FOR MANAGEMENT OF SEVERE HEAD INJURY IN THE NEURO-INTENSIVE CARE UNIT

1. **Reassess airway and ventilation**

   In general, patients in stupor or coma (those unable to follow commands because of a depressed level of consciousness) should be intubated for airway protection. If there is no evidence of increased ICP, ventilatory parameters should be set to maintain P_{CO_2} at 40 mm Hg and the minimal amount of F_{iO_2} to achieve a P_{O_2} at least 80 mm Hg.

2. **Monitor BP**

   If the patient shows signs of hemodynamic instability (hypotension or hypertension), monitoring is best accomplished with an arterial catheter. Because autoregulation is frequently impaired with acute head injury, mean arterial pressure (MAP) must be carefully maintained to avoid hypotension (mean BP < 65 mm Hg), which can lead to cerebral ischemia, or hypertension (mean BP > 130 mm Hg), which can exacerbate cerebral edema.

3. **Consult neurosurgery to insert an ICP monitor in patients with a Glasgow Coma Scale score of 8 or less**

   Because severe ICP elevations (Lundberg A waves or plateau waves) occur suddenly and without warning, a monitor should be inserted even if the patient does not currently show signs of increased ICP. Ventricular catheters are advisable if significant intraventricular hemorrhage with hydrocephalus is present; otherwise, a parenchymal monitor may be used.

4. **Fluid management**

   Only isotonic fluids (normal saline or Plasma-Lyte solution) should be administered to patients with head injury because the extra free water in half-normal saline or D5W can exacerbate cerebral edema.

5. **Nutrition**

   Severe head injury leads to a generalized hypermetabolic and catabolic response, with caloric requirements that are 50% to 100% higher than normal. Enteral feedings via a nasogastric or a nasoduodenal tube should be instituted as soon as possible.

6. **Temperature management**

   Fever (temperature >101°F) exacerbates cerebral injury and should be aggressively treated with acetaminophen or temperature-modulating devices with a core temperature feedback control.

7. **Anticonvulsants**

   Phenytoin or **fosphenytoin (20 mg/kg IV loading dose, then 300 mg/day IV)** reduces the frequency of early (i.e., first week) posttraumatic seizures from 14% to 4% in patients with intracranial hemorrhage but does not prevent later seizures. If the patient has not experienced a seizure, then phenytoin should be discontinued after 7 to 10 days. Levels should be monitored closely because subtherapeutic levels frequently result from hypermetabolism of phenytoin. A reasonable alternative for seizure prophylaxis is levetiracetam 1-2 g BID IV. Levetiracetam has minimal drug interactions, but levels cannot be easily followed and it can aggravate agitation.

8. **Steroids**

   Steroids have *not* been shown to favorably alter outcome in patients with head injury and may lead to increased risk of infection, hyperglycemia, and mortality. Large doses of steroids actually increase the risk of death from these complications. For this reason, *steroids such as dexamethasone have no role in the treatment of traumatic brain injury.*

9. **Prophylaxis for DVT**

   Pneumatic compression boots are routinely used in immobilized patients to protect against lower extremity DVT and the associated risk of pulmonary thromboembolism. **Heparin 5000 U subcutaneously (SC) every 8 hours or enoxaparin**

40 mg SC once a day should be started 24 hours after injury even in the presence of intracranial hemorrhage.

10. **Prophylaxis for gastric ulcer**

Patients on mechanical ventilation or with coagulopathy are at increased risk of gastric stress ulceration and should receive **pantoprazole 40 mg PO/IV once daily.**

11. **Antibiotics**

The routine use of prophylactic antibiotics in patients with open skull injuries is controversial. Penicillin may reduce the risk of pneumococcal meningitis in patients with CSF otorrhea, rhinorrhea, or intracranial air but may increase the risk of infection with more virulent organisms.

12. **Follow-up CT scan**

In general, a follow-up head CT scan should be obtained 24 hours after the initial injury in patients with intracranial hemorrhage to assess for delayed or progressive bleeding.

SELECTED COMPLICATIONS OF SEVERE HEAD INJURY

1. **CSF leaks**

CSF leaks result from disruption of the leptomeninges and occur in 2% to 6% of patients with closed head injury. CSF leakage ceases spontaneously with head elevation alone after a few days in 85% of patients; a lumbar drain may speed this process by limiting flow through the dural fistula in persistent cases. Although patients with CSF leaks are at increased risk for meningitis (usually from pneumococci), administration of prophylactic antibiotics is not indicated. Persistent CSF otorrhea or rhinorrhea or recurrent meningitis is an indication for operative repair.

2. **Carotid cavernous fistulae**

Carotid cavernous fistulae, characterized by the triad of *pulsating exophthalmos, chemosis, and orbital bruit,* may develop immediately or several days after injury. Angiography is required to confirm the diagnosis. Endovascular balloon occlusion is the most effective means of repair and can prevent permanent visual loss resulting from retinal venous hypertension.

3. **Diabetes insipidus**

Diabetes insipidus may result from traumatic damage to the pituitary stalk, resulting in cessation of antidiuretic hormone secretion. Patients excrete large volumes of dilute urine, resulting in hypernatremia and volume depletion. **Arginine vasopressin (Pitressin) 5 to 10 U IV,** intramuscularly **(IM), or SC every 4 to 6 hours** or **desmopressin acetate (DDAVP) SC 2 to 4 mg or IV every 12 hours** is given to control urine output to less than 200 mL/h, and volume is replaced with hypotonic fluids (D5W or 0.45% saline) depending on the severity of hypernatremia.

4. **Posttraumatic seizures**

Posttraumatic seizures may be **immediate** (occurring within 24 hours), **early** (occurring within the first week), or **late** (occurring after the first week). Immediate seizures do not predispose to late seizures; early seizures, however, indicate an increased risk of late seizures, and these patients should be maintained on anticonvulsants. The overall incidence of late posttraumatic epilepsy (recurrent, unprovoked seizures) after closed head injury is 5%; the risk is as high as 20% in patients with intracranial hemorrhage or depressed skull fractures.

PROGNOSIS

The outcome after head injury is often a matter of great concern, particularly in patients with serious injuries. The admission Glasgow Coma Scale score has substantial prognostic value; however, long-term prognostication should not be done at the time of admission. Often, examinations are dynamic, and secondary complications can occur early in the course of injury that can change the outcome. Prognostication should be done only after resuscitation and a period of close observation. Tests such as MRI, electroencephalography (EEG), or somatosensory evoked potential (SSEP) can provide additional useful information. *Postconcussion syndrome* refers to a chronic profile of headache, fatigue, dizziness, inability to concentrate, irritability, and personality changes that develops in many patients after head injury. Often, there is overlap with symptoms of depression.

Focal Mass Lesions

Introduction

Focal brain masses are a common reason for neurologic consultation, particularly in the inpatient setting. The main etiologic considerations include malignancy, infection, and, less commonly, inflammatory disease. The management of the brain mass varies widely depending on the etiology. This chapter will focus on the initial diagnostic evaluation and initial management of focal brain lesions.

PHONE CALL

Questions

1. **Is the patient fully awake and alert?**
   A stuporous patient is at risk for airway compromise.
2. **What are the vital signs?**
   Hypertension with or without bradycardia (Cushing syndrome) is a sign of increased intracranial pressure.
3. **Does the patient have any preexisting medical conditions?**
   In particular, a prior history of cancer or immunocompromised state can help narrow the differential diagnosis.
4. **Has the patient traveled recently?**
   This raises concern for fungal/parasitic infections (see the following).
5. **Does the patient have any neurologic symptoms (e.g., headache, weakness, visual complaints, speech difficulty)?**
   If so, approximately how long have these symptoms existed? Symptoms occurring over the course of days would raise concern for infection, whereas symptoms occurring over weeks to month would be more consistent with a cancer.

Orders

1. If there is clinical concern for increased intracranial pressure, the following measures should be implemented: (a) elevate the head of the bed to 30 degrees and (b) administer osmotherapy with either 20% mannitol 1g/kg intravenously (IV) or 30 mL of 23.4% hypertonic saline (this requires dental venous access).
2. If there is concern that the patient cannot protect his or her airway, the patient should be intubated and hyperventilated to a $Paco_2$ of 30mm Hg.
3. Rapid HIV test.
4. Complete blood count (CBC) with differential, basic metabolic panel (BMP), coagulation tests.
5. Chest X-ray (CXR).

ELEVATOR THOUGHTS

What is the differential diagnosis for focal mass lesions? The main two considerations are **malignancy** (metastatic or primary) or **infection** (abscesses or cerebritis). Other etiologies include autoimmune/inflammatory and vascular.

Before seeing the patient, the neurologist should visually review the imaging of concern. Usually, the imaging of concern is a computed tomography (CT) scan. Most brain masses are hypodense on CT scan. A divergence from this can be helpful in narrowing the differential diagnosis:

1. *Hyperdense signal mixed into the hypodense mass:*
   • Tumor with hemorrhage (e.g., glioblastoma), tumor with calcification (e.g. oligodendroglioma) or abscess
2. *Homogenous hyperdense signal:*
   • Melanoma, medulloblastoma, or meningioma.
3. *Punctate calcification:*
   • Ependymomas > meningiomas > medulloblastomas. Tuberculomas have a pathognomonic "target sign" resulting from central calcification surrounded by a hypodense area with peripheral ring enhancement with IV contrast.

Differential Diagnosis of Focal Intracranial Mass Lesions

Neoplasms

1. **Brain Metastases**
   • *Most common*: lung (small cell), breast (especially HER2 protein +/estrogen receptor [ER] −), melanoma, renal cell cancer, and colorectal cancer
   • Typically multiple lesions are seen
   • Metastases (Fig. 10.1) tend to localize at the gray-white junction of cerebral hemispheres (80%)

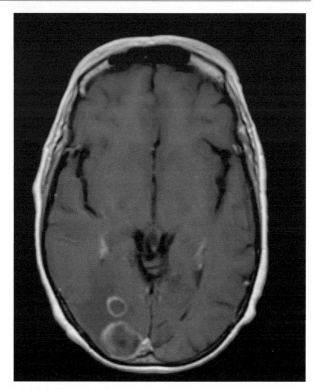

FIG. 10.1 Metastatic brain tumors.

- Diagnostic evaluation: Whole body CT and PET, mammo-gram, or skin exam demonstrating a primary tumor con-firms the diagnosis

2. **Gliomas**
   - *Most common*: glioblastoma (GBM, peak >50 years), ana-plastic astrocytoma (peak 40-50 years), oligodendroglioma (<40 years)
   - GBM (Fig. 10.2) shows most often as a combination of edema, enhancement, cystic components and necrosis (DWI restriction). A Cho/AA ratio >2.2 on MR spectroscopy is consistent with a high-grade malignant tumor.

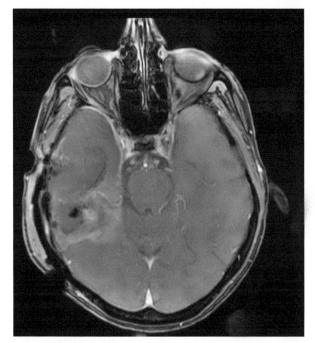

FIG. 10.2 Glioma in adult.

- Oligodendroglioma shows calcification (60%), enhancement (60%), cystic components (20%), hemorrhage (20%), and rarely edema.
- Anaplastic astrocytoma shows modest enhancement but no necrosis

3. **Meningioma**
   - Most often in middle-aged (40-60 years) women (2:1 ratio of women to men)
   - Presents as dense and homogeneous enhancement of a solitary dural-based mass (Fig. 10.3)
   - Can be associated with substantial surrounding brain edema

4. **Primary CNS Lymphoma**
   - Immunocompromised patients (i.e. AIDS) are at increased risk
   - On MRI T1 is hypointense and T2 is hyperintense, core diffusion weighted imaging (DWI) is restricted indicating necrosis, and there is diffuse enhancement.

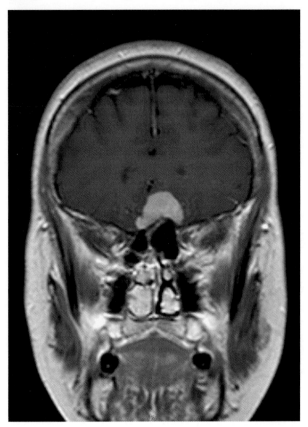

FIG. 10.3 Meningiomas.

- PCNSL have a predilection for the periventricular white matter and deep gray matter, but are notorious for presenting with a wide variety of locations and distributions.
5. **Pituitary tumors**
   - *Most common*: pituitary adenoma, Rathke cyst, craniopharyngioma
   - Pituitary adenomas are hypointense on T1 imaging and show delayed enhancement on dynamic gadolinium contrast imaging
   - Rathke cysts are nonenhancing, whereas craniophayngiomas are often calcified

- *Diagnostic evaluation*: serum prolactin, FSH, LH, cortisol, T3/T4, TSH, growth hormone, and visual field testing

Infections

1. **Bacterial abscess**
   - Presents as solitary or multiple ring-enhancing lesions (Fig. 10.4).
   - *Most common*: Gram (+) agents
   - Often occurs in the setting or recent dental work or endocarditis
   - Core DWI restriction on MRI is consistent with central necrosis
   - *Diagnostic evaluation*: blood cultures, transesophageal echocardiogram, LP

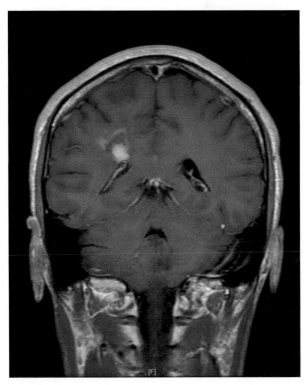

FIG. 10.4 Bacterial abscess in immunocompetent patient.

2. **Fungal abscess**
   - Presents as ring-enhancing lesions
   - *Most common*: Cryptocossus, aspergillosis, *Candia*, mucormycosis, *Nocardia*
   - Typically the patient is immunocompromised
   - DWI restriction occurs in wall of the abscess (rather than core as with bacterial abscess)
3. **Viral encephalitis**
   - Focal swelling and patchy enhancement of temporal lobe can be seen with *Herpes Simplex virus (HSV)* encephalitis
   - *Diagnostic evaluation:* CSF HSV polymerase chain reaction (+)
4. **Tuberculoma**
   - Can be multiple and military (multiple small ring enhancing lesions) or solitary and tumor-like (tuberculoma)
   - "Target sign" on CT (central calcification surrounded by hypodense area and peripheral enhancement) is pathognomonic
   - May be associated with diffuse nodular meningeal enhancement
   - *Diagnostic evaluation:* chest CT, LP, purified protein derivative (PPD) skin testing, quantiferon gold
5. **Parasitic infections**
   - *Cysticercosis* often presents as multiple cysts of varying ages, which can be non-enhancing and cystic (dormant), inflamed and enhancing, or chronic and calcified. Endemic in Latin America and sub-Saharan Africa. Most common helminthic infection
   - *Toxoplasmosis* presents as ring-enhancing granulomatous encephalitis. Common in AIDS. May be single or multiple. Most common protozoal infection. Diagnosis confirmed by radiographic response (lesion shrinkage) to empiric therapy (see Chapter 22)
   - *Diagnostic evaluation:* serum IgG antibodies can confirm prior exposure.

Inflammatory Diseases

1. **Sarcoidosis**
   - Peak frequency at age 30-50 years
   - Mass lesions may or may not enhance
   - Often associated with nodular meningeal enhancement on MRI with gadolinium.
   - *Diagnostic evaluation*: CSF and serum ACE activity, chest CT, gallium scan, lacrimal gland biopsy
2. **Tumefactive multiple sclerosis (Marburg variant)**
   - Peak age 30-40 years, often with prior symptoms consistent with MS

- By definition lesions are typically >2 cm in diameter with mass effect and edema
- MR may show partial ring enhancement with incomplete ring adjacent to gray matter

MAJOR THREATS TO LIFE

1. Increased intracranial pressure
2. Abscesses, particularly bacterial abscess, are often associated with endocarditis or bacteremia

BEDSIDE

Focused History

1. **History of presenting illness**
   (a) **Age**: Different brain tumors affect different age groups. Among the common pediatric brain tumors, ependymoma tends to affect children under age 5, whereas medulloblastomas and pilocytic astrocytomas generally affect children ages 5 to 10. The common adult tumors are also distributed by age. Oligodendrogliomas have a peak incidence at age 40, anaplastic astrocytomas at age 50, and glioblastomas at age 65. Pituitary adenomas tend to occur in young adulthood (age 20 to 50), and meningiomas tend to occur in middle adulthood (age 40 to 60).
   (b) **Gender**: Meningiomas and pituitary adenomas are more common in women.
   (c) **Time course** of symptoms: Hours to days would be consistent with a bacterial meningitis, days to weeks would be the time course of a fungal meningitis, and weeks to months would be fitting with a malignancy.
2. **Neurological review of systems**
   (a) **Recent seizure like activity**: This will affect the decision about starting antiepileptics.
   (b) **Headache:** Headaches, particularly those worse with recumbency, are concerning for increased intracranial pressure.
   (c) Prior history of **transient (days) neurological symptoms**, in particular transient vision loss and pain, should raise suspicion for tumefactive multiple sclerosis.
3. **Systemic review of systems/past medical history**
   (a) Screen for the **common systemic cancers** that tend to metastasize to the brain: persistent cough (lung cancer), smoking history (lung cancer), breast lumps (breast cancer), last mammogram (breast cancer), skin changes (melanoma), blood in stool (colorectal cancer), stomach

discomfort (colorectal cancer), weight loss, any prior cancer history.

    (1) If the patient does endorse a prior history of cancer, certain follow-up questions will be helpful. If it is a history of lung cancer, inquire as to if it was non–small-cell lung cancer (NSCLC) or small-cell lung cancer (SCLC). The former metastasizes to the brain in 7% of cases, as opposed to the latter, which metastasizes in 50% of cases. If the patient had a breast cancer history, inquire about the receptor status. HER2+/estrogen receptor (ER)- tumors are more likely to metastasize to the brain. If there is a melanoma history, inquire as to the location of the melanoma; head/oral/neck lesions are more likely to spread to the brain.

(b) Screen for **immunocompromised state,** e.g., HIV and HIV risk factors, transplant history, chemotherapy use, diabetes, and steroid use. HIV increases the risk for primary central nervous system lymphoma (PCNSL) and toxoplasmosis. Neutropenia and chronic steroid use increase the risk for certain fungal infections (aspergillosis, *Candida*, mucormycosis, and *Nocardia*).

(c) Query about **systemic inflammatory diseases**: Sarcoid in particular can present with focal mass lesions.

(d) Inquire about history of **tuberculosis and syphilis**, both of which can cause mass lesions in the brain.

(e) **Systemic symptoms** such as weight loss can suggest an occult malignancy, fevers and chills can suggest infection, and night sweats combined with weight loss can indicate central nervous system (CNS) lymphoma or tuberculosis.

(f) Prior distant history of **radiation** increases risk for meningiomas and malignant glioma. Recent history of radiation can result in radiation necrosis, which presents as a focal mass lesion.

4. **Recent travel:** Certain fungal and parasitic infections have different geographic predilections. Blastomycosis and histoplasmosis are endemic in Midwestern United States, *Coccidioides* in Western United States, histoplasmosis and *Coccidioides* in Central/South America, and cysticercosis in Central/South America and sub-Saharan Africa.

5. If the mass is in the **suprasellar region**, then screen for symptoms of pituitary dysfunction (amenorrhea, galactorrhea, gynecomastia, erectile dysfunction, impotence, decrease in body hair, gigantism, or hyperthyroidism).

Selective Physical Examination

General Physical Examination

1. **Vitals**
   (a) Hypertension with/without bradycardia is known as Cushing reflex and is a sign of increased intracranial pressure.
   (b) Fever is a sign of infection.
   (c) Weight loss can be a sign of malignancy.
2. **General exam:**
   (a) Cardiac murmur, petechiae, splinter hemorrhages, Janeway lesion, and Osler nodes are all concerning for endocarditis.
   (b) Neck stiffness is a sign of bacterial meningitis

Neurologic Examination

1. **Mental status:**
   (a) Inattention can be a sign of impending herniation and is a useful sign to follow while awaiting implementation of definitive treatment.
   (b) Focal impairments in mental status (aphasia, neglect, visual spatial functioning, or amnesia) can support the localization that was already visualized on imaging but may also indicate broader dysfunction.
2. **Cranial nerves:**
   (a) Pale discs, red desaturation, and/or an afferent pupillary defect raises the suspicious for multiple sclerosis.
   (b) Papilledema and abducens palsy(ies) are signs of increased intracranial pressure.
   (c) An unreactive, dilated pupil ("blown pupil") indicates damage to the parasympathetic fibers of the oculomotor nerve and is a sign of herniation.
   (d) Lower motor neuron dysfunction in multiple cranial nerves should raise concern for a leptomeningeal process in addition to the focal mass lesion.
3. **Motor Exam:**
   (a) Increased tone on the ipsilateral side of the lesion is concerning for herniation and compression of the contralateral cerebral peduncle.
4. **Reflexes**
   (a) As previously mentioned, increased *reflexes* on the ipsilateral side of the lesion are concerning for herniation and compression of the contralateral cerebral peduncles

Further Diagnostic Workup

1. **Magnetic resonance imaging (MRI) brain:** If the initial image is a CT, an MRI brain should be obtained to radiographically characterize the lesion better, unless there is a contraindication (e.g., patient hemodynamically unstable, implanted device).

2. An **MR spectroscopy** can sometimes add further clarity as to the underlying etiology. An elevated choline/N-acetyl-aspartate (Cho/NAA) ratio (>2.2) is suggestive of a high-grade brain tumor. Lactate can be elevated in infections and necrotic tumors.

3. A brain **positron emission tomography (PET)** scan can help assess the grade of a tumor; a high-grade tumor would show increased metabolism. The brain PET scan can also distinguish between a recurrent high-grade tumor and radiation necrosis; the former will be hypermetabolic and the latter will be hypometabolic.

4. A whole body PET/CT is indicated when there is clinical concern for metastatic disease.

5. Lumbar puncture:
   (a) Lumbar puncture is indicated when there is clinical concern for
      (i) Infectious meningitis/cerebritis,
      (ii) Inflammatory etiology for focal mass lesions (e.g., sarcoid, multiple sclerosis), or
      (iii) Lymphoma, leukemia, carcinomatous meningitis, or germ cell tumor.
   (b) If there is concern for impending herniation, then a lumbar puncture is contraindicated
   (c) The preferred diagnostic modality for brain abscesses is CT-guided drainage and culture and that for brain tumors is tissue biopsy $\pm$ partial/total debulking.

MANAGEMENT

1. If there is radiographic concern for **impending herniation** from tumor or an abscess, then steroids should be administered (one dosing regimen often used is dexamethasone 10 mg IV × 1 followed by a standing regimen of 16 to 24 mg/day divided into four times a day dosing). See Chapter 13 for more information on management of increased intracranial pressure.

2. If there is radiographic concern for **lymphoma** and there is no evidence of impending herniation, then steroids should be withheld until a diagnostic biopsy is performed. Corticosteroids can adversely affect the sensitivity of tissue biopsy analysis. See Chapter 23 more more details.

3. If there is clinical and radiographic concern for **toxoplasmosis** (e.g., AIDS patient, serum toxoplasma antibody positive, basal ganglia lesions, multiple lesions) and no evidence of impending herniation, then the most commonly used approach is to initiate a 2-week empiric toxoplasmosis treatment course and monitor for radiographic and clinical improvement (see Chapter 22 for more details).

Gait Failure

The control of gait and posture involves numerous components of the nervous system. Gait ataxia implies decomposition in the coordinated control of posture and gait that are typically controlled by the cerebellum and other subcortical structures.

A call for a patient with gait failure requires consideration of a broad differential diagnosis. Successful evaluation begins with an assessment of the time course of the symptoms. Associated signs on examination will help with anatomic localization. Management may range from emergent neurosurgical decompression of a cerebellar hematoma to a thorough laboratory evaluation to seek a cause for a chronic degenerative disease.

PHONE CALL

Questions

1. **When did the patient last walk normally?**

   This is a key question from which your route of investigation and management begins.

   Acute Onset: If the patient was known to have been walking normally within the past 24 hours, you must rule out stroke (Chapter 6), spinal cord compression (Chapter 7), traumatic brain injury (Chapter 9), or a mass lesion in the posterior fossa (Chapter 10). These are medical emergencies.

   Subacute Onset: A subacute course (days to weeks) suggests an infectious, inflammatory, or neoplastic process.

   Chronic Onset: If the gait deterioration has occurred over weeks to months, your differential diagnosis will be weighted toward degenerative processes, either inherited or acquired.

2. **Has there been any trauma to the head, neck, or back?**

   A traumatic subdural hematoma or injury to the spinal cord or peripheral nerves may alter gait.

3. **What is the patient's level of consciousness?**

   Is the patient alert and awake, agitated, or confused? If a patient has an abnormal mental status in combination with ataxia or gait failure, acute intoxication or significant brain injury is likely.

4. **What are the vital signs?**

Irregular heart rhythm may suggest cardioembolic stroke; fever may suggest an infectious process.

Orders

1. Maintain the patient at bed rest.
2. Use a chest restraint, if necessary, to prevent patients from injuring themselves.
3. If there has been trauma to the head or neck, stabilize the cervical spine with a cervical collar (see Chapter 7, Spinal Cord Compression).

ELEVATOR THOUGHTS

What is the differential diagnosis of gait failure?

Gait failure may occur as a result of damage to almost any part of the neural axis. Your initial examination of the patient will help establish whether you are dealing with disturbance of motor, sensory, or cerebellar function. Table 11.1 is an outline of the categories of diseases that cause gait dysfunction and the characteristic features of the gait disturbance. Table 11.2 provides a more detailed differential diagnosis of ataxia.

TABLE 11.1	Clinical Features of Gait Disturbances
Disease Category	**Features of Gait Failure**
Focal brain injury (hemiparesis)	Spastically extended leg Spastically flexed arm Circumduction of paretic limb
Spinal cord injury (paraparesis)	Stiff, effortful movements at knees and hips Bilateral circumduction Toe-walking or scissoring gait
Peripheral or central deafferentation (sensory ataxia)	Wide-based stance and gait High-stepping gait Positive Romberg sign
Cerebellar disease	Titubation (unsteady, oscillating posture) on sitting or standing Wide-based stance and gait Difficulty turning Ataxia: staggering or lurching (unilateral or bilateral)
Normal-pressure hydrocephalus	"Magnetic," shuffling gait Many steps taken to turn 180 degrees Turning en bloc Increased sway in stance Start hesitation and freezing of gait Slow gait speed with short steps

TABLE 11.1	Clinical Features of Gait Disturbances—cont'd

Disease Category	Features of Gait Failure
Lower motor neuron disease	Distal weakness (e.g., foot drop) High-stepping gait
Myopathy	Proximal leg weakness Difficulty arising from seated position Difficulty climbing stairs
Parkinsonism	Stooped posture Shuffling gait Retropulsion Difficulty initiating and terminating Freezing of gait "festinating gait" Variable stepping Slow, narrow base of support during gait Reduced arm swing during gait
Congenital/ perinatal (cerebral palsy)	Hypertonic extended legs Hypertonic flexed arms Scissoring gait Adventitial movements (abnormal posturing or movements of one or more limbs)
Multiple sclerosis	Slow gait Reduced endurance Reduced stride length and joint motion May see foot drop caused by weakness
Concussions	Slow gait Increased sway in frontal plane Impairments worsen during divided attention (dual-task gait)
Dementia (vascular)	Gait disorder occurs early in disease Slow gait, short steps, and rigidity Wide support base
Dementia (Alzheimer's disease)	Gait disorder occurs later in disease Slow speed, short steps Greater time on both feet Variable stepping, especially when performing cognitive dual task
Cautious gait	Slow speed, short steps Extremely long time on both feet "Walking on ice": stiff lower limbs, outstretched arms Linked with increased fear of falling

TABLE 11.2	Differential Diagnosis of Gait Failure by Mode of Onset
Mode of Onset	**Disease Process**
Acute (minutes to hours)	Cerebellar hemorrhage Cerebellar infarction Acute intoxication Head trauma Basilar migraine Dominant periodic ataxia (in children) Benign paroxysmal positional vertigo
Subacute (hours to days)	Posterior fossa tumor Posterior fossa abscess Multiple sclerosis Toxins/intoxications Hydrocephalus Miller-Fisher variant of Guillain-Barré syndrome Viral cerebellitis (mostly in children)
Chronic (days to weeks)	Alcoholic cerebellar degeneration Paraneoplastic cerebellar syndrome Foramen magnum compression Chronic infection (e.g., Jakob-Creutzfeldt disease, rubella, panencephalitis) Hydrocephalus Hypothyroidism Vitamin E deficiency Inherited ataxias (autosomal recessive or dominant) Idiopathic degenerative ataxias
Episodic	Recurrent intoxications Multiple sclerosis Transient ischemic attacks Dominant periodic ataxia (children)

Modified from Harding AE. Ataxic disorders. In Bradley WG, Daroff RB, Fenichel GM, Marsden CD, eds. *Neurology in Clinical Practice.* Boston, MA: Butterworth-Heinemann; 1991.

MAJOR THREAT TO LIFE

- **Cerebellar hemorrhage or infarction**

    Hematoma or infarction in the posterior fossa may progress to herniation and death if the lesion is large. It may require emergent neurosurgical evacuation.
- **Acute intoxication**

    Intoxication with sedatives such as barbiturate or alcohol may present initially as ataxia and may lead to respiratory failure.

BEDSIDE

Quick-Look Test

Is the patient awake and alert?

A decreased level of consciousness in the presence of ataxia is more serious than ataxia alone.

Is there any evidence of head or neck trauma?

Head trauma rarely presents as ataxia alone but may require more immediate management. Vertebral artery dissection may result from trauma to the neck.

Has the patient been vomiting?

Nausea, vertigo, and vomiting are common symptoms that accompany posterior fossa disease.

Selective History and Chart Review

The diagnosis for the etiology of gait failure often can be made on the history alone. If the patient is unable to give a history, get the history from a relative, nurse, or other witness. In the absence of a witness on hand, review the chart.

1. When did the gait disturbance begin?
2. Was the onset sudden or gradual?
3. Why was the patient unable to walk? Was it because of weakness, imbalance, pain, or numbness?
4. Were there any accompanying symptoms?

    Diplopia, dysarthria, vertigo, or nausea suggests posterior fossa involvement. Unilateral weakness or numbness implies focal hemispheric brain injury (e.g., stroke). Urinary or fecal incontinence suggests spinal cord involvement. Pain radiating into the legs implies nerve root disease.

5. *Is the patient taking any medications that might cause ataxia?*

    Most of the effects of medications are dose dependent (Table 11.3).

TABLE 11.3	Medications Known to Cause Ataxia
Aminoglycoside antibiotics	Cyclobenzaprine
Amiodarone	Cyclosporine A
Angiotensin-converting enzyme inhibitors	Cytosine arabinoside
	Dextromethorphan
Baclofen	Divalproex
Barbiturates	Ethosuximide
Benzodiazepines	Felbamate
Beta-adrenergic blockers	Flucytosine
Carbamazepine	Fluorouracil
Carbonic anhydrase inhibitors	Gabapentin
Carboplatin	Isoniazid
Chloral hydrate	Histamine H1-receptor
Cisplatin	antagonists

TABLE 11.3	Medications Known to Cause Ataxia—cont'd
Lamotrigine	Paraldehyde
Lithium	Phenothiazines
Methocarbamol	Phenytoin
Methosuximide	Primidone
Methysergide	Reserpine
Methotrexate	Tacrolimus
Metronidazole	Thiothixene
Monoamine oxidase inhibitors	Tricyclic and tetracyclic
Nitrofurantoin	antidepressants
Opioid agonists and	Valproate
agonist-antagonists	Zolpidem
Paclitaxel	

Adapted from Brust, JCM. *Neurotoxic Side Effects of Prescription Drugs*. Boston, MA: Butterworth-Heinemann; 1996.

Selective Physical Examination I
General Physical Examination

Vital signs	Fever may suggest an infectious etiology, such as abscess, viral cerebellitis, or fungal infection
	Fever may also occur in some of the inherited metabolic ataxias (mostly in children)
	Irregular heart rhythm may suggest cardioembolic stroke
HEENT	Look for signs of head or neck trauma
	Subdural or epidural hematoma may produce hemiparesis
Abdomen	Look for signs of chronic alcohol use, such as hepatomegaly, caput medusae, or ascites
	Hepatosplenomegaly may also appear in Wilson disease and in some inherited metabolic ataxias

HEENT, Head, ears, eyes, nose, and throat.

Neurologic Examination

- **Mental status:** Establish level of alertness and attentiveness by asking the patient to count backward from 20 to 1 or to recite the months of the year backward.
- **Cranial nerves: Gait failure with almost any cranial nerve finding means there is brain stem or cerebellar involvement.**
  1. **Pupils:** Pinpoint pupils may suggest *opiate intoxication*; asymmetric pupils may be a part of Horner syndrome (miosis, ptosis, and anhidrosis), which, in combination with ataxia and contralateral pain and temperature sensation loss,

makes up Wallenberg (lateral medullary) syndrome. Small, irregular pupils that react to accommodation but not to light (Argyll Robertson pupils) may be a sign of *central nervous system (CNS) syphilis, brain stem encephalitis, or mass effect on the midbrain.*

2. **Extraocular movements: Nystagmus, particularly if vertical or dysconjugate, is a sign of injury to the brain stem or cerebellum.** Vertical (upbeat or downbeat) nystagmus is a reliable indicator of cerebellar or brain stem damage (see Chapter 14 for a more detailed discussion of nystagmus). Horizontal gaze palsies localize disease to a large hemispheric or small pontine lesion. Impaired upgaze, particularly in combination with retraction nystagmus and loss of pupillary accommodation, implies pressure on or damage to the tectum of the midbrain and can be seen in pineal region tumors or in hydrocephalus (Parinaud phenomenon). Cranial nerve (CN) 6 palsies may be a nonspecific sign of increased intracranial pressure (ICP). Oculoparesis, in combination with ataxia and areflexia, makes the diagnosis of the *Miller-Fisher variant of Guillain-Barré syndrome.*

3. **CN 7:** Upper motor neuron facial paresis may be part of a hemiparesis or may indicate brain stem involvement if CN 6 is affected on the same side.

4. **CN 8:** Tinnitus or hearing loss with ataxia suggests a *peripheral vestibular neuropathy or labyrinthitis*, particularly if there is a rotational component to the nystagmus.

5. **CN 9 to CN 12:** Dysphagia, nasal speech, dysarthria, or tongue deviation may suggest a *brain stem stroke* or *mass lesion at the skull base*, producing spastic paraparesis and gait failure in addition to the lower cranial nerve findings.

- **Cerebellar testing:** Rapid, repetitive finger-thumb opposition (rapid alternating movements [RAM]) and finger-nose-finger (FNF) movements are two sensitive screening tests for cerebellar function. Irregular rhythm (dysdiadochokinesis) on finger tapping or ataxia of movements as the finger approaches the target on the FNF test suggests cerebellar dysfunction. The heel-knee-shin test is the equivalent of the FNF test for the lower extremities. Figure 11.1 illustrates three common cerebellar tests: FNF, RAM, and HKS. **Unilateral limb ataxia implies ipsilateral cerebellar hemisphere damage** because the cerebellar circuits that coordinate movement cross twice, once while descending in the frontopontocerebellar pathway and a second time while ascending in the dentatothalamic, dentatorubral, and dentatocortical pathways. Titubation (truncal ataxia) on sitting or standing or gait ataxia in the absence of limb ataxia suggests midline cerebellar damage.

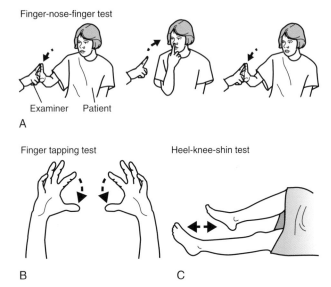

FIG. 11.1 Cerebellar function tests. (A) Finger-nose-finger test. Patient touches the finger of the examiner and his or her own nose sequentially. (B) Finger tapping test. Patient taps index finger and thumb as rapidly as possible. (C) Heel-knee-shin test. Patient runs the heel up and down the opposite shin as accurately and rapidly as possible.

If the patient is able to stand, the gait evaluation is a crucial part of the examination for anatomic localization and determination of the underlying pathophysiology. Table 11.1 reviews the features of gait dysfunction that characterize different disease processes. The gait should be tested with the patient walking normally, walking on the toes, walking on the heels, and doing a tandem walk. Observe for symmetry of balance, stride, and arm swing.

- **Motor:** Test for strength by confrontation and look for pronator drift with the arms extended and palms up (pronator drift may be the only sign of a subtle hemiparesis.) Evaluate for presence of tremor at rest (indicative of Parkinson disease). Evaluate for increased tone (spastic or rigid).
- **Sensory:** Temperature and vibration are the most sensitive parameters for testing sensory loss. Proprioceptive loss may indicate damaged posterior columns, as occurs in *vitamin B₁₂ deficiency* (subacute combined degeneration) or *tabes dorsalis* (a now rare, late complication of syphilis). Look for a sensory

level, which suggests a spinal cord lesion, or saddle anesthesia, which suggests conus medullaris syndrome (Chapter 1).

- **Reflexes:** Unilateral hyperreflexia usually accompanies hemiparesis, bilateral hyperreflexia may indicate myelopathy, and areflexia is seen in peripheral neuropathy and in the *Guillain-Barré syndrome.*
- **Presence of Babinski sign (upgoing/hyperextended toe)** implies an upper motor neuron lesion (caused by spinal cord injury or stroke)

MANAGEMENT

Acute ataxia, particularly with any accompanying signs or symptoms of posterior fossa disease or increased ICP, must be treated with utmost urgency.

1. **Obtain a noncontrast head computed tomography (CT) or magnetic resonance imaging (MRI) scan.**

    If cerebellar hematoma or infarction is identified, proceed with the next steps.

2. **Admit the patient to an intensive care unit.**

3. **Consult with the neurosurgery service.**

    If there is hematoma near the brain stem or if the hematoma is large, rapid, and irreversible, neurologic deterioration may occur. Delayed deterioration may be the result of a rebleed or reactive edema formation. *Surgical evacuation of cerebellar hematoma greater than 3 cm in diameter has been shown to reduce morbidity and mortality rates for these patients.* Consideration for surgical evacuation is warranted, particularly if the patient is relatively young and is following a deteriorating course. *It may be necessary to place an intraventricular drain if hydrocephalus develops.*

4. **Cerebellar hematomas smaller than 3 cm may be managed medically with reasonably good results.**

    Therapy is largely supportive, with blood pressure (BP) control to a target maximum systolic BP (SBP) of 160 to 180 mm Hg and control of coagulopathy with fresh frozen plasma if necessary. Hydrocephalus can develop even with smaller hematomas, necessitating neurosurgical placement of an intraventricular drain.

5. **Cerebellar infarction, if large, may produce the same syndrome of rapid progression to coma as does cerebellar hematoma.**

    As the infarcted territory becomes edematous, compression of the fourth ventricle may produce *obstructive hydrocephalus*, leading to further increase in ICP. Cerebellar infarction in the posterior inferior cerebellar artery territory carries a worse prognosis than infarction in the anterior inferior cerebellar artery or superior cerebellar artery territories. *Surgical evacuation of a large cerebellar infarction may be lifesaving.* As noted in the previous item 3, placement of an intraventricular drain may become necessary with cerebellar infarction if hydrocephalus develops.

Other causes of gait failure that require immediate management include cord compression or acute myelopathy (see Chapter 7), **subdural or epidural hematoma from head trauma** (see Chapter 9), **acute cerebral infarction** (see Chapter 6), or **acute intoxication** (see Chapter 5).

Selective Physical Examination II

Once posterior fossa lesions have been ruled out by imaging, further examination for systemic signs associated with chronic ataxic disorders should be performed:

Hair	Alopecia may be a sign of *thallium poisoning, hypothyroidism, or adrenoleukomyeloneuropathy*
Skin	Telangiectasias, particularly in the conjunctivae, nose, and ears, or flexures, may be seen in *ataxia-telangiectasia*
	Pigmentation may be seen in adrenoleukomyeloneuropathy
HEENT	Kayser-Fleischer rings appear as a brown border at the edge of the iris in *Wilson disease*
	Retinal angiomas seen on fundoscopic examination may be a part of *von Hippel-Lindau disease*, which also includes cerebellar hemangioblastomas
	Deafness in combination with short stature is often a sign of *mitochondrial encephalopathy*
Heart	Cardiomegaly, murmurs, arrhythmias, and heart failure may accompany *Friedreich's ataxia*
	Conduction defects on ECG may be present in mitochondrial encephalopathy
Musculoskeletal	Short stature is characteristic of mitochondrial encephalopathy and ataxia-telangiectasia. Other skeletal deformities may be a part of hereditary ataxias and hereditary motor and sensory neuropathy. Joint swelling or erythema can indicate an underlying arthritis (degenerative or inflammatory).

ECG, Electrocardiogram; *HEENT,* head, ears, eyes, nose, and throat.

Diagnostic Testing

LABORATORY INVESTIGATION

Laboratory investigation should begin with an attempt to diagnose treatable or reversible causes of ataxia or gait failure. Laboratory tests to be performed include the following blood tests:

1. Chemistry panel, including electrolytes, glucose, and liver function tests
2. Urine and serum toxicology screen
3. Vitamin B_{12} and folate levels
4. Venereal Disease Research Laboratory (VDRL) test
5. Thyroid function tests
6. Anticonvulsant levels if the patient is taking anticonvulsants
7. Lithium level if the patient is taking lithium
8. Anti-Yo serum antibodies to investigate paraneoplastic cerebellar degeneration from ovarian, lung, or breast carcinoma, or Hodgkin lymphoma (see Chapter 23)
9. Ceruloplasmin levels (Wilson disease)

Other Diagnostic Tests

1. **Chest radiograph**

   A chest radiograph may disclose occult neoplasm, raising the possibility of metastatic disease or a paraneoplastic cerebellar degeneration.

2. **Transcranial Doppler ultrasonogram or MR angiogram**

   Vertebrobasilar transient ischemic attacks (TIAs) or vertebrobasilar insufficiency may be suggested if there is stenosis of the basilar or vertebral arteries.

3. **Visual evoked responses**

   Delayed P100 suggests multiple sclerosis.

4. **Lumbar puncture**

   Oligoclonal bands are present in multiple sclerosis. Abnormal cerebrospinal fluid (CSF) cell count, protein, or glucose may point to an infectious or neoplastic process. Elevated CSF protein without pleocytosis is found in the Miller-Fisher variant of Guillain-Barré syndrome. Cytology may be performed if a CNS-based or meninges-based tumor is suspected.

5. **Electromyography (EMG)/nerve conduction studies (NCS)**

   The Miller-Fisher variant of the Guillain-Barré syndrome includes ataxia, oculoparesis, and areflexia. A typical demyelination pattern of slowed conduction velocities and prolonged F waves supports this diagnosis. Gait failure on the basis of neuropathy can also be diagnosed with EMG/NCS.

Treatment of Some of the Reversible Causes of Ataxia

1. **Acute sedative intoxication:** Administer **naloxone (Narcan) 0.4 to 2 mg intravenously (IV)** for opiate overdose and **flumazenil (Romazicon) 0.5 mg IV** for benzodiazepine overdose. Admit for observation and supportive therapy.

2. **Anticonvulsant overdose:** Stop administering the anticonvulsant, admit for observation and cardiovascular monitoring, and follow anticonvulsant levels.

3. **Hypothyroidism:** Administer **Synthroid 0.05 to 0.15 mg every day.**

4. **Lithium toxicity:** Admit patient for cardiac monitoring, adjust dose, and follow lithium and electrolyte levels.

5. **Paraneoplastic disorder:** Treating the underlying malignancy may reverse the symptoms in some patients. Immunosuppressive therapy and plasmapheresis have not been proved to be effective.

6. **Vertebrobasilar TIAs:** Admit patient for workup for etiology of TIAs. Anticoagulation may be required (see Chapter 24).

7. **Multiple sclerosis:** Treat with IV methylprednisolone and beta interferon (see Chapter 21).

8. **CNS infections:** Treat with appropriate antimicrobial agents (see Chapter 22).

9. **Miller-Fisher variant of Guillain-Barré syndrome:** A several-day course of plasmapheresis or IV immunoglobulin (IVIG) early in the disease may be effective in halting progression and speeding recovery (see Chapter 16).

10. Treatment of **benign positional vertigo** with Epley maneuver (refer to Chapter 14).

Acute Visual Disturbances

Few symptoms may be as disturbing or dramatic to a patient as acute visual loss. Although acute ocular diseases such as uveitis, retinal detachment, and some forms of glaucoma may require urgent evaluation by an ophthalmologist, a high percentage of acute visual disturbances fall within the province of the neurologist. Neurologic visual symptoms may be reported as blurriness, double vision, focal obscurations or shadows, vision loss, or positive visual phenomena such as flashes of light or visual hallucinations. Because the visual pathway from the retina to the calcarine cortex and eye movement control centers are constant from individual to individual, anatomic localization can be made on physical examination with a high degree of accuracy. The time course and progression, associated symptoms and signs, and clinical setting will help you make the correct diagnosis and suggest the proper acute management.

PHONE CALL

Questions

The following questions will need to be repeated during your selective history and physical examination of the patient. Nonetheless, these questions, asked prior to your arrival at the bedside, will form the starting point for your diagnostic and management algorithm.

1. **Is the visual disturbance in one or both eyes?**

   This is the first point for anatomic localization. Visual disturbances affecting only one eye indicate pathology between the cornea and the optic chiasm. Binocular disturbances suggest lesions in the visual pathway between (and including) the chiasm and the calcarine cortex. Keep in mind that patients sometimes misinterpret asymmetric binocular vision loss as vision loss in only one eye, so it is important to examine both eyes carefully when you see the patient. In the case of double vision, neurologic causes should resolve when either eye is covered.

173

2. **What is the nature of the visual disturbance?**

   This is an elaboration of question 1. Vision can be altered in one of the following ways: monocular visual loss (temporary or persistent), bilateral visual loss (temporary or persistent), a homonymous hemifield cut, diplopia, scotomata, or positive phenomena (e.g., flashes or lines). The first description of the disturbance will assist with localization and categorization of the vision loss into specific disease entities.

3. **How old is the patient?**

   Certain disorders, such as ischemic optic neuropathy, retinal artery occlusion, or transient monocular vision loss (TMVL; also called amaurosis fugax), are rare in patients under 45 years of age, whereas a first presentation of multiple sclerosis (MS) with optic neuritis, idiopathic intracranial hypertension (IIH), or migraine is much more common in a younger patient.

4. **Is the patient still experiencing the visual symptom?**

   Although persistent acute visual loss may require immediate, specific therapy, transient visual loss in one or both eyes may be no less ominous as a warning sign for further visual, cerebrovascular, or inflammatory events.

5. **When did the visual disturbance begin?**

   Acute monocular or binocular blindness is a neuroophthalmologic emergency. Ischemia in the retina resulting from a central retinal artery occlusion (CRAO) and ischemia in the occipital lobes may be irreversible without acute emergent intervention. Furthermore, even if the patient presents many hours after the onset of visual loss, efficient and accurate diagnosis may prevent contralateral visual loss caused by temporal arteritis or stroke from carotid or vertebrobasilar artery disease.

6. **Was there any trauma or injury to the eyes?**

   Eye injury will nearly always require ophthalmologic evaluation. Because a dilated fundoscopic examination by an ophthalmologist will interfere with your ability to get an accurate assessment of pupillary reactivity, you should try to perform your assessment first.

Orders

If there has been eye trauma, if there is a preexisting ophthalmologic condition such as glaucoma, if the patient is experiencing a great deal of flashing lights in one eye indicating retinal detachment, or if you are unable to visualize the fundus in a patient with vision loss, call the ophthalmology service for consultation.

Inform RN

"Will arrive at the bedside in…minutes."

ELEVATOR THOUGHTS

What is the differential diagnosis of acute visual disturbance?

The differential diagnosis of acute visual disturbance can be divided into processes affecting one eye or both eyes.

1. **Monocular visual loss**

    Table 12.1 lists the most common causes of painless monocular visual loss.

    - **Retinal ischemia (CRAO or branch retinal artery occlusion [BRAO])**

        This occlusion is usually caused by an embolus from the ipsilateral internal carotid artery or from the heart or aortic arch. If the symptoms are transient (TMVL or amaurosis fugax), the mechanism may be hemodynamic rather than embolic. Hemodynamic TMVL may be caused by perfusion failure in the retinal artery from high-grade carotid stenosis. Patients with vascular causes for retinal ischemia usually have risk factors for cerebrovascular disease, such as hypertension, diabetes, or a history of smoking. Temporal arteritis is occasionally a cause of CRAO or TMVL.

    - **Optic nerve head ischemia (anterior ischemic optic neuropathy [AION])**

        Although its pathophysiology is uncertain, this entity is often associated with arteritis. Younger patients may have systemic lupus erythematosus, polyarteritis nodosa, sickle cell trait, or polycythemia. In patients over 60 years of age, the most common associated arteritis is giant cell (temporal) arteritis, which must be treated emergently. There is a nonarteritic form of AION, but arteritic forms must be ruled out on an emergent basis.

TABLE 12.1	Most Common Causes of Monocular Visual Loss

Amaurosis fugax (transient monocular vision loss caused by ischemia/hypoperfusion)

Anterior ischemic optic neuropathy (arteritic from temporal arteritis versus nonarteritic)

Retinal artery occlusion (CRAO or BRAO)

Central retinal vein occlusion

Optic neuritis

Papilledema (intracranial mass lesion, cerebral venous sinus thrombosis, meningitis, idiopathic intracranial hypertension)

Compressive optic neuropathy (tumor, thyroid eye disease)

Ocular: glaucoma, cataract, diabetic maculopathy, vitreous hemorrhage, retinal detachment

BRAO, Branch retinal artery occlusion; *CRAO*, central retinal artery occlusion.

- **Inflammatory/demyelinating optic neuritis**

    The most common cause for optic neuritis in a patient under 40 years of age is demyelination, which could be the first attack of MS, but neuromyelitis optica should also be considered. Idiopathic optic neuritis and sarcoid optic neuritis also can occur.

- **Retrobulbar mass lesion**

    The lesion may be a tumor, such as optic glioma, neurofibroma, meningioma, or metastasis, or a giant aneurysm in the cavernous segment of the carotid. Such lesions usually present with progressive subacute vision loss, but they can present acutely.

- **Idiopathic intracranial hypertension**

    This can mimic an intracranial mass lesion, causing papilledema and visual loss in young women who are often obese. Visual loss may begin unilaterally.

2. **Binocular visual loss**

    Binocular involvement with visual field defects implies pathology at or behind the optic chiasm. Acute binocular visual loss affecting the chiasm, the optic tracts, the thalamus (lateral geniculate body), the optic radiations, or the calcarine cortex is nearly always caused by an anatomic lesion such as a *tumor, abscess, or stroke. Migraine* is a notable exception, in which "spreading depression" (a wave of depolarization) is thought to produce neuronal deactivation that moves slowly across the cortex and produces scintillating scotomata in both visual fields, although many patients report its presence in only one eye. *Pituitary adenomas* often produce bitemporal visual field defects because pressure from the mass disrupts midline-crossing fibers from both nasal retinae (Fig. 12.1). Although vision loss is often slowly progressive with adenomas, acute vision loss may occur in one or both eyes with pituitary apoplexy (a true emergency). The farther back along the visual pathway the lesion is located, the more congruous is the visual field defect. Table 12.2 lists unusual visual syndromes associated with occipital cortex lesions.

3. **Diplopia**

    Double vision implies a position misalignment between the two eyes. If diplopia persists when one eye is covered, the etiology is likely an ophthalmologic condition such as uncorrected refractive error, dislocated lens, or keratoconus. Factitious disorder is also in the differential, but it is a diagnosis of exclusion. For true binocular diplopia, the lesion in emergency settings is often in the brain stem or involving cranial nerve (CN) 3, CN 4, or CN 6. The most common conditions affecting the brain stem are *stroke* and *MS*, although *brain stem tumors* may rarely present with diplopia. Most often, with such entities the diplopia

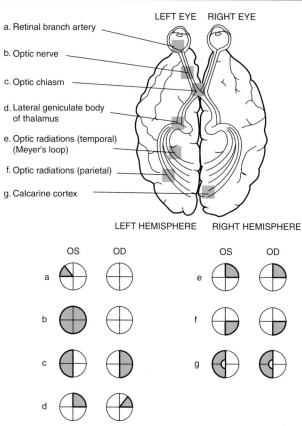

FIG. 12.1 Visual field cuts produced by lesions at different points along the visual pathway. *a.* Monocular segmentanopia produced by a branch retinal artery occlusion in the left eye. *b.* Monocular blindness produced by a lesion in the left optic nerve. *c.* Bitemporal hemianopia produced by a mass lesion at the optic chiasm. *d.* Right segmentanopia produced by a lesion in the lateral geniculate body of the left thalamus. *e.* Right upper quadrantanopia produced by a lesion in the left temporal optic radiation (Meyer loop). *f.* Right lower quadrantanopia produced by a lesion in the left parietal optic radiation. *g.* Left homonymous hemianopia produced by a lesion in the calcarine cortex of the right occipital lobe. Note that macular vision is sometimes spared because of middle cerebral artery collateral blood flow to the occipital pole. *L*, left; *OD*, Oculus dexter; *OS*, oculus sinister; *R*, right.

TABLE 12.2	Unusual Visual Syndromes Associated With Occipital Cortex Lesions	
Syndrome	**Localization**	**Description**
Anton syndrome	Bilateral calcarine	Bilateral loss of vision in which the patient denies blindness
Balint syndrome	Bilateral occipital	Simultanagnosia, optic parietal ataxia, and ocular apraxia
Charles Bonnet syndrome	Unilateral or bilateral calcarine, severe vision loss	Visual hallucinations in the absence of delirium and in the presence of vision loss
Dyschromatopsia	Lingual gyrus	Abnormal color perception contralateral to lesion
Palinopsia	Incomplete injury or recovery in parietal cortex	Visual persistence of afterimages
Prosopagnosia	Right or bilateral lingual gyrus	Inability to recognize faces

will be accompanied by other brain stem symptoms. Ocular motor cranial nerves may be affected in isolation by microvascular ischemia. A *berry aneurysm* of the posterior communicating artery may produce diplopia by stretching CN 3 as it passes over the artery on its way forward toward the cavernous sinus. Invasive or metastatic *tumor in the cavernous sinus region, meningitis, and temporal arteritis* may cause ocular motor disturbances. Unilateral or bilateral CN 6 palsies can be a false localizing sign of *increased intracranial pressure* (see Chapter 13). *Hyperthyroidism* may cause diplopia by mechanical limitation of infiltrated, fibrotic ocular muscles. Weakness of the extraocular muscles because of *myasthenia gravis* must be considered in the differential diagnosis of diplopia, particularly if the symptoms fluctuate or appear with fatigue.

Diagnoses for which immediate, specific therapy may arrest loss or restore vision are the following:

- CRAO
- Intracranial hypertension with severe papilledema
- Pituitary adenoma with or without apoplexy
- Acute glaucoma

Diagnoses for which urgent management may prevent further vision loss, stroke, or major morbidity/mortality are the following:

- TMVL with carotid stenosis
- Retrobulbar mass lesion (aneurysm or tumor)

- Ischemic optic neuropathy, TMVL, or diplopia from temporal arteritis
- CN 3 palsy from a posterior communicating artery aneurysm

MAJOR THREAT TO LIFE

Acute visual loss in the absence of other neurologic signs is rarely life-threatening. Visual emergencies with the greatest threat to life include pituitary apoplexy and CN 3 palsy from a posterior communicating artery aneurysm.

BEDSIDE

Quick-Look Test

1. *Are there any signs of trauma?*
2. *Is the patient in any pain or discomfort?*
3. *Is one eye affected or are both?*

Selective History and Chart Review

Some of the questions asked in the initial telephone interview should be discussed with the patient.

1. **Is one eye affected or both?**

    It may be difficult for a patient to distinguish between hemianopia visual field loss and monocular vision loss. A patient will often refer to "the left eye" as being defective when in fact the left hemifield is affected. Ask if the symptoms resolve if "the bad eye" is covered.

2. **When and how did the visual disturbance begin?**

    Ask the patient to describe the onset of the symptoms, with particular reference to the location and pattern of the visual disturbance. An obscuration that moves across the visual field "like a shade coming down" is a common description of a retinal arterial occlusion. An altitudinal defect is common with the nonarteritic form of AION. An expanding blind spot or episodes of vision loss lasting only a couple of seconds may suggest worsening papilledema. Slowly marching lights, particularly the jagged-edged "scintillating scotomata," is a common description of migraine, whether or not it is followed by headache. Sudden loss of vision over minutes suggests a vascular cause. Progression over hours to days may suggest ischemic optic neuropathy, demyelination, mass lesion, or papilledema.

3. **Is there pain?**

    Headache is common in temporal arteritis, intracranial hypertension, and migraine. Masticatory claudication and other myalgias may be a tip-off for temporal arteritis. Pain with eye movement is the rule for the inflammatory optic neuritis of MS, but pain is usually absent with retinal embolism and ischemic optic neuropathy. The exception is in carotid artery dissection, which may cause pain in the side of the head or jaw, with radiation into the orbit.

4. **Are there any associated neurologic symptoms?**

Dysarthria, vertigo, nausea, vomiting, and ataxia suggest stroke or mass lesion in the posterior fossa. Urinary incontinence, ataxia, diplopia, and patchy weakness or sensory loss can be other presenting symptoms of MS. Pulsatile tinnitus may suggest raised intracranial pressure.

Selective Physical Examination
General Physical Examination

- **Vital signs:**

  Fever may be a feature of temporal arteritis. Cardiac arrhythmia and hypertension are risk factors for cerebrovascular disease.

- **HEENT:**

  Palpate the temporal arteries just anterior and superior to the ear and along the side of the head. Exquisite tenderness strongly suggests temporal arteritis. Listen for *carotid bruits*.

- **Eye examination:**

  Check for *proptosis* by viewing the orbits from above. A retrobulbar mass lesion may cause the eye to protrude. Gentle palpation of the globe may disclose more resistance to posterior motion. The high pressure of glaucoma may also be detected, if present.

Neurologic Examination

- **Mental status**

  Aphasia or hemineglect may rarely accompany a disruption of optic radiations through the parietal lobe.

- **Cranial nerves**

  Check the following:

  1. **Visual acuity.** Has the patient read the smallest line on a near card. If the patient is older than 50 and does not have reading glasses with them, punch holes in an index card or piece of paper with a pin and have the patient read the chart through the holes. Determination of the patient's best corrected visual acuity in each eye separately is critical.

  2. **Pupillary reactivity.** Examine each pupil's direct and consensual response to light. Use low ambient light and a bright flashlight for the stimulus. A relative or absolute *afferent pupillary defect (APD)* may be detected by swinging the flashlight from one eye to the other. If the pupil enlarges when the flashlight swings to that eye, an APD *(Marcus Gunn pupil)* is present and pathology is suspected in the optic nerve.

3. **Visual fields.** Test visual fields by having the patient visually fix on your nose and by holding your hands in two of the four visual quadrants at an arm's length from the patient. Move a finger or briefly display a number of fingers on one or both hands. Test all four quadrants. More subtle visual field loss may be tested by comparing the brightness of a small red object in each quadrant. Red desaturation may occur without frank blindness. Be sure to check macular vision in the central 6 degrees of vision. Figure 12.1 illustrates the visual field defects expected with lesions at various points along the visual pathway.

4. **Fundoscopic examination.** This can reveal a specific pathology, although an examination adequate to make a definitive diagnosis may require pharmacologic dilation of the pupil. Table 12.3 lists the fundoscopic features of the most important diagnoses of monocular vision loss. *Hollenhorst (cholesterol) plaques* in retinal arteries are a sign of cholesterol emboli from atherosclerotic plaque in the aortic arch or carotid arteries (Table 12.3).

TABLE 12.3	Fundoscopic Features of Some Neuroophthalmologic Entities
Diagnosis	**Fundoscopic Appearance**
Central retinal artery occlusion	White, edematous, ground-glass retina "boxcar segmentation" (clumped red blood cells) in retinal veins (<1 h)
	Macular cherry-red spot (hours to days)
Branch retinal artery occlusion	Embolic material (bright calcium flecks or lipid yellow Hollenhorst plaques) at arterial branch points
	Arcuate band of retinal infarction (whitened retina)
Ischemic optic neuropathy	Disc head edema acutely, often in the superior or inferior half only
Papilledema	Swollen optic discs with obscuration of disc margins and vasculature
	Superficial flame hemorrhages
Glaucoma	Optic disc cupping
Optic neuritis	Normal optic disc or mild disc edema acutely
Idiopathic intracranial hypertension	Papilledema
Foster Kennedy syndrome	Optic atrophy ipsilateral to a retrobulbar mass
	Papilledema in contralateral eye caused by increased intracranial pressure

5. Check **ocular motility** with the following steps:
   A. **Have the patient follow your finger through horizontal and vertical range of motion.** Note impaired eye movement range if it occurs. Simple observation of the eye movements may be sufficient to diagnose a CN 3 or CN 6 lesion.
   B. **Latent or subtle eye misalignment may be revealed by the cover–uncover test.** Ask the patient to fix on one point such as your finger. Cover one eye, then uncover it. Repeat with the other eye. If the covered eye shifts when it is uncovered, there is an ocular misalignment. Although a positive cover–uncover test may suggest brain stem or cranial nerve pathology, benign congenital eye misalignments may cause a positive test.
   C. **Evaluate subtle ocular misalignments using a Maddox rod.** If there is preexisting amblyopia or if the patient is suppressing one eye's image, it may be difficult to identify diplopia without isolating different images between the two eyes. To check for horizontal diplopia, have the patient place the Maddox rod, with the slats oriented horizontally in front of the right eye (by convention), and then have the patient fixate on a point light source with both eyes. Two images should be seen: a vertical red line will be seen by the right eye and a point of light by the left eye. If the gaze is conjugate, then light should bisect the red line. As you move the light laterally, the light and line will move farther apart if there is a paresis of lateral gaze in one eye. This occurs as the image is projected onto the retina, away from the macula in the affected eye. Fig. 12.2 diagrams the use of the Maddox rod. The same procedure can be used to check for a vertical ocular misalignment by orienting the slats of the Maddox rod vertically (making the visualized red line horizontal) and moving the light up or down. Impairment of abduction may indicate CN 6 or lateral rectus palsy. Impairment of adduction may indicate CN 3 or medial rectus palsy. If adduction palsy is accompanied by abduction nystagmus in the opposite eye, then this is likely an *internuclear ophthalmoplegia*, suggesting MS in a younger patient or a paramedian midbrain infarct in an older person. *Nystagmus* is discussed in Chapter 14.

- **Coordination and gait**
  Ataxia or dysdiadochokinesis may be a sign of MS or may suggest posterior circulation infarction affecting the cerebellum and the occipital cortex.

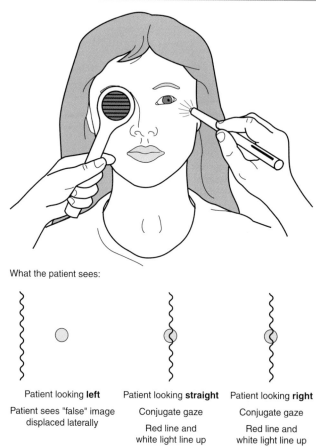

What the patient sees:

Patient looking **left**	Patient looking **straight**	Patient looking **right**
Patient sees "false" image displaced laterally	Conjugate gaze	Conjugate gaze
	Red line and white light line up	Red line and white light line up

FIG. 12.2 Use of the Maddox rod in a patient with a right cranial nerve (CN) 3 palsy. Patient sees the red line to the left of the white light on left gaze. This occurs because the red line projects farther laterally onto the retina of the abnormal eye, giving a false image that appears displaced laterally. The gaze is conjugate on primary gaze and on rightward gaze. Right CN 3 palsy would be confirmed by holding the Maddox rod so that the red line is oriented horizontally and asking the patient to look upward. The red line would then appear above the white light.

- **Sensation**

  Unilateral sensory loss may accompany visual field cuts produced by lesions in the thalamus or parietal lobe.

- **Reflexes**

  Asymmetry may be a subtle sign of brain injury.

MANAGEMENT

Order the following blood tests:

1. Erythrocyte sedimentation rate (ESR) and C-reactive protein (CRP) (when temporal arteritis is suspected)
2. Complete blood count (CBC) with platelet count
3. Prothrombin time (PT)/international normalized ratio (INR) and partial thromboplastin time (PTT)
4. Chemistry panel including glucose and cholesterol levels

If there is monocular vision loss or any suspicion of injury to the eye, have someone call for an ophthalmologic consultation to follow your assessment.

1. **Central retinal artery occlusion (CRAO)**

   No current treatment intervention has been shown in randomized trials to improve visual outcome compared with the natural history of CRAO, thus the most critical management should be focused on secondary prevention of additional vascular events.

   Efforts have been made to focus hyperacute intervention on reperfusion or dislodgment of the embolic particle. Data are lacking on the time window for reperfusion, and restoration of complete vision is unlikely. Permanent retinal ischemia is theoretically preventable only within the first 120 minutes after the occlusive event. Reversal of blindness has been reported up to 12 hours after embolus. Local intraarterial thrombolysis with tissue plasminogen activator (tPA) may be possible within 6 to 12 hours of vision loss, but consideration must be given to complication risk. At longer windows of treatment up to 20 hours after onset, intraarterial (IA) tPA did not demonstrate benefit over standard therapy in a large randomized trial. Treatment using intravenous (IV) tPA within less than 3 to 6 hours may be beneficial, although further studies are needed.

   Although randomized trials have not demonstrated reliable benefit, a classic therapeutic intervention performed to dislodge the embolus has included ocular massage (laying the patient flat and intermittently, pressing firmly on the globe for 10–20 minutes). Anterior chamber paracentesis has also not demonstrated reliable benefit in randomized trials.

   CRAO should raise suspicion for concurrent cerebral or myocardial infarctions, and it requires a search for an embolic source. Obtain brain magnetic resonance imaging (MRI) to evaluate for cerebral stroke because this is seen in 24% of patients with acute retinal ischemia, even without other neurologic symptoms. Search for a cardioembolic source with an MR angiography (MRA) of the head and neck (carotids, aortic arch), an echocardiogram and cardiology consultation, and hypercoagulable laboratory tests in the young, and use cardiac monitoring including electrocardiogram and blood pressure. Duplex Doppler ultrasonography of the carotid arteries can be performed urgently when MRA is not immediately available. If a cardioembolic source is known, **IV heparin at 800 U/h (no bolus), with a PTT target of 1.5 to 2.0 times the control value,** may be given as a bridge to oral anticoagulation, provided there are no contraindications to anticoagulation therapy. Long-term anticoagulation with warfarin (Coumadin) is indicated if a cardioembolic source such as atrial fibrillation or an intracardiac thrombus is identified or if the patient has a hypercoagulable state such as anticardiolipin antibody syndrome. **Patients with ipsilateral carotid stenosis greater than 70% should be referred for carotid endarterectomy or carotid angioplasty** and stenting to reduce the risk of cerebral infarction.

2. **Arteritic ischemic optic neuropathy**

Identifying temporal arteritis is of utmost importance. Because the prognosis for recovery of vision is less than 15% for the first eye, and because contralateral blindness is likely to occur, early recognition is important. Realistically, if visual loss is the presenting symptom, then therapy is aimed at preventing involvement of the contralateral eye. Anorexia, fever, myalgias, and jaw claudication accompanying visual loss and headache in a patient over 65 years of age strongly suggest the diagnosis clinically. Less typical presentations are possible. ESR, CRP, and fibrinogen levels are usually markedly elevated. For acute visual loss the treatment of choice is **IV methylprednisolone 1 g per day** for three days **followed by a very slow oral prednisone taper (begin with 1 mg/kg).** Unilateral temporal artery biopsy on the affected side should be arranged within a week. When there is visual loss steroid therapy should never be delayed pending the results of a biopsy. Corticosteroids generally have to be continued for 1 to 2 years. The ESR and CRP can be used as markers of disease activity.

3. **TMVL**

Patients with painless TMVL, particularly those with risk factors for cerebrovascular disease, should be evaluated emergently for cardioembolic sources and risk of stroke. TMVL is a classic warning sign for high-grade carotid stenosis. As in CRAO, the patient should be referred for duplex Doppler ultrasonography, echocardiography, and MRI/MRA of the head and neck. Maintaining the patient on an antiplatelet agent when a cardioembolic source is not found is recommended, along with vascular risk factor control. In the presence of a high-grade carotid stenosis, antiplatelet treatment while awaiting imminent endarterectomy will reduce the risk of stroke or recurrent transient ischemic attack (TIA) (see Chapter 24). Most interventional neuroradiologists favor a combination of 81 mg ASA (Aspirin) and 75 mg clopidogrel in preparation for carotid stenting.

4. **Retrobulbar mass lesion**

In a patient with a suspected retroorbital mass, high-quality imaging is the key to accurate diagnosis. *MRI orbits with fat suppression and with gadolinium contrast enhancement* will help define soft-tissue masses. *Computed tomography (CT) scan with thin cuts through the orbits* can help define any bony erosion. Appropriate *surgical referral* to an ophthalmologist or neurosurgeon should be made.

5. **Inflammatory optic neuritis**

Optic neuritis is the presenting symptom for MS in approximately 15% of patients, and it occurs at some point in the course of the disease in approximately 50% of patients. Optional treatment of optic neuritis is **IV methylprednisolone 1 g for 3 days, but it may be longer if additional new MS-related focal deficits co-occur, or if MRI of the neuraxis with gadolinium shows additional areas of enhancement.** Steroid treatment does not improve visual outcome over the natural history of optic neuritis. IV steroids are sometimes followed by a tapering dose of oral prednisone. Immunomodulatory therapies may be indicated, but they are generally not started in the emergent setting (see Chapter 21). **Oral prednisone as a first-line treatment for acute optic neuritis is associated with a higher risk of recurrent optic neuritis and should not be used.**

6. **Idiopathic intracranial hypertension (IIH)**

Prior to diagnosis of IIH, patients should have an MRI and MR venography (MRV) to evaluate for cerebral mass lesions, venous sinus thrombosis, and transverse sinus narrowing. A lumbar puncture performed in the lateral decubitus position will give an accurate opening pressure (expected to be 25 cm H_2O or higher in IIH) with normal composition cerebrospinal fluid (CSF).

Visual loss is the most significant and dreaded complication of IIH. Papilledema may occur with or without decreased acuity, but once visual loss begins, urgent therapy is imperative to prevent progression to blindness. Visual disturbance usually begins with an expanding blind spot or with nasal constriction of the peripheral fields. *Formal visual field testing is essential in patients with papilledema, because confrontation visual field tests may not detect vision loss.* For mild visual loss, give **acetazolamide 500 mg PO two times a day, and this may be increased by 250 mg weekly up to 4 g per day to achieve efficacy.** For severe visual loss, the addition of **methylprednisolone 250 mg IV four times a day** as a temporizing measure until surgical intervention is available may be vision saving. For patients whose visual loss is unresponsive to or progressive despite medical therapy, consult an ophthalmologist for *optic nerve sheath fenestration or a neurosurgeon for ventriculoperitoneal shunting.* Periodic lumbar punctures may be a good treatment option for a pregnant patient.

Increased Intracranial Pressure

Increased intracranial pressure (ICP) is not a symptom; rather, intracranial hypertension is a pathologic state common to a variety of serious neurologic illnesses (Table 13.1). All conditions that result in increased ICP are characterized by an increase in intracranial volume. Accordingly, all therapies for ICP (hyperventilation, mannitol, etc.) are directed toward reducing intracranial volume.

Normal ICP is less than 20 cm H_2O, or 15 mm Hg. Because elevations beyond these levels can rapidly lead to brain damage and death, prompt recognition and treatment are essential. This chapter will be most useful in cases in which the pathology is known, and increased ICP is the suspected cause of clinical deterioration.

PHONE CALL

Questions
1. **What is the patient's underlying neurologic problem?**
2. **Why is increased ICP suspected?**
3. **What is the patient's current level of consciousness?**

BEDSIDE

Quick-Look Test
Does the patient have clinical signs of increased ICP?

Increased ICP should be suspected in patients with known or suspected intracranial pathology (e.g., stroke, trauma, neoplasm) who exhibit the following symptoms and signs.

Signs that are almost always present:
- Depressed level of consciousness (lethargy, stupor, coma)
- Hypertension, with or without bradycardia

TABLE 13.1	Conditions Associated With Increased ICP

Intracranial Mass Lesions
Subdural hematoma
Epidural hematoma
Intracerebral hemorrhage
Brain tumor
Cerebral abscess

Increased CSF Volume (or Resistance to Outflow)
Hydrocephalus
Benign intracranial hypertension (pseudotumor cerebri)

Increased Brain Volume (Cytotoxic Cerebral Edema)
Cerebral infarction
Global hypoxia-ischemia
Reye syndrome
Acute hyponatremia

Increased Brain and Blood Volume (Vasogenic Cerebral Edema)
Head trauma
Meningitis
Encephalitis
Lead encephalopathy
Eclampsia
Hypertensive encephalopathy
Dural sinus thrombosis
Subarachnoid Hemorrhage

CSF, Cerebrospinal fluid; *ICP,* intracranial pressure.

Symptoms and signs that are sometimes present:
- Headache
- Vomiting
- Papilledema
- Cranial nerve (CN) 6 palsies

Remember, however, that these signs may be nonspecific. For this reason, the only way to confirm the diagnosis and properly treat increased ICP is to measure it.

Does the patient have clinical signs of herniation?

Clinical signs of herniation, listed here, result from *brain stem compression:*
- Loss of pupillary reactivity
- Impairment of eye movements
- Hyperventilation
- Motor posturing (flexion or extension)

When ICP is differentially increased across the tentorium (as is usually the case with hemispheric mass lesions), pressure gradients lead to downward displacement of brain tissue into the posterior fossa. Herniation is often rapidly fatal but can be reversed in some cases by treatments that reduce intracranial volume and ICP.

BOX 13.1	Emergency Treatment for Elevated Intracranial Pressure in an Unmonitored Patient

1. Elevate head of bed 30–45 degrees
2. Intubate and hyperventilate (target Pco_2 is 28–32 mm Hg)
3. Insert a Foley catheter
4. Administer mannitol (20%) 1 to 1.5 g/kg IV rapid infusion
5. Administer normal saline (0.9%) at 100 mL/h (avoid hypotonic fluids)
6. Consult the neurosurgery service

IV, Intravenous; *Pco_2*, partial pressure of carbon dioxide.

MANAGEMENT I

Emergency Measures for Reduction of Intracranial Pressure

If the clinical signs of potentially increased ICP are identified in a comatose patient, the emergency measures listed in Box 13.1 can "buy time" prior to computed tomography (CT) scan and a definitive neurosurgical procedure (craniotomy, ventriculostomy, or placement of an ICP monitor).

Placement of an Intracranial Pressure Monitor

Most clinicians would not treat a patient with suspected high blood pressure (BP) without measuring it. However, empirical therapy for increased ICP (i.e., repeated doses of mannitol) without monitoring is used all the time to the great disadvantage of the patient. This approach is unsatisfactory because most ICP treatments are effective for a short time only, lose their efficacy with prolonged use, and have side effects. Optimally, therapy should be given when ICP is high and should be withheld when it is normal. Only the use of an ICP monitor can make this possible.

Indications for ICP monitoring (all three conditions should be met):
1. **The patient is in a coma (Glasgow Coma Scale score of <8).**
2. **Brain imaging shows intracranial mass effect or global brain edema.**
3. **The prognosis is such that aggressive treatment in the intensive care unit (ICU) is indicated.**

Intracranial Pressure Monitors

If the decision has been made to treat the patient for suspected ICP, and surgical reduction of intracranial volume (i.e., ventriculostomy, craniotomy) is not feasible, an ICP monitor should be placed. There are two main types of monitors, shown in Fig. 13.1.

1. **Ventricular catheter**
   Once inserted, a ventricular catheter is connected to both a pressure transducer and an external drainage system via a

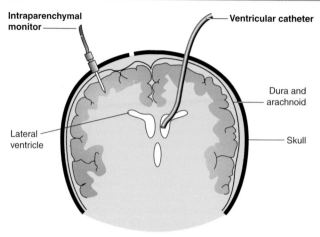

FIG. 13.1 ICP monitoring devices.

three-way stopcock. The major advantage to ventricular catheters is that they allow treatment of increased ICP via drainage of
cerebrospinal fluid (CSF). The main disadvantage is the high
infection rate (10%–20%), which increases dramatically after
5 days.

2. **Intraparenchymal probe (Camino, Codman, Raumedic)**
   These devices are easy to insert and very accurate, and the
   infection rate is exceedingly low (approximately 1%).

ELEVATOR THOUGHTS

What are the physiologic principles of ICP?
   If you are caring for a patient with increased ICP, a firm understanding of intracranial physiology is essential.

Intracranial Anatomy

There are three principal components of volume within the cranium of the normal adult: brain (1400 mL), blood (150 mL),
and CSF (150 mL). CSF is produced by the choroid plexus within
the ventricles at a rate of approximately 20 mL/h, resulting in the
formation of almost 500 mL/day. Normal ICP ranges from 50 to
200 mm H_2O (4–15 mm Hg). CSF is reabsorbed across the convexity of the meninges into the venous circulation via arachnoid gran-
ulations. These pathways normally offer little resistance to CSF

outflow. For this reason, jugular venous pressure is normally the principal determinant of ICP.

Intracranial Compliance

Because the cranial vault is a rigid, fixed container, any increase in intracranial volume can lead to increased ICP. In clinical practice, the most common mechanisms of increased intracranial volume are **extrinsic mass lesions, hydrocephalus, and cerebral edema (brain swelling)**. Initially, as volume is added to the intracranial space, increases in pressure are minimal because of the highly compliant nature of the intracranial contents; as intracranial volume increases, CSF is displaced through the foramen magnum into the paraspinal space, and blood is displaced from compressed brain tissue. When these mechanisms are exhausted, however, intracranial compliance decreases, and further increases in intracranial volume lead to dramatic elevations of ICP (Fig. 13.2).

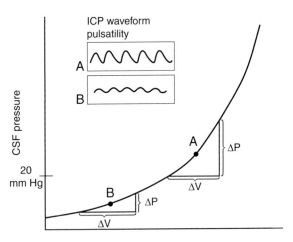

FIG. 13.2 Intracranial pressure (ICP)-volume curve. At low pressures *(B)* the intracranial compartment is compliant, meaning that large increases in volume (ΔV) lead to small increments in pressure (ΔP). At higher pressures *(A)* the intracranial space becomes less compliant. As a result, the amplitude and pulsatility of the arterial reflection in the ICP waveform increases *(inset)*. CSF, Cerebrospinal fluid.

Cerebral Perfusion Pressure

Cerebral perfusion pressure (CPP) is routinely monitored in conjunction with the ICP because it is an important determinant of cerebral blood flow (CBF). CPP is defined by the equation

$$CPP = MABP(mean\ arterial\ blood\ pressure) - ICP$$

When autoregulation is intact, CBF is maintained at a constant level across a wide range of CPPs (50–150 mm Hg). However, in injured brain with impaired autoregulation, CBF approximates a straight-line relationship with CPP; that is, reductions of CBF are more severe at any given level of reduced CPP (Fig. 13.3). *CPP should be closely regulated within 60 to 100 mm Hg in patients with increased ICP* because reductions below this level can lead to secondary hypoxic-ischemic damage and trigger ICP plateau waves, whereas excessive increases can lead to "breakthrough" hyperperfusion and aggravation of cerebral edema.

Intracranial Pressure Waveforms

The normal ICP waveform (see Fig. 13.2) reflects a transient surge in cerebral blood volume that occurs with each heartbeat. As ICP rises and intracranial compliance decreases, the amplitude of the ICP waveform increases, and superimposed pathologic ICP elevations can occur. Two types of pathologic ICP waves have been described (Fig. 13.4):

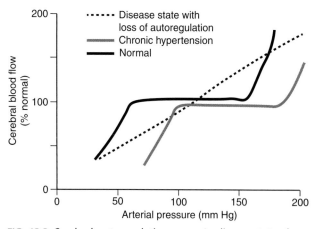

FIG. 13.3 Cerebral autoregulation curve. In disease states (e.g., vasospasm or ischemia), cerebral blood flow becomes pressure passive *(dotted line)*. With chronic hypertension, the autoregulatory curve shifts to the right.

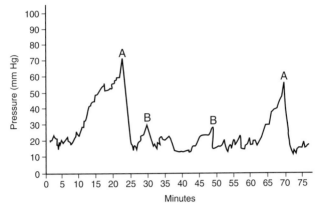

FIG. 13.4 Pathologic intracranial pressure elevations. *A* = Lundberg A (plateau) waves; *B* = Lundberg B waves. (Redrawn from Chestnut RM, Marshall LF. Treatment of abnormal intracranial pressure. *Neurosurg Clin North Am.* 1991;2:267–284.)

1. **Lundberg A waves (plateau waves):** Plateau waves are dangerous elevations of ICP; they can reach levels of 20 to 80 mm Hg and generally last more than 10 minutes. When severe, they are associated with reduced CPP (less than 60 mm Hg) and CBF, leading to global hypoxic-ischemic injury.

2. **Lundberg B waves:** These waves are of lesser amplitude (10–20 mm Hg) and duration (1–5 minutes) than plateau waves and thus are less dangerous. Clinically, they are a useful marker of abnormal autoregulation and reduced intracranial compliance.

MANAGEMENT II

General Measures for Treating Patients with Increased Intracranial Pressure

1. **Elevate head of bed by 30 to 45 degrees and maintain a straight head position.**

   Head elevation reduces ICP by reducing jugular venous pressure and by enhancing venous outflow. Sharp head angulation should be avoided because it may cause jugular venous compression, increased venous backpressure, and increased ICP.

2. **Prevent seizures.**

   Seizures can lead to profound elevations of CBF, intracranial blood volume, and ICP, even in patients who are paralyzed.

Levetiracetam (500–2000 mg intravenously [IV] twice a day) is the preferred agent for seizure prophylaxis.

3. **Treat fever aggressively.**

Fever can exacerbate ICP, and it lowers the threshold for neuronal death. Treatment with **acetaminophen (650 mg every 4 hours), indomethacin (25 mg every 6 hours),** or a **cooling blanket** can be effective.

Steps for Treating an "Intracranial Pressure Crisis" in an Intubated, Monitored Patient

Proper treatment of increased ICP requires an organized, stepwise approach (Box 13.2). Brief elevations of ICP (lasting only 1–5 minutes) occur frequently with suctioning, coughing, and repositioning and do not require aggressive treatment. **In general, the following measures should be instituted only when the ICP is elevated above 20 mm Hg for a period of 10 or more minutes.**

TIER I INTERVENTIONS: WHAT TO DO FIRST

These are the first measures to take when called to the bedside for ICP elevation. In many patients at baseline a ventricular drain has been placed and is open, the patient is sedated, and orders for CPP parameters are written at baseline.

Step 1. **Removal of intracranial mass or drainage of CSF**

Remember that reduction of intracranial volume is the only definitive treatment for increased ICP. In patients with

BOX 13.2	Stepwise Treatment Protocol for Elevated Intracranial Pressure in a Monitored Patient (Intracranial Pressure > 20 mm Hg for >10 Minutes)

Tier 1
- ✓ Emergent craniotomy or ventriculostomy
- ✓ Sedate patient to attain a quiet, motionless state
- ✓ Optimize cerebral perfusion pressure with vasopressors to maintain >60 mm Hg, or with blood pressure-lowering agents maintain <100 mm Hg

Tier 2
- ✓ Bolus osmotherapy with mannitol or hypertonic saline
- ✓ Hyperventilate to maintain P_{CO_2} between 28 and 32 mm Hg
- ✓ Paralyze with neuromuscular blocking agents

Tier 3
- ✓ Pentobarbital infusion
- ✓ Hypothermia to 32°C–34°C
- ✓ Decompressive craniectomy

acute mass lesions, obstructive hydrocephalus, or both, physical decompression is the first step in gaining control of ICP. If a ventricular catheter is in place, make sure that it is not occluded by checking for a waveform and for waveform "fling" when the manipulating the line. If the drain is clamped for ICP monitoring, then the system should be opened to drainage, and 5 to 10 mL of CSF should be removed.

Step 2. **Sedation and paralysis**

In patients with reduced intracranial compliance, physical agitation or fighting the ventilator can lead to elevated ICP because of increased intrathoracic, jugular venous, and arterial pressures. *Before further measures are instituted, agitated patients with increased ICP should be sedated to the point at which they are motionless and quiet.*

Note: IV sedatives cause apnea and hypotension and thus require intubation and intravascular BP monitoring. The following agents can be used:

- **Morphine IV** is an opioid with sedative-hypnotic and analgesic effects. The dose is **2 to 5 mg IV push (IVP) every hour.**
- **Fentanyl IV** (supplied as 50 µg/mL) is also an opioid and is 100 times more potent than morphine. For rapid control of agitation, give **25 to 100 µg IVP**. For sustained sedation, give **fentanyl IV infusion 4 mg/250 mL normal saline (NS).** Start at 5 mL/h (1.33 µg/min); the range is 8 to 23 mL/h (2–6 µg/min).
- **Propofol IV (10 mg/mL)** is a powerful sedative-hypnotic drug whose effect is more rapidly reversible than that of fentanyl. The typical maintenance dose is **5 to 50 µg/kg/min (0.3–3 mg/kg/h);** this translates into 2 to 20 mL/h for a 70-kg person.

Step 3. **CPP optimization**

If ICP remains elevated in a sedated patient, optimization of CPP should be attempted using vasoactive agents *before* mannitol and hyperventilation are administered.

- If CPP is >100 mm Hg and ICP is >20 mm Hg, then BP should be lowered. *However, CPP should not be allowed to fall to <60 mm Hg.* Agents for controlling hypertension include the following:
  1. **Labetalol IV (5 mg/mL)** is a combined alpha-1 and beta-1 blocker. For immediate control of BP, **push 20 to 80 mg every 10 to 20 minutes**. Once the desired BP is attained, start **200 mg/200 mL NS (1 mg/mL) at 2 mg/min (120 mL/h) and titrate.**

2. **Nicardipine IV** is a rapidly titratable calcium channel blocker. Start with **25 mg/250 mL NS at 50 mL/h (5 mg/hr) and titrate**.

- If CPP is <60 mm Hg and ICP is >20 mm Hg, then mean arterial pressure (MAP) and CPP should be elevated; this can lead to a reflex reduction of ICP by reducing the cerebral vasodilatation that occurs in response to inadequate perfusion. Pressor agents for raising CPP include

1. **Norepinephrine (4 mg/250 mL N5NS) infusion starting at a dose of 8 µg/min (30 mL/h),** adjusted to maintain desired target CPP (range 2–12 µg/min).

2. **Phenylephrine (10 mg/250 mL)** is a pure alpha agonist. Start at **15 mL/h (10 µg/min)** and titrate upward to a maximum of 200 µg/min.

Note that when ICP is measured via a ventricular drain, the pressure transducer for ICP and arterial BP should both be set at head level (i.e., level of the tragus), especially when the head is elevated. Measuring ICP at head level and BP at the level of the heart with the head up can lead to serious underestimation of ICP.

TIER II: NAVIGATING INTRACRANIAL PRESSURE CRISIS

ICP crisis refers to intracranial hypertension that is excessive (>30 mm Hg), prolonged (>30 minutes), or both.

Step 4. **Bolus osmotherapy**

In general there are two frequently used options for bolus osmotherapy: **20% mannitol** solution and **23.4% hypertonic saline.** Mannitol, an osmotic diuretic, is preferable when there is no central venous access, or in patients who are fluid overloaded or have congestive heart failure. Hypertonic saline volume expands and raises BP. It is preferred when patients are hypotensive or hypovolemic, but its administration requires central access.

Mannitol lowers ICP via its cerebral dehydrating effects. The effects of mannitol are biphasic. Rapid infusion immediately creates an osmotic gradient across the blood–brain barrier, resulting in movement of water from brain to the intravascular compartment. The result is decreased brain tissue volume and, hence, reduced ICP. The secondary effect of mannitol results from its action as an osmotic diuretic. As mannitol is cleared by the kidneys, it leads to free water clearance and increased serum osmolality. As a result, even after the mannitol is gone, an intracellular dehydrating effect is maintained as water flows down the osmotic gradient, from the intracellular to the extracellular space.

- **The initial dose of mannitol 20% solution is 1 to 1.5 g/kg, followed every 1 to 6 hours with doses of 0.25 to 1.5 g/kg, repeated as needed.** The effect on ICP is maximal when mannitol is given rapidly (over 10 minutes).
- The effect of mannitol on ICP begins in 10 to 20 minutes, reaches its peak between 20 and 40 minutes, and lasts for 3 to 6 hours.
- Adverse effects of mannitol therapy include exacerbation of congestive heart failure (because of the initial intravascular volume load), volume contraction (after prolonged use), hypokalemia, acute kidney injury (because of excessive hyperosmolality), and profound hyperosmolality (after prolonged use). Osmotic demyelination is a rare complication that can occur when osmolality is raised very quickly to very high levels.
- Patients treated repeatedly with mannitol require measurements of serum electrolytes and osmolality every 6 hours and careful measurement of intake and output. Volume lost through urine should be replaced with NS (0.9%) to avoid volume depletion.
- The *osmolar gap* is the difference between measured and calculated osmolality ($= 2$ Na + glucose/18 + blood urea nitrogen (BUN)/2.8). The osmolar gap should typically be about 10. Levels >20 indicate retention of mannitol, which is a sign of mannitol-induced acute kidney injury; in this case mannitol should be switched to hypertonic saline.

Hypertonic saline comes in a wide variety of concentrations, but the most commonly used concentration for acute ICP elevation is 23.4%. This solution comes in 30-mL vials or "bullets," and are slowly injected by hand via a central line over approximately 5 minutes. Care must be taken to not inject too quickly or a paradoxical drop in BP can result.

- **The dose of 23.4% saline is 0.5 to 2.0 mL/kg, repeat as needed**. To attain this dose, 2, 3, or 4 bullets can be "stacked" back to back over 20 to 30 minutes.
- The effect on ICP is very similar to that of 1 g/kg of mannitol, with a peak reduction in ICP in 20 to 40 minutes and a variable duration of effect ranging from 3 to 6 hours

- Adverse effects when given properly are mostly related to fluid overload or congestive heart failure when used repeatedly, especially in patients with reduced left ventricular function. Hypernatremia and hyperosmolality can occur after prolonged, repeated use.
- As with mannitol, patients receiving repeated doses of hypertonic saline should have close monitoring of sodium, osmolality, and fluid intake and output.

  Osmotherapy mythology is belief in systems or practices that simply are not true.

- *One common myth about bolus osmotherapy is that both mannitol and hypertonic saline stop working, or should not be used, once serum osmolality exceeds 320 mOsm/L.* This is simply not true; just see for yourself the next time you give one of these agents when ICP exceeds 20 mm Hg and the osmolality exceeds 320 mOsm/L. The ICP will go down, and the osmolality will simply go up further.
- A second common myth is that of the ICP *rebound effect.* This concept maintains that when the osmotherapy wears off, the ICP will rebound to an even higher level than it was at baseline. This does not happen; instead the therapy simply wears off and ICP rebounds to its baseline level.

Step 5. **Hyperventilation**

By acutely lowering the P_{CO_2} level to 28 to 32 mm Hg, *hyperventilation can lower ICP within minutes.* The alkalosis caused by hypocarbia leads to cerebral vasoconstriction, reduced cerebral blood volume, and decreased ICP.

- Hyperventilation is best accomplished by increasing the ventilatory rate (16–20 cycles/min) in mechanically ventilated patients, or by using bag-valve-mask ventilation in nonintubated patients.
- *The peak effect of hyperventilation on ICP is generally reached within 30 minutes.* Over the next 1 to 3 hours, the effect may gradually diminish as compensatory acid–base buffering mechanisms correct the alkalosis, but exceptions can occur.
- Once ICP is stabilized, hyperventilation should be tapered slowly over 6 to 12 hours, because abrupt cessation can lead to vasodilatation and rebound increases in ICP.

  Note: Beware that prolonged severe hyperventilation (P_{CO_2} less than 25 mm Hg) may actually exacerbate cerebral ischemia by causing excessive vasoconstriction.

Step 6. **Paralysis with a neuromuscular blocking agent**

After repeated doses of bolus osmotherapy and hyperventilation have been started, if ICP crisis persists, consideration should be given to starting an infusion of a neuromuscular blocking agent in a patient who is already deeply sedated. These agents lower ICP by reducing intrathoracic pressure, jugular and central venous pressure, and cerebral blood volume (primarily on the venous side). Two commonly used agents include:

- Rocuronium 0.5 to 1.0 mg/kg/hr via continuous infusion
- Vecuronium 50 to 70 µg/kg/hr via continuous infusion

TIER III: SALVAGE INTERVENTIONS

These three therapeutic options are sometimes used as a "last ditch" to try and save the life of a patient when ICP is refractory to all of the previously mentioned interventions. The problem is that all three also carry considerable risks.

Option 7. **Pentobarbital**

High-dose barbiturate therapy, given in doses equivalent to those inducing general anesthesia, can effectively lower ICP in many patients refractory to the steps outlined previously. The effect of pentobarbital is multifactorial but most likely stems from coupled decreases in cerebral metabolism, blood flow, and blood volume. In addition, pentobarbital causes profound hypotension and usually requires the use of vasopressors to maintain CPP at or higher than 60 mm Hg.

- **Pentobarbital typically requires a loading dose of 5 to 20 mg/kg, given in repeated 5-mg/kg boluses,** until a state of flaccid coma with preserved pupillary reactivity is attained. IV pressors (dopamine, phenylephrine) should be ready at the bedside to maintain BP and CPP.
- **Maintenance doses are usually 1 to 4 mg/kg/h (order as 500 mg/250 mL NS, starting at 35 mL/h).** Continuous or intermittent electroencephalography (EEG) monitoring should be used, with the infusion rate titrated to a burst–suppression pattern.
- If ICP is adequately controlled with pentobarbital, it is generally maintained for 24 to 48 hours. It can then be discontinued abruptly, with a washout period lasting from 24 to 96 hours.
- Complications include hypotension; immunosuppression; a rare "metabolic infusion syndrome"

characterized by lactic acidosis, vasodilatory shock, and renal failure; and severe critical illness neuromyopathy caused by prolonged immobilization in the majority of patients.

- Failure of ICP to respond to pentobarbital is an ominous sign. If ICP remains markedly elevated (higher than 30 mm Hg), then decompressive craniectomy (or withdrawal of life-sustaining therapy) should be considered.

Option 8. **Hypothermia**

Lowering body temperature to 33°C can reduce ICP elevations that are refractory to CPP optimization, osmotherapy, and hyperventilation, as an alternative to pentobarbital anesthesia. In general this technique should be applied by experienced intensivists. Advanced feedback-controlled technology to rapidly and precisely cool the patient, in the form of an adhesive surface cooling system or endovascular heat exchange catheter, is typically required. After cooling, the patient can be gradually rewarmed to 37°C at a rate of 0.20°C to 0.33°C per hour. An example of a critical care checklist for therapeutic temperature modulation (TTM) is shown in Table 5.5.

- Complications of hypothermia include shivering, immunosuppression, coagulopathy, cardiovascular depression, arrhythmias, hyperglycemia, ileus, and rebound hyperkalemia during rewarming.
- These complications are severe, and may explain why mortality is increased when cooling is started early in the course of ICP elevation after traumatic brain injury.

Option 9. **Decompressive craniectomy**

The ultimate step to take when confronted with medically refractory ICP is to decompress the cranial vault. Decompression of the cranium allows the brain to swell out of the skull defect, and it is the definitive intervention for severe ICP. In severe TBI patients who have suffered ICP > 25 mm Hg for 12 to 24 hours despite Tier I and II therapy, proceeding to craniectomy results in reduced mortality (approximately 25% versus 50%) compared with continued medical therapy including escalation to pentobarbital. Decompressive craniectomy should only be used as a salvage intervention, however. Another trial that randomized TBI patients to surgery at the very first sign of ICP elevation actually resulted in increased disability with no effect on mortality.

Dizziness and Vertigo

Dizziness and vertigo are among the most common neurologic complaints. The etiology of these conditions may range from the relatively benign, such as labyrinthitis, to the potentially serious, such as cardiac syncope or life-threatening cerebellar hemorrhage. *Vertigo* may be defined specifically as a sensation of movement, either of the environment or of the patient. A spinning sensation is most commonly described, but feelings of acceleration or other movement may also be reported. *Dizziness*, on the other hand, is a term that may be used to mean vertigo, but it also may mean light-headedness, fatigue, or a general sense of illness.

PHONE CALL

Questions

1. **Does the patient have a normal level of consciousness?**
   Vertigo followed by a decreased level of consciousness may be a sign of impending herniation, which is a neurologic emergency.
2. **When did the dizziness or vertigo begin?**
   In general, a more acute onset requires a greater urgency in making a diagnosis.
3. **What are the vital signs?**
   Rapid, slowed, or irregular heart rhythm may suggest cardiac syncope or cardioembolic stroke. Low blood pressure will cause dizziness. Fever may suggest infection. Tachypnea may be a sign of heart failure or an anxiety attack.

Orders

1. **Obtain a finger-stick glucose.**
2. **Obtain orthostatic blood pressure.**
3. **Obtain an electrocardiogram (ECG).**

Inform RN

"Will arrive at the bedside in…minutes."

ELEVATOR THOUGHTS

What is the differential diagnosis of dizziness and vertigo?

The most common causes of dizziness and vertigo are orthostatic hypotension, medication side effect, benign paroxysmal positional vertigo (BPPV), and labyrinthitis. A more complete differential diagnosis follows.

V   Vascular: brain stem stroke (most often pontine, brachium pontis, or cerebellar), cerebellar hemorrhage, arteriovenous malformation (rare), brain stem TIAs resulting from vertebrobasilar stenosis ("insufficiency") or embolism, vasodepressor syncope, hypotension, postural hypotension, cardiac arrhythmia

I   Infectious: viral labyrinthitis (including herpes zoster oticus = Ramsay Hunt syndrome), syphilis, viral or bacterial meningitis, otitis media with vestibular extension, Lyme disease involving the vestibular cranial nerve, viral cerebellitis (mostly in children)

T   Traumatic: head trauma with brain or vestibular injury, temporal bone fracture, postconcussion syndrome

A   Autoimmune: multiple sclerosis

M   Metabolic/toxic: diabetes with hypoglycemia, dehydration, drug toxicity (Table 14.1)

I   Idiopathic/iatrogenic: benign paroxysmal positional vertigo (BPPV), Meniere disease, migraine, vestibular neuralgia, superior semicircular canal dehiscence

N   Neoplastic: neurofibroma, schwannoma, meningioma of the acoustic nerve; brain stem glioma; posterior fossa metastasis, leptomeningeal carcinomatosis

S   Seizure/psychiatric: seizure, anxiety, panic attack

MAJOR THREAT TO LIFE

1. Cardiac arrhythmia
2. Cerebellar infarction or hemorrhage

BEDSIDE

Quick-Look Test

Is there hypotension or evidence of arrhythmia?
Is the patient awake and alert?

Lethargy may indicate a brain stem or cerebellar stroke with potential for herniation or progression to coma.

Selective History and Chart Review

1. **Is the dizziness lightheadedness or true vertigo?**

   Lightheadedness, a swimming sensation, faintness, or other similar symptoms, points to a systemic disorder such as cardiac syncope, postural hypotension, or systemic infection. True vertigo, on the other hand, suggests neurologic or ear dysfunction. However, both the patient and the physician may have trouble distinguishing between vertigo and lightheadedness. Associated symptoms, the time course (acute, subacute, or chronic; isolated or recurrent), triggers (head motion, arising), and the physical examination (associated neurologic symptoms) will help to distinguish peripheral causes of vertigo from central nervous system (CNS) causes and clarify the differential diagnosis.

2. **What is the time course of the symptoms?**

   As previously noted, an acute onset of vertigo may indicate posterior fossa stroke or hemorrhage or BPPV or labyrinthitis. Rapid onset of lightheadedness can occur with cardiac disease. A more gradual onset may suggest medication toxicity, infection, tumor, or demyelinating disease. If this is an episode in a series of recurrences, then migraine, Meniere disease, or BPPV may be the cause.

3. **Do the symptoms change with changes in head position?**

   Dizziness on standing may indicate orthostatic hypotension; vertigo specifically with head turning may be a sign of BPPV.

4. **Has the patient begun any new medications recently?**

   Table 14.1 shows common medications that cause vertigo. Dizziness without true vertigo is one of the most common side effects of medication. Refer to the *Physician's Desk Reference* for medications not listed in the table.

TABLE 14.1	Common Medications That Cause Vertigo and Dizziness[a]

Anticonvulsants: carbamazepine, phenytoin, primidone, ethosuximide, methsuximide
Antidepressants: nortriptyline and other tricyclic antidepressants
Antihypertensives: enalapril
Antihistamines: ranitidine, cimetidine
Antiarrhythmics: flecainide
Antibiotics: streptomycin, tobramycin, gentamicin
Analgesics: propoxyphene (Darvocet), naproxen, indomethacin
Neuroleptics: phenothiazines
Tranquilizers: diazepam, chlordiazepoxide, meprobamate
Aspirin
Digoxin

[a]Many medications have dizziness as a side effect; this is only a partial list.

5. **Are there any accompanying symptoms?**

Ask about symptoms specific to the brain stem, including diplopia, dysarthria, and ataxia. Hearing loss or tinnitus may localize the problem to the inner ear. Hearing loss can also accompany stoke in the territory of the anterior inferior cerebellar artery. If there is posterior neck or head pain, consider vertebral artery dissection and stroke.

Selective Physical Examination

General Physical Examination

Head, ears, eyes, nose, and throat (HEENT): Be sure to look into the external auditory canal for vesicles of herpes zoster. Unilateral hearing loss and tinnitus are usual signs of injury outside the brain stem.

Neurologic Examination

- **Mental status:** Ensure that the patient is awake, alert, and attentive. Decreased attentiveness may suggest drug toxicity or metabolic disarray. If there is vertigo with decreased alertness, see Chapter 5 for further management.
- **Cranial nerves:** Any cranial nerve abnormality such as diplopia, dysarthria, facial motor or sensory asymmetry, decreased gag response, or asymmetry of tongue protrusion in combination with dizziness or vertigo should be considered a sign of brain injury until it is proved otherwise.

Head impulse test: An abnormal head impulse test (or head thrust) is a reliable indicator of peripheral vestibular dysfunction. The patient is instructed to fixate on the examiner's nose and then the examiner rotates the patients head horizontally a small amount but quickly. A normal response is that the eyes remain fixated on the examiner's nose. In a peripheral vestibular deficit the eyes lag behind and a corrective saccade is needed to refixate. Remember that a normal response is seen in normal examination *or* a central lesion causing vertigo.

Look for Skew: This is a vertical separation of the eyes that usually indicates a central lesion and is easily evaluated by alternately covering each eye.

Look for Nystagmus: When vestibular input to the brain stem is disrupted (e.g., damage to the vestibular nerve or inner ear apparatus), the eyes will drift toward the affected side. Repeated corrective saccades result in jerk nystagmus, with the fast phase away from the lesion. The sensation of movement experienced with vertigo is the illusion of environmental drift because the eyes move through the slow phase of nystagmus in the other direction. Corrective saccades are suppressed by visual tracking systems so that there is a sensation of continued field shift in one direction. Oscillopsia (the illusion of the environment jumping or oscillating) is actually quite rare and most commonly seen after bilateral vestibular injury. Nystagmus subtypes are listed in Table 14.2. A common and crucial differential diagnosis that arises in almost every case of vertigo is whether the process is peripheral, and less alarming, or whether it represents a lesion in the brain stem or cerebellum. Certain characteristics of nystagmus can help identify the site of pathology (Table 14.3).

- Look for nystagmus in the primary gaze by having the patient fix on your finger. More subtle nystagmus can be seen by looking for oscillations of the fundus on indirect ophthalmoscopy, which eliminates fixation. Remember that the back of the eye is moving in the opposite direction from of the eye; therefore the nystagmus is in the opposite direction of what you see.
- Have the patient follow your finger through the full range of horizontal and vertical gaze. The hand should be kept at a distance of 2 to 3 feet to minimize convergence, which should be tested separately. Look for nystagmus in each field of gaze. Peripheral nystagmus always beats in the same direction and increases when looking away from the side of the lesion or toward the fast phase. Peripheral nystagmus also decreases with fixation.

Perform Provocative tests: these can be helpful in distinguishing peripheral from central injury.

- Nystagmus should be looked for with the patient in different positions, particularly if the patient notes a positional component to the vertigo. The Dix-Hallpike maneuver is essential in evaluating for BPPV (Fig. 14.1). Upbeat nystagmus with a rotational component after a latency of a few seconds, and a lessening of the magnitude of the response with subsequent trials, all suggest posterior canal BPPV. Horizontal nystagmus can be seen in the less common horizontal canal variant.
- Irrigating the ear on the side of an intact vestibular pathway (see Fig. 5.3) with cold water will result in nystagmus, with the fast component beating away from the stimulus. If the patient is comatose, cold water will induce the ipsiversive gaze with no contralateral corrective saccades. Be sure you view an intact tympanic membrane before attempting this test. Also, be warned that the stimulus may produce nausea in an awake patient.
- **Motor/sensory:** Evaluate for any focal deficit.
- **Cerebellar:** Evaluate for limb ataxia and gait ataxia. The patient must be walked.

TABLE 14.2	Subtypes of Nystagmus

Jerk Nystagmus

Gaze-evoked: Nystagmus at the extremes of gaze beating in the direction of gaze

Physiologic: Fine nystagmus, usually fatigues

Drug/medication: Often seen with sedatives and anticonvulsants

Brainstem/cerebellar lesions: May be sustained

Rebound nystagmus: After looking eccentrically for approximately 1 minute on return to primary gaze there is nystagmus beating in the other direction, associated with brainstem or cerebellar lesions

Brun's nystagmus: Slow large-amplitude nystagmus in one direction and rapid small-amplitude nystagmus in the other direction suggests a cerebellopontine angle lesion on the side of the slow, large-amplitude nystagmus

Horizontal Nystagmus

Peripheral nystagmus: Nystagmus only beats in one direction, away from the affected side, which obeys Alexander's law, usually mixed with torsion, and inhibited by fixation

Central nystagmus: Nystagmus may change directions, may be purely horizontal, does not obey Alexander's law, fixation does not inhibit

Periodic alternating nystagmus: Nystagmus alternating directions every 1–2 minutes, associated with lesions at the cervicomedullary junction or in the cerebellum

Dissociated nystagmus: Nystagmus differing between the eyes, seen with internuclear ophthalmoplegia or mimicked by myasthenia gravis

Downbeat nystagmus: Nystagmus usually increases on down and lateral gaze, seen with involvement of the dorsal medulla or the cerebellar flocculus or projections, associated with lesions at the cervicomedullary junction, medications (lithium, carbamazepine, phenytoin), alcohol, hypomagnesemia, thiamine deficiency, paraneoplastic syndromes, cerebellar degenerations, and others

Upbeat nystagmus: Associated with brain stem and cerebellar lesions, most commonly the medulla

Congenital nystagmus: Often a mixture of jerk and pendular nystagmus

Convergence-retraction nystagmus: Part of Parinaud dorsal midbain syndrome, convergence and retraction of the eyes

Positional nystagmus: Seen with specific head motions

Pendular Nystagmus

Acquired: Seen with brain stem and cerebellar lesions

Congenital: Often a mixture of jerk and pendular nystagmus

Spasmus Nutans: Infant onset, nystagmus is asymmetric and rapid, often associated with head nodding and head turning, usually resolves

See-Saw nystagmus: Opposite conjugate vertical and torsional movements, associated with mesencephalic or parasellar lesions

Oculopalatal myoclonus: Rhythmic 2- to 3-Hz movements seen late after lesion of Mollaret triangle

Oculomasticatory myorhythmia: Rhythmic movements of eye convergence and contraction of masticatory or other muscles, seen in 20% of patients with Whipple disease

TABLE 14.3 | Peripheral Versus Central Nystagmus

	Peripheral	Central
Appearance	Combined torsional, horizontal, and vertical Nystagmus beats away from the affected side	Often pure vertical, horizontal, or torsional, any trajectory
Fixation	Inhibits	No effect
Gaze	Obeys Alexander's law (nystagmus increases when looking toward the side of the fast phase)	May change direction, does not obey Alexander's law,

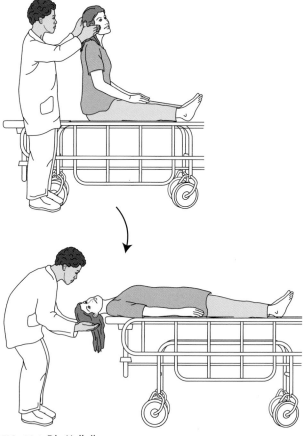

FIG. 14.1 Dix-Hallpike maneuver.

MANAGEMENT

1. **Identify and correct hypotension or cardiac arrhythmia**

2. **Rule out a posterior fossa mass lesion.**

   Because the consequences of missing a cerebellar hematoma or posterior fossa tumor can be serious, imaging should usually be obtained in first-time vertigo, particularly in the elderly, and certainly if there is any evidence of brain stem involvement. Noncontrast CT will identify hemorrhage but is poor at identifying smaller lesions and infarcts in the posterior fossa. Magnetic resonance imaging (MRI) is preferable.

3. **Correct any obvious metabolic disorder, or discontinue, taper, or substitute any toxic medication.**

4. **Identify a possible peripheral cause of vertigo.**

   Common peripheral causes of vertigo include labyrinthitis (usually viral), migraine, Meniere disease (recurrent attacks of severe vertigo, tinnitus, and hearing loss), and BPPV. On follow-up, an electronystagmogram and audiogram may be helpful in diagnosis. Symptomatic medications for peripheral vertigo commonly include antihistamines and benzodiazepines. First-line therapy is **meclizine (Antivert) 12.5 to 25 mg PO three times a day**.

5. **Treat BPPV with repositioning exercises.**

   BPPV results from loose particulate debris most often found in the posterior semicircular canal. Particular head positions or head movement may cause the particles to inappropriately move, stimulating the vestibular system, which results in vertigo. Posterior canal BPPV, the most common type, is best diagnosed by performing the Dix-Hallpike maneuver with complaints of vertigo and visualization of upbeating and torsional nystagmus when the affected side is down. It is best treated with the modified Epley maneuver, which attempts to reposition the particles (Fig. 14.2). Less common forms of BPPV involving the horizontal canal or rarely the anterior canal result in different types of nystagmus on positioning and are treated with different maneuvers. If the history and examination are typical for BPPV, then imaging is not usually needed.

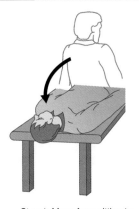

Step 1: Move from sitting to reclining position with the head extended 45 degrees over the end of the table, turned with the "bad" ear down (e.g., left)

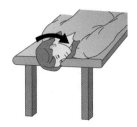

Step 2: Turn the head to the right slowly over 1 minute

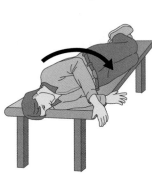

Step 3: Roll over onto the right side, with the head looking down at the floor

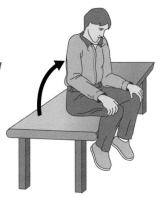

Step 4: Slowly return to sitting position with the chin tilted down

FIG. 14.2 Modified Epley maneuver.

Headache

Headache is one of the most common complaints presented to neurologists. This symptom can be caused by two broad categories of disorders. One group comprises the **primary headache disorders**, including migraine, tension-type headache, cluster headache, and other trigeminal autonomic cephalalgias (TACs). **Secondary headache disorders** include those attributed to trauma or injury to the head; vascular and nonvascular intracranial lesions; systemic diseases; or local diseases of the eye, sinuses, or nasopharynx. The goal of a headache consultation is to (1) identify red flags for secondary headaches and evaluate these possibilities in a timely manner; or (2) establish a primary headache diagnosis and initiate effective treatment.

PHONE CALL

Questions

1. **Does the headache reach full intensity instantly or gradually?**

   Sudden onset of severe headache is suggestive of subarachnoid hemorrhage, intracerebral hemorrhage, reversible cerebral vasoconstriction syndrome (RCVS), arterial dissection, or cerebral venous thrombosis. Primary headaches, such as headache associated with sexual activity, can occasionally have a "thunderclap" presentation, but the more ominous causes need to be excluded first, starting with subarachnoid hemorrhage.

2. **When did the headaches begin? Has there been a change in frequency, severity, or clinical features?**

   Headaches with a recent onset or with progressive worsening over time suggest a symptomatic etiology such as brain tumor, subdural hematoma, or brain abscess. A stable headache pattern over years is almost always indicative of a primary headache. Remember, having a primary headache such as migraine does not grant an individual immunity to developing tumors or infections. Worsening of a preexisting headache type without an identifiable trigger should raise concern over the development of a secondary headache.

TABLE 15.1	Protocol for the Emergency Room Treatment of Migraine

Mild-To-Moderate Migraine
Administer sumatriptan 6 mg SC or ketorolac 60 mg IM

Prolonged, Refractory, or Severe Migraine
1. IV hydration with NS for persistent vomiting
2. **Prochlorperazine** 10 mg IV, or **metoclopramide** 10 mg IV infused over 15 min; monitor for symptoms of akathisia and acute dystonia; treat with IV diphenhydramine 20–50 mg or midazolam 2 mg; if dopamine receptor antagonists are contraindicated, use **ondansetron** 8 mg IV
3. Ketorolac 30 mg IV infused over 10–15 min
4. If no response, administer **dihydroergotamine** 0.5 mg, infused over 30 min to avoid nausea, with a second dose of 0.5 mg over 30 min if well tolerated; it is contraindicated in patients with cardiovascular, cerebrovascular, and peripheral vascular disease and use of any triptan or ergot in the prior 24 h
5. Consider **magnesium sulfate** 1–2 g IV infused slowly to avoid burning at IV site; consider particularly for patients with migraine with aura; contraindicated with history of neuromuscular disease, renal impairment, AV block, and now pregnancy
6. Give **dexamethasone** 10 mg IV infused over 10–15 min; particularly helpful for status migrainosus and prevention of headache recurrence
7. Consider **valproate sodium** 15–20 mg/kg IV infused over 15–30 min

AV, Atrioventricular; *IM,* intramuscularly; *IV,* intravenously; *NS,* normal saline; *SC,* subcutaneously.

3. **What are the vital signs?**

Significant hypertension can signal hypertensive emergency, stroke, increased intracranial pressure (ICP), or preeclampsia. Fever suggests an infection and concern for meningitis.

Orders

1. Stat computed tomography (CT) head if concern for subarachnoid hemorrhage or mass lesion.
2. If you are confident that the headache represents a long-standing, recurrent, and previously diagnosed migraine disorder, place the patient in a quiet, darkened room. The patient can be treated with a nonopioid agent that has previously relieved the headache, or with injectable **sumatriptan**, intravenous (IV) **metoclopramide**, or **ketorolac** (see dosages in Table 15.1).

ELEVATOR THOUGHTS

What causes headache?

Disorders marked with as asterisk can present as sudden-onset or thunderclap headache. Disorders marked with a plus sign are at increased risk during pregnancy and immediate postpartum.

Primary Headache Disorders

1. Migraine, including with and without aura, chronic migraine
2. Tension-type headache
3. Cranial autonomic cephalalgia
   - Cluster headache
   - Paroxysmal hemicrania
   - SUNCT (Short-lasting Unilateral Neuralgiform headache with Conjunctival Tearing and injection);
   - SUNA (Short-lasting Unilateral Neuralgiform headache with cranial Autonomic symptoms)
   - Hemicrania continua
4. Primary cough (or other Valsalva maneuver) headache, exercise headache*, headache with sexual activity*, thunderclap headache*, stabbing headache
5. Hypnic headache

Secondary Headache Disorders

1. Vascular
   - Subarachnoid hemorrhage*+
   - Subdural hematoma
   - Intracerebral hemorrhage*
   - Carotid or vertebral dissection*
   - Cerebral venous thrombosis*+
   - Cerebral infarction, particularly posterior circulation*+
   - Arteritis, including giant cell arteritis
   - RCVS*+
   - Pituitary apoplexy*+
   - Acute hypertensive crisis*
   - Preeclampsia and eclampsia*+
   - Dural arteriovenous fistula, carotid cavernous fistula
2. Infectious
   - Meningitis*
   - Sinusitis particularly with barotrauma*
   - Infections remote from the nervous system
3. Posttraumatic headache
4. Increased ICP
   - Intracranial mass lesions (tumor, hemorrhage, abscess, etc.)
   - Idiopathic intracranial hypertension (IIH; pseudotumor cerebri)
   - Hydrocephalus*
5. Decreased ICP
   - Spontaneous intracranial hypotension*
   - Post lumbar puncture (LP) headache
6. Chiari malformation type I
7. Noninfectious inflammatory
   - Aseptic meningitis

- Syndrome of transient headache and neurological deficits with cerebrospinal fluid lymphocytosis (HaNDL)

8. Substance exposure or withdrawal
   - Caffeine withdrawal
   - Overuse of any analgesics used to treat headache attacks
   - Nitric oxide exposure
   - Alcohol induced, immediate and delayed
   - Monosodium glutamate induced

9. Medical and other
   - High-altitude headache
   - Sleep apnea
   - Hypothyroidism
   - Cardiac cephalalgia
   - Cervicogenic headache
   - Acute glaucoma*
   - Temporomandibular disorder

Painful Cranial Neuropathies and Other Facial Pain

1. Trigeminal neuralgia
2. Trigeminal neuropathy including caused by acute herpes zoster or post-herpetic, trauma, multiple sclerosis
3. Glossopharyngeal neuralgia
4. Nevus intermedius neuralgia
5. Occipital neuralgia
6. Idiopathic facial pain

What red flags suggest secondary headache disorders?

A helpful mneumonic is to "SNOOP" for causes of secondary headaches (Box 15.1)

BOX 15.1	SNOOP Mneumonic for Secondary Causes of Headache

Systemic symptoms (fever, chills, weight loss)
Systemic disease (HIV, history of cancer)
Neurologic symptoms and signs (loss of vision, change in mental status, seizure, abnormal exam)
Onset (acute, sudden, split seconds)
Older patient (>50 with new or progressive headache)
Previous headache history that is different (new headache, change in attack frequency, severity, clinical features)
Progressive headache
Precipitated by Valsalva maneuver
Postural headache
Pregnancy

MAJOR THREAT TO LIFE

- *Subarachnoid hemorrhage*
  Aneurysmal subarachnoid hemorrhage, if not properly diagnosed, can lead to fatal rebleeding.
- *Bacterial meningitis*
  Bacterial meningitis must be recognized early if antibiotic treatment is to be successful.
- *Herniation from intracranial mass lesions*
  Herniation may occur as a result of a tumor, subdural or epidural hematoma, brain abscess, or any other mass lesion.

BEDSIDE

Quick-Look Test

Does the patient look well (comfortable), sick (uncomfortable), or critical (about to die)?

Amid a severe migraine, patients may appear sick because of severe photophobia and nausea. Patients with subarachnoid hemorrhage or meningitis look sick. Any sign of depressed level of consciousness or nuchal rigidity suggests these secondary headache disorders and urgency.

Airway and Vital Signs

What is the body temperature?

Fever associated with headache suggests meningitis. Headache can also represent a nonspecific reaction to a systemic febrile illness or be a symptom of giant cell arteritis.

What is the blood pressure (BP)?

Contrary to popular belief, headache is rarely caused by hypertension, unless the hypertension is both acute and severe (systolic pressure greater than 180 mmHg and/or diastolic pressure greater than 120 mmHg). Hypertension may also reflect subarachnoid hemorrhage, acute stroke, or increased ICP from an intracranial mass lesion.

Selective History and Chart Review

A detailed, well-focused history is the most important tool in diagnosing the cause of headache. In addition to reassessing questions 1 and 2 from the Phone Call section with the patient, the following questions are important:

1. **What triggered this episode?**
   Head injury or neck hyperextension suggest posttraumatic headache; for further evaluation, review Chapter 9. Recent change in medications may suggest medication effect. Stress

or stress letdown, rapid estrogen level fall such as with menstruation, insufficient sleep, alcohol, or fasting may suggest migraine. Cough or other Valsalva maneuvers may precipitate headache because of Chiari I malformation or a dural tear and low cerebrospinal fluid (CSF) pressure, cervical vessel dissection, or a primary headache. Sexual activity or exertion may precipitate RCVS or aneurysmal rupture, or be primary.

2. **Are there any changes in vision?**

   Double vision or transient visual obscuration suggests increased ICP. Evaluate for mass lesions, cerebral venous thrombosis, and IIH. Intermittent or progressive loss of vision in an older patient is concerning for giant cell arteritis. Visual aura with migraine has a gradual onset, gradual spread through the visual field with scintillations, and scotoma lasting less than 1 hour.

3. **Does the headache change depending on position?**

   Pain substantially worsened with standing may suggest low CSF pressure or a CSF leak. Look for recent history of LP (within 5 days), history of connective tissue disease, or minor trauma. However, with severe chronic migraine, patients prefer to remain reclined as well. Pain exacerbated by being reclined and worst headache in the mornings suggest increased ICP and consideration for a mass lesion or IIH.

4. **How long do headache episodes last without treatment?**

   This is a key diagnostic characteristic for various primary headache disorders. Migraine lasts at least 4 hours. A migraine ongoing for at least 3 days is called *status migrainosus*. A cluster headache lasts 15 to 180 minutes. Other cranial autonomic cephalalgias are shorter lasting, seconds in the case of SUNCT to minutes in the case of paroxysmal hemicrania. Tension-type headache can last 30 minutes to days.

5. **Are any symptoms associated with the headache?**

   Nausea, vomiting, photophobia and phonophobia, osmophobia, and movement sensitivity are suggestive of migraine. Asking if patients prefer to lie down in a dark and quiet room or stop looking at a bright computer screen helps identify these symptoms. Tearing, conjunctival injection, ptosis or miosis, nasal congestion, eyelid edema, and ear fullness are cranial autonomic symptoms ipsilateral to pain that occur prominently with trigeminal autonomic cephalgias (TACs) such as cluster headache, but they also can be seen in migraine.

6. **What is the pattern of the headache?**

   The characteristics of quality, location, and severity on their own are not sufficient for diagnosis; primary headache disorders have different patterns that should be sought out. In addition to timing and associated symptoms, laterality of pain and variability in laterality is the most helpful of the characteristics. Migraine may be unilateral or bilateral and throbbing, moderate to severe, and importantly be associated with migrainous features. Unilateral and side-locked, fluctuating but ever-present headache with autonomic symptoms warrants an indomethacin treatment trial for hemicrania continua. Cluster headache is strictly unilateral, typically orbital or temporal, severe, occurring from every other day to eight times per day and more frequently at night, disturbing sleep, and associated with autonomic features. Tension-type headaches are typically bilateral tightening, and they have mild to moderate intensity and usually no associated symptoms; therefore they are rarely seen in hospital consultation.

7. **Are there any associated focal deficits?**

Differentiating between migraine aura and transient ischemic attack (TIA) is important; prior diagnosis of migraine with aura is a risk factor for stroke. Migraine with aura is preceded or accompanied by one or more transient neurologic symptoms that, unlike a TIA, have (1) gradual onset, spread, and resolution; (2) involve positive and negative phenomena; and (3) can occur in succession. The most common is visual aura, which may consist of a scintillating scotoma; sensory aura is a spread of tingling followed by numbness over the face or limb. Aphasic aura symptoms can range from expressive to global. Each symptom of an aura lasts 5 minutes up to 1 hour, although in practice it may last slightly longer, particularly when the aura consists of multiple symptoms. Hemiplegic migraine aura is a rare form of aura, with hemiparesis that may last up to 72 hours and is associated with other classical aura symptoms. On presentation of hemiplegia or first-time aphasia, complete stroke workup must occur first. More sudden or on negative predominant presentation of scotoma, numbness also should be evaluated as a TIA. Remember, posterior circulation strokes can present with a visual field cut or sensory loss and notably headache.

Selective Physical Examination

In most patients with headache, the neurologic and physical examinations are normal. The primary purpose of the initial screening examination is to check for signs of meningismus, increased ICP, disorders of the head and neck, and neurologic focality.

Head	Sinus tenderness (sinusitis); temporal artery tenderness, swelling, reduced or absent pulses (giant cell arteritis); locking of jaw, limited opening

	of jaw, crepitus and tenderness over the temporomandibular joint (TMJ dysfunction); Tinel sign with pressure over occipital nerves found one-third and two-thirds of the way along an imaginary line between occipital protuberance and mastoid process (occipital neuralgia)
Eyes	Funduscopic exam: presence of spontaneous venous pulsations versus papilledema (disc elevation, blurring of disc margin, obscuration of vessels crossing the disc margin, venous distention, peripapillary hemorrhage), retinal hemorrhage (presence in peripheral retina not only immediately near optic disc suggests malignant systemic hypertension);
	Conjunctival injection (cluster or migraine headache); subtle signs of corneal clouding (acute angle closure glaucoma)
Neck	Nuchal rigidity with inability to flex neck so that chin touches the chest, Kernig or Brudzinski sign (Fig. 15.1) (subarachnoid hemorrhage or meningitis) versus cervical muscle spasm with tender trigger points (tension-type headache or migraine)
Vascular	Cranial bruit (arteriovenous malformation)
	Carotid bruit (dissection)

Selective Neurologic Examination

1. Level of consciousness and orientation, more detailed exam with report of aphasic aura, or other related symptoms.
2. Complete cranial nerve examination with attention to pupillary symmetry, signs of Horner syndrome (increased pupillary asymmetry in the dark, dilation lag, mild ptosis with lower lid "reverse" ptosis), in addition to trigeminal sensory exam observe trigger ability of paroxysmal pain with stimulation of each distribution or other structures.
3. Pronator drift.
4. Deep tendon and plantar reflexes.
5. Gait: hemiparetic, ataxic, observe arm swing at the same time.

Diagnostic Testing

Radiologic testing is *not* necessary if the patient has a long history of headache characteristic of migraine, a normal neurologic examination, and no fever or meningismus.

1. **Obtain head CT in patients with the following:**
   - Severe headache reaching full intensity instantly (thunder-clap headache).

A

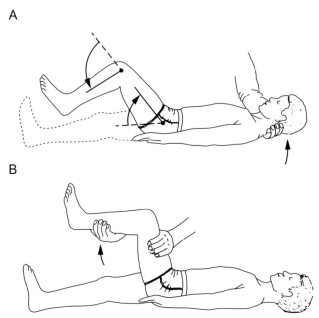

B

FIG. 15.1 (A) Brudzinski sign. The test result is positive when the patient actively flexes the hips and knees in response to passive neck flexion by the examiner. (B) Kernig sign. The test result is positive when pain or resistance prevents full extension of the knee from the 90-degree hip/knee flexion position. (From Marshall SA, Ruedy J. *On Call: Principles and Protocols,* 4th ed. Philadelphia, PA: Elsevier; 2004.)

- Headache with progressive onset over days to weeks that is not similar to previous headaches.
- Altered mental status, focal neurologic signs, or papilledema.

2. **If subarachnoid hemorrhage (SAH) or meningitis is suspected and the CT scan is negative, a follow-up LP is mandatory.**

   Head CT, if performed within 6 hours of onset of headache, has over 98% sensitivity in detecting subarachnoid hemorrhage. The sensitivity falls as time from onset of symptoms increases. Imaging may miss a small bleed and, if clinical suspicion is high, an LP is indicated to assess for xanthochromia and red blood cells that are not attributed to a traumatic tap. See Chapter 24 for further management of SAH.

   When bacterial meningitis is suspected (headache, fever, neck rigidity), head CT should be obtained for patients with risk factors for a mass lesion, including those who are immunocompromised, have depressed level of consciousness or focal neurologic deficits, papilledema, or new-onset seizure. Empiric antimicrobial therapy and dexamethasone (if indicated) should not be delayed for the workup. If imaging does not reveal alternate etiology of symptoms and LP is not contraindicated, proceed with CSF analysis. Without risk factors, an LP may be performed without head CT. See Chapter 22 for further management of meningitis.

3. **Obtain further imaging when concerned for the following:**
   - Cerebral venous thrombosis: Magnetic resonance imaging (MRI) brain and MR venography (MRV) or CT venography (CTV) of the head
   - RCVS with recurrent thunderclap headache episodes over a few weeks and negative workup for subarachnoid hemorrhage: MRI brain and MR angiography (MRA) head or CTA head for segmental vasoconstriction; repeat vessel imaging 1 to 2 weeks from onset of symptoms because imaging may be normal within the first week
   - Cervical carotid dissection with side locked headache and ipsilateral Horner syndrome: MRA with T1 proton-density weighted fat-suppressed sequences or CTA neck
   - Low CSF pressure headache: MRI brain with contrast, may need to follow with MRI spine with contrast for additional evidence, and radioisotope cisternography if the previous study is inconclusive
   - TAC: MRI brain with contrast to evaluate for pituitary tumors and other posterior fossa lesions that can mimic the phenotype

4. **Obtain LP for opening pressure** (OP) with headache and signs of increased ICP including papilledema or abducens palsy, and no other etiology for increased ICP identified with imaging previously described, to confirm diagnosis of IIH

5. **Laboratory testing**
   - With suspicion for giant cell arteritis obtain erythrocyte sedimentation rate (ESR), C-reactive protein (CRP), complete blood count (CBC), and consider temporal artery biopsy
     1. Ophthalmology consultation with suspicion for acute angle closure glaucoma, detailed visual field testing for IIH, question of papilledema versus pseudopapilledema

MANAGEMENT

Migraine

Migraine is the most common disabling primary headache disorder, with a 12% prevalence in the United States. The diagnosis of migraine is based on headache duration, features, associated

TABLE 15.2	Common Migraine Triggers

- Stress or stress letdown
- Hormonal fluctuations (menstrual association)
- Sleep deprivation or excess
- Skipped meals and dehydration
- Physical exertion
- Alcohol (particularly red wine)
- Caffeine withdrawal
- MSG (found in Chinese cuisine, bouillon cubes, certain chips, and seasoning mixes)
- Environmental factors (weather changes, high altitude, bright lights, loud noises, odors)

MSG, Monosodium glutamate.

symptom, and a recurrent pattern to the attacks (at least five for diagnosis). Common triggers of the attacks are listed in Table 15.2.

Migraine Without Aura

Migraine without aura is defined by the following criteria:
1. Recurrent headaches of 4 to 72 hours' duration with at least two of the following characteristics:
   - Unilateral location
   - Pulsating quality
   - Moderate or severe pain intensity
   - Aggravation by routine physical activity
2. In addition, at least one of the following characteristics must be present:
   - Nausea or vomiting
   - Photophobia and phonophobia

Note: Migraine pain does not have to be unilateral or pulsatile.

Migraine With Aura

Up to one-third of patients with migraine have symptoms of a migraine aura, which was previously termed "classic migraine." These are transient, completely reversible neurologic symptoms with gradual onset and spread over at least 5 minutes that are followed by headache, but they can occur at any point during a headache or without headache. Headache associated with aura may not fulfill criteria for the migraine previously mentioned, but it is still considered migraine because of the association. Each symptom of an aura may last up to an hour and may occur in succession. Aura symptoms are more likely to consist of positive (flashing) or positive and negative (scintillating scotoma) symptoms than purely negative symptoms. The symptoms correspond to a cortical spreading depression wave of activation followed by the suppression of neurons of eloquent areas.

Typical ("classical") aura symptoms:

- **Visual:** Most common of all aura symptoms. Described as sparkling objects forming a growing spot, or a zigzag figure enlarging and spreading to the periphery. Patients have a hard time describing these symptoms and find it helpful to see images they can relate to, such as Fig. 15.2. Description of monocular, rather than homonymous, visual disturbance is a common mistake: patients should be asked to describe how they visualize a face or a clock and asked to test eyes individually with future episodes.
- **Sensory:** Pins and needles followed by numbness spreading over one side of face or body. Numbness may be the only symptom, but gradual spread is an important feature.
- **Aphasic:** May range from mild to dense, and expressive aphasia is more common than receptive or complete.

The following rare forms of aura should be identified and closely worked up for secondary etiologies including stroke, ophthalmic pathology, and, if brief, seizures. Triptan and ergot therapy is contraindicated in patients with these auras.

Hemiplegic aura:

- Fully reversible weakness, typically unilateral, that may last up to 72 hours, in rare cases up to weeks, along with at least one typical aura symptom above. Mutations in genes responsible for facilitating cortical spreading depression, including CACNA1A,

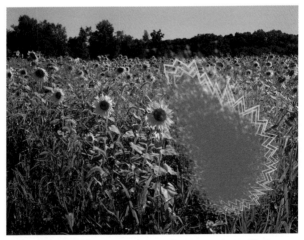

FIG. 15.2 Visual aura of migraine consisting of scintillating scotoma with fortification spectra front.

ATP1A2, SCN1A, may be causative. In patients with mutations, attacks can be triggered by mild head trauma. In 50% of families, progressive cerebellar ataxia may occur independent of migraine attacks.

Retinal aura:

- Monocular visual disturbance similar to typical visual aura but affecting only a single eye. Must first evaluate causes of transient monocular visual loss (see Chapter 12).

Brain Stem aura:

- Previously described as basilar artery migraine, this exceedingly rare aura consists of at least one of typical aura symptoms listed previously in addition to at least two brain stem symptoms of the following: dysarthria, vertigo, tinnitus, hyperacusis, diplopia, ataxia, and decreased level of consciousness. Many of these symptoms may occur with anxiety and hyperventilation, and careful history should be obtained.

Chronic Migraine

The term *chronic migraine* is habitually misused to describe a long history of migraines. This diagnosis should be reserved for the specific condition based on the frequency of headaches experienced by the patient, such as headache occurring on 15 or more days per month for more than 3 months with migraine headaches on 8 or more days of the month. In addition to asking patients how often they have migraines, it is important to assess frequency of additional less debilitating headaches. *An appropriate diagnosis should lead to assessment of modifiable risk factors for migraine chronification including:*

- Medication and caffeine overuse
- Anxiety
- Depression
- Sleep disorders, including obstructive sleep apnea
- Obesity

It also should lead to management with the most effective therapies, including **onabotulinum toxin A** or **topiramate.**

Status Migrainosus

A debilitating migraine attack lasting more than 3 days is called status migrainosus. Brief remissions in pain with medications or sleep can occur. In some cases, treatment for status migrainosus may require outpatient or inpatient IV therapy.

TREATMENT

In an outpatient setting, treatment includes identifying and eliminating triggers (see Table 15.2), counseling about healthy habits (regular sleep schedule, healthy regular meals, stress management), and addressing risks for migraine chronification listed previously.

Medication overuse with simple analgesics, triptans, combination medications, and caffeine can make preventive therapy ineffective.

Acute therapy for migraine headache includes **nonsteroidal antiinflammatory drugs** (NSAIDs), **triptans** (serotonin (5-$HT_{1B/1D}$) receptor agonists), and an older class of **ergot derivatives**. Agents are listed in Table 15.3. Triptans and ergots are contraindicated in patients with cardiovascular, cerebrovascular,

TABLE 15.3	Selected Medications Used for Acute Treatment of Migraine
Triptans	
• Sumatriptan (Imitrex)	6 mg SC, repeat once after 1 h PRN, maximum 12 mg QD; 50–100 mg PO, repeat once after q2h PRN, maximum 200 mg QD; 20 mg single intranasal spray, repeat once after q2h PRN, maximum 40 mg QD
• Naratriptan (Amerge)	2.5 mg PO repeat once after 4 h PRN, maximum 5 mg daily
• Rizatriptan (Maxalt)	5–10 mg PO repeat once after 2 h PRN, maximum 30 mg daily
• Zolmitriptan (Zomig)	2.5–5 mg PO, repeat once after 2 h PRN, maximum 10 mg daily; 5 mg single intranasal spray, repeat once after 2 h PRN
• Frovatriptan (Frova)	2.5 mg PO, repeat once after 2 h PRN, maximum 5 mg daily
• Eletriptan (Relpax)	20–40 mg PO, repeat once after 2 h PRN, maximum 80 mg daily
• Almotriptan malate (Axert)	6.25–12.5 mg PO, repeat once after 2 h PRN, maximum 25 mg daily
NSAIDs and Acetaminophen (Listed in Order of Increasing Half-Life)	
• Acetaminophen (Tylenol)	650–1000 mg PO q4–6h, maximum 3250 mg daily
• Diclofenac potassium (Cambia powder)	100 mg PO at onset, then 50 mg PO q8h 50 mg powder diluted in 1 oz water PO q8h
• Ibuprofen (Motrin, Advil)	400–800 mg PO q6h
• Aspirin	500–1000 mg PO q6h
• Indomethacin	25–50 mg PO q8h
• Ketorolac (Toradol, Sprix)	60 mg IM one dose, or 30 mg q6h IM/IV, maximum 120 mg daily 15.75 mg/spray, 1 spray in each nostril q6–8 h, maximum 8 total sprays daily, limit to 5 days per month
• Naproxen sodium (Aleve, Anaprox)	440–550 mg PO q12h
• Nabumetone	500–750 mg PO q12h
• Piroxicam	10–20 mg PO daily

TABLE 15.3	Selected Medications Used for Acute Treatment of Migraine—cont'd

Antiemetics (Listed in Order of Increasing Potential for Dyskinesia)

• Ondansetron (Zofran)	4–8 mg PO q12h PO; 8 mg q12h IV
• Promethazine (Phenergan)	12.5–25 mg q8–12h PO
• Metoclopramide (Reglan)	5–10 mg q 8–12h PO; 10 mg q8h IV
• Prochlorperazine (Compazine)	5–10 mg q8-12h PO; 10 mg q8h IV 25 mg q12h per rectum
• Chlorpromazine (Thorazine)	10–25 mg q8–12 h PO; 12.5–25 mg q8h IM/IV

Ergot Derivatives

• Dihydroergotamine (DHE, Migranal nasal spray)	1 mg IM/SC, repeat q1h PRN, maximum 3 mg IM/SC QD; 0.5 mg 1 spray to each nostril, may repeat once in 15 min, maximum daily dose of 3 mg or 6 sprays
• Ergotamine tartrate (Ergomar, sublingual)	2 mg sublingual, may repeat after 30 min up to three tablets, maximum 6 mg daily, maximum 10 mg in any week

IM, Intramuscularly; *IV,* intravenously; *NSAIDs,* nonsteroidal antiinflammatory drugs; *PO,* by mouth; *PRN,* as needed; *q,* every; *QD,* every day; *SC,* subcutaneously.

and peripheral vascular disease. NSAIDs should be avoided in patients with poor kidney function or peptic ulcers. The overriding principle of acute migraine therapy is to treat early in the attack and with a sufficiently high dose of medication. Triptans are usually only effective in the first few hours of a migraine, after that NSAID therapy is preferred.

Seven triptans are available in the United States, all in tablet form. **Sumatriptan** is also available in injectable formulation, which has an advantage over tablets when nausea or vomiting is prominent or the headache grows in severity rapidly and rapid time of peak plasma concentration is important. **Zolmitriptan** is available as an intranasal formulation and has a similar advantage in context of nausea. Triptans can be combined with NSAIDs for increased efficacy.

Adjunctive therapy with antiemetics such as metoclopramide, and others in Table 15.3, may be added to reduce nausea and vomiting, and they may enhance absorption of other acute therapies. These medications should be infused, not bolused, in the acute setting, to reduce risk of akathisia. Monitoring for acute dystonic reaction and counseling about tardive dyskinesia with prolonged use are necessary.

Butalbital-containing medications have a high likelihood of causing medication-overuse headache and are not recommended for management of headache disorders.

Those with frequent attacks (more than four per month) or disabling attacks (not responsive to acute medications or not candidates for acute medications) are candidates for preventive therapy. Agents commonly used for migraine prevention fall into categories of BP agents, antidepressants, and antiepileptic drugs, and they are listed in Table 15.4. Preventives are selected based on comorbidities and desired and undesired side effects. For example, an overweight patient may benefit from **topiramate** (which has side effect of weight loss), a patient with insomnia may benefit from **amitriptyline** (which is a sedating tricyclic antidepressant

TABLE 15.4	Selected Treatments Used for Prevention of Migraine

Beta-Blockers
Contraindicated with brittle diabetes, Raynaud syndrome, beta-1 selective agents can be considered at lower doses and cautiously with history of bronchospastic disease

• Propranolol	40–320 mg daily in one to two doses with long-acting or regular formulation
• Nadolol	40–240 mg daily
• Atenolol[a]	25–100 mg daily
• Metoprolol[a]	50–200 mg daily in one to two doses a day with long-acting or regular formulation

Antidepressants TCA/SNRIs
Monitor ECG for QT prolongation, caution with cardiovascular disease

• Amitriptyline	20–100 mg at night
• Nortriptyline	20–100 mg at night
• Venlafaxine	75–150 mg daily

Anticonvulsants
Topiramate is contraindicated with history of kidney stones and acute angle closure glaucoma, monitor for hyperchloremic metabolic acidosis, multiple serious side effects with divalproex detailed in formulary

• Topiramate (Topamax, Qudexy, Trokendi)	50–200 mg daily in one to two doses a day with long-acting or regular formulation
• Divalproex sodium (Depakote)	500–1500 mg daily in one to two doses a day with long-acting or regular formulation

Other Classes

• Candesartan (angiotensin receptor blocker)	8–16 mg daily
• Verapamil (calcium channel blocker) may be helpful for migraine with aura	240 mg daily

TABLE 15.4	Selected Treatments Used for Prevention of Migraine—cont'd
• Cyproheptadine (antiserotonin)	2–4 mg daily
• Onabotulinum toxin A (Botox) for chronic migraine only	155 units injected IM in 31 sites in head and neck (PREEMPT protocol)
• Supraorbital/supratrochlear transcutaneous electrical nerve stimulation (Cefaly)	20 minutes nightly
• Magnesium	500–600 mg daily
• Riboflavin (vitamin B$_2$)	200 mg BID

[a]Beta-1 selective agents.

BID, Twice a day; *ECG,* electrocardiogram; *IM,* intramuscularly; *PREEMPT,* phase 3 research evaluating migraine prophylaxis therapy; *SNRI,* serotonin-norepinephrine reuptake inhibitor; *TCA,* trigeminal autonomic cephalalgia.

used at significantly lower doses for migraine prevention than treatment of depression), a patient with comorbid depression warrants consideration for **venlafaxine**, and patients with high BP may be treated with **propranolol** or **candesartan**. Common side effects should be carefully discussed; for instance, topiramate can cause paresthesias in up to 50% of patients and can cause cognitive symptoms such as word-finding difficulty. Medications are started at low doses and increased slowly to help adjust to side effects and help find the lowest effective dose. Preventive therapies in migraine may have a latency period of several weeks up to 3 months before they become effective.

A new class of migraine preventives is based on antagonism of the calcitonin gene-related peptide (CGRP) or its receptor. CGRP is a proinflammatory and neuromodulatory peptide released from trigeminal ganglion fibers with a crucial role in headache pathophysiology: (1) CGRP blood levels are increased in patients during acute migraine and cluster attacks, (2) infusion of CGRP has been used to trigger migraine-like headaches, and (3) its levels are elevated in patients with chronic migraine outside of migraine attacks. At this time there are three CGRP antagonists available for migraine prophylaxis: **Erenumab 70 mg SQ** once a month (some patients may benefit from **140 mg** once a month); **Fremanezumab 225 mg SQ** monthly (or **675 mg** every 3 months); and **Galcanezumab 240 mg SQ** as a single loading dose, followed by **120 mg** once monthly. Trial results thus far are showing significant relief in chronic and frequent episodic migraine without serious side effects. **Ubrogepant,** a small molecule CGRP receptor antagonist, is currently not approved but in phase 3 clinical trials for acute treatment of migraine.

Protocols for the emergency room treatment of severe migraine are shown in Table 15.1. In most cases, those seeking care in the emergency room have prolonged attacks, or status migrainosus, and the usual oral therapies are not likely to be effective. IV hydration is important for those with intractable vomiting. A stepwise treatment with antiemetic, **ketorolac, dihydroergotamine (DHE)**, **dexamethasone**, and **valproate sodium** can break the exacerbation in most patients. The use of DHE is contraindicated within 24 hours of the use of a triptan (and vice versa). Dexamethasone may be helpful for prevention of recurrence of headache. If the initial stepwise treatment is ineffective, admission for repetitive administration of IV **DHE** every 8 hours, for up to 5 days and a total of 11.25 mg is considered according to the modified Raskin protocol.

During pregnancy, the focus should be on nonpharmacological prevention of migraine because the risk of teratogenicity is not completely known with most medications. For instance, **magnesium** is no longer recommended as a daily preventive or status migrainosus therapy: high-dose magnesium has been associated with bone abnormalities in the fetus, and the exact dose of this effect is not known. Luckily, the majority of women find spontaneous improvement in migraine during pregnancy: over 45% improve in the first trimester, and over 80% improve in later trimesters. Improvement is more likely in women with migraine without aura. For women with persistent or occasionally worsened migraines, healthy habits, trigger avoidance, and behavior treatment for stress reduction such as relaxation training and biofeedback may be helpful. Noninvasive neuromodulation is frequently used for prevention of severe or high-frequency migraines when pharmacological prevention is contraindicated. Transcutaneous stimulation of supraorbital and supratrochlear nerves with a mild electric current through a small device with a self-adhesive electrode placed over the forehead (**Cefaly**) is thought to modulate the trigeminal nociceptive threshold and have a sedative effect. It is approved for prevention of migraine and is under investigation for acute migraine treatment. Mechanistically, there are no concerns during pregnancy. Another modality that can be considered is single-pulse transcranial magnetic stimulation (TMS). A handheld device (**sTMS mini**) abutted occipitally delivers 0.9T magnetic field pulse to the cerebral cortex, which is thought to disrupt cortical spreading depression and modulate corticothalamic circuits involved in induction of central pain. It is approved for acute treatment of pain of migraine with aura and may help on a preventive basis. Postmarket pilot program of the device included pregnant patients in second and third trimesters without any adverse effects; magnetic field strength near a fetus is as low as several exposures to a microwave oven, although extensive safety studies are not available. Interventional strategy includes occipital nerve blocks with lidocaine for prevention of frequent migraines and for treatment of status migrainosus. **Cyproheptadine** may be considered preventively with caution for sedation and weight gain. Acute therapies include **metoclopramide** for associated nausea and **acetaminophen** for pain, in limited quantities. Based on triptan registry studies, prenatal exposure has not been associated with large increased rates of major congenital malformations, although studies are limited by relatively low numbers of patients for rare effects to be definitively ruled out, and there may be increased risk of spontaneous abortion with triptan exposure.

Tension-Type Headache

Tension-type headache is the most common headache disorder, but because of a lower level of associated disability, it is not often seen by neurologists. Headache may last anywhere from 30 minutes to a week, and have at least two of the following features: bilateral location, pressing or pulsating quality, mild-to-moderate intensity, and no aggravation by routine physical activity. These headaches are not associated with migrainous or cranial autonomic symptoms. They never occur with nausea or vomiting and should not have more than one of either photophobia or phonophobia. The chronic form of this disorder, with unremitting headache lasting hours or days occurring on at least 15 days per month over several months, is the most likely to present for medical evaluation.

TREATMENT

Most patients respond to relaxation techniques and NSAIDs (see Table 15.3). Tricyclic antidepressants, independent of their antidepressant effect, may be helpful for prevention of the chronic tension-type headache.

Medication-Overuse Headache

Those suffering from frequent headaches, most commonly migraines, with frequent use of acute medications to obtain pain relief, can transform their episodic attacks into much more frequent (at times daily) headache. Medications ranging from acetaminophen and other over-the-counter simple analgesics to triptans and most notably combination medications that contain butalbital and caffeine can result in overuse headache. The frequency of use of these medications can range from 15 days per month for simple analgesics to as little as 10 days per month for the latter group. Medications with shorter half-lives and more rapid onset of action are more likely to cause overuse. Medication-overuse headaches are much less likely to respond to preventive therapy unless overuse is addressed, and additional acute therapies are likely to perpetuate the problem.

Treatment involves initiation of preventive therapy that is appropriate for the prior episodic headache disorder and withdrawal of the overused medication. Bridge therapies to support withdrawal headaches include a course of long-acting NSAIDs, steroids, and occipital nerve blocks. Withdrawal from butalbital-containing medications should be gradual to avoid seizures.

Cluster Headache and Other Trigeminal Autonomic Cephalalgias

Cluster headache is characterized by excruciating unilateral head pain often localized to the orbit or temple. The pain is described as boring and piercing and occurs in attacks lasting 15 minutes to 3 hours. Headaches are associated with autonomic, predominantly parasympathetic, symptoms of ipsilateral facial flushing, Horner syndrome, tearing or conjunctival injection, ear fullness, nasal congestion or rhinorrhea, or a sense of restlessness or agitation. Although migraineurs prefer to lie in bed in a dark room with attacks, cluster patients pace relentlessly. The headaches occur in "clusters," during which sufferers develop one or more attacks daily for a period of weeks to months, interspersed by headache-free intervals lasting from months to years. Cluster headaches occur most commonly late at night, often awakening the person out of sleep, and they frequently occur with regularity at a particular time of day. Alcohol can trigger attacks during active cluster periods but not outside of these periods. A chronic form of the disorder afflicts patients when no headache-free intervals occur for over a year. Secondary etiologies of cluster headache warranting workup include posterior fossa lesions such as pituitary tumors and **acute angle closure glaucoma**. The latter may present as intermittent eye or periorbital pain with trace conjunctival injection, precipitated by dark lighting, prolonged near-work, or being prone.

In addition to cluster headache, the family of TACs includes the rarer **paroxysmal hemicrania** and **short-lasting unilateral neuralgiform headache attacks** (with **c**onjunctival injection and **t**earing called SUNCT, or with other **a**utonomic symptoms called SUNA). Attacks with these disorders are shorter in duration, lasting seconds to minutes. Diagnoses are based on the presence of severe unilateral (frequently orbital) headache with at least one prominent ipsilateral autonomic symptom, and different durations of attacks, compared in Table 15.5 along with treatment suggestions. These headache disorders, with pathophysiology tied to the hypothalamus, are not to be confused with trigeminal neuralgia, which is a disorder of nerve compression or traction and ephaptic transmission (discussed further in Chapter 18, Pain Syndromes). Although both types of disorders consist of brief stabbing episodes of pain, with TACs, autonomic symptoms are much more prominent and there is no refractory period after an episode is

TABLE 15.5	Comparison of Trigeminal Autonomic Cephalalgias

Disorder	Timing	First-Line treatment
Cluster headache	15-min to 3-h attacks occurring every other day up to eight per day	• Preventive therapy: verapamil (240–720 mg divided in three doses), galcanezumab 300 mg SQ at cluster onset and monthly there after • Short-term prevention: 10- to 21-day prednisone taper or occipital nerve block • Acute therapy: sumatriptan 6 mg SC, zolmitriptan 5 mg IN, or 100% oxygen for 15–20 min
Paroxysmal hemicrania	2- to 30-min episodes occurring 5–30 times per day	Indomethacin titrated from 25 mg TID up to 75 mg TID for up to 2 weeks for complete suppression of pain and confirmation of diagnosis
SUNCT/SUNA	1-s to 10-min episodes occurring up to hundreds of times per day on at least half of the days	Lamotrigine 150–200 mg daily
Hemicrania continua	Continuous headache lasting over 3 months with moderate or severe exacerbations lasting variable times	Indomethacin titrated from 25 mg TID up to 75 mg TID for up to 2 weeks for complete suppression of pain and confirmation of diagnosis

IN, Intranasally; *SC,* subcutaneously; *TID,* three times a day. SUNCT (Short-lasting Unilateral Neuralgiform headache with Conjunctival Tearing and injection); SUNA (Short-lasting Unilateral Neuralgiform headache with cranial Autonomic symptoms)

triggered as is the case with trigeminal neuralgia. Importantly, secondary etiologies to workup and treatments are different.

TREATMENT

Cluster headache treatment differs substantially from that of migraine. For acute attacks, first-line treatments include:

1. **Sumatriptan 6 mg SC**, and 4 mg SC may be considered for more frequent attacks because the maximum daily dose is

12 mg. **Zolmitriptan** 2.5 to 5 mg intranasally can be used as an alternative, with a maximum daily dose of 10 mg.

2. **Oxygen 100% at 10 to 12 L/min** using a nonrebreather mask should be initiated as soon as the attack begins, for 15 to 20 minutes. Many cluster patients are smokers and need to be advised of the dangers of smoking while using oxygen.

3. **DHE 1 mg IV or intramuscularly (IM)/SC** may be used in place of triptans.

4. Noninvasive portable vagus nerve stimulation (**gammaCore**) was approved by the FDA in 2017 for treatment of episodic, but not chronic, cluster attacks. Three 2-minute doses delivered transcutaneously to the neck ipsilaterally to pain can be repeated after 3 minutes and used to treat up to four attacks per day.

In many cluster headache patients, unless a pattern of short cluster bouts with less than 1 to 2 attacks per day is established, prophylactic medications are necessary. **Verapamil, particularly immediate release formulation, should be started at 40 to 80 mg TID** and titrated up every 2 weeks with reduced frequency/severity of episodes typically under 400 mg, but up to 720 mg in some cases. Careful monitoring for development of electrocardiogram (ECG) abnormalities is necessary. Alternatives for cluster headache prophylaxis include galcanezumab (Table 15.5) **topiramate** or **lithium**.

A short-term preventive "bridge" treatment is indicated if attacks are frequent at onset while titrating verapamil or other preventive medication to a therapeutic range, or for short-lasting cluster periods. These include:

1. **Prednisone 60 to 80 mg per day,** slowly tapered over 10 to 21 days

2. **Occipital nerve block** with a combination of 1% to 2% lidocaine and methylprednisolone 80 mg.

After several weeks, when the patient appears to be free from attacks, the prophylactic medications are slowly withdrawn.

Hemicrania Continua

Frequently misdiagnosed as chronic migraine, this disorder falls into the category of cranial autonomic cephalalgias and is one of the more common disorders in the group. Unlike other paroxysmal disorders in the class, hemicrania continua is a strictly unilateral *persistent* headache with exacerbations that can be short or long associated with ipsilateral autonomic symptoms akin to cluster. Migrainous symptoms are not uncommon with this disorder, as is comorbidity with migraine. Photophobia may be prominent ipsilateral to headache. In obtaining the history of frequent episodes of unilateral headaches, asking "is there a constant low-level discomfort between your bad headaches on the same side of your head?"

can help identify this disorder. As with other cranial autonomic cephalalgias, secondary etiologies, including pituitary tumors, should be sought out.

TREATMENT

The diagnosis is confirmed by a treatment trial with **indomethacin. Starting with 25 mg TID, the dose is increased every 5 to 7 days up to 50 mg TID, and if the pain does not completely resolve, it is increased to 75 mg TID for up to 2 weeks.** Smaller maintenance doses are used after that for treatment. If headache does not resolve with high-dose indomethacin, alternative diagnosis, most likely side-locked chronic migraine, should be considered.

Posttraumatic Headache

New headache, or substantial exacerbation in prior headache disorder, that starts within a week of having sustained head trauma or whiplash injury is categorized as posttraumatic headache. For details of initial evaluation and management of head injury, see Chapter 9. Headache can occur in isolation, or as part of postconcussion syndrome, which includes dizziness and imbalance, poor concentration and mild memory problems, irritability and mood disturbance, and insomnia. Headache symptoms are usually comparable to migraine or tension-type headache, but they may be consistent with another primary headache disorder and should be treated as such. Most headaches resolve in the first 3 months, although some patients develop chronic headaches.

TREATMENT

Initially, acute treatment with NSAIDs (see Table 15.3) is appropriate, with caution to avoid medication overuse. It is important to address each additional symptom of postconcussion syndrome including insomnia, vestibular symptoms (with vestibular rehabilitation), and mood symptoms with counseling or medications because these can exacerbate headache. With a prolonged headache course, preventive therapy with **tricyclic antidepressants** is first-line treatment. With posttraumatic migraine, caution is advised with the use of topiramate if there are underlying cognitive symptoms and with beta-blockers for athletes.

Idiopathic Intracranial Hypertension

Also known as "pseudotumor cerebri," this is a disorder of increased ICP in the absence of an intracranial mass lesion or other secondary etiologies. It is characterized by papilledema and headache that may be associated with transient visual obscurations (loss of vision lasting <30 seconds in one or both eyes), diplopia, or with pulsatile tinnitus, or it may be exacerbated by reclining. The main hazard in IIH is visual loss that results from optic nerve damage and can be permanent. Visual field testing with perimetry shows enlarged blind spots, constriction of peripheral fields, and, less commonly, central or paracentral scotomas.

The disorder occurs most commonly in young obese women. Recent exposure to tetracyclines, excessive vitamin A or retinoids such as isotretinoin, and hypoadrenalism or hypoparathyroidism are other risk factors for developing IIH. Depressed level of consciousness or other neurologic exam abnormalities do not occur except for abducens nerve palsy, which represents a nonspecific sign of increased ICP.

Before establishing the diagnosis, other causes of increased ICP must be excluded. MRI of the brain with and without contrast should be performed for all patients, and MRV should be performed for those who are not a known risk group for IIH (female and obese) to rule out a mass lesion, communicating or obstructive hydrocephalus, and cerebral venous thrombosis. An elevated LP OP, ≥ 250 mm H_2O in adults and ≥ 280 mm H_2O in children, with normal CSF composition and the presence of papilledema are the other two criteria for diagnosis. The LP should be obtained during exacerbation of symptoms to capture elevated pressure, and the OP should be measured in the lateral decubitus position. Sedation for the procedure may cause hypercapnia and artifactually elevated CSF pressure. Without evidence of papilledema, diagnosis can be made based on the previously criteria and the presence of unilateral or bilateral abducens nerve palsy. In the absence of papilledema and abducens palsy, a diagnosis can be suggested with history and LP findings and at least three of the following neuroimaging criteria: empty sella, flattening of posterior aspect of the globe, distension of the perioptic subarachnoid space with or without tortuous optic nerve, and transverse sinus stenosis.

TREATMENT

Many patients may respond to repeated LPs and removal of CSF performed every few days to every few weeks; however, the benefit of these practices is uncertain. In obese patients, weight reduction and low-salt diet are recommended. **Acetazolamide 500 mg twice a day** up to 2 g per day and in some higher, if tolerated, is the first-line treatment for reduction of CSF production and ICP. Another carbonic anhydrase inhibitor that often causes weight loss and may help with headache with migrainous symptoms is **topiramate, starting at 50 to 200 mg twice a day** can be used. Furosemide 40 to 80 mg daily may be used as adjunctive therapy. All patients need to have baseline visual field and acuity testing and serial visual field testing. If visual loss progresses despite medical therapy, a lumboperitoneal shunt or optic nerve sheath fenestration may be necessary.

Spontaneous Intracranial Hypotension

This disorder resembles post-LP headache, and it is characterized by headache that worsens after standing or with Valsalva maneuvers and is relieved by laying down. Associated symptoms include nausea, tinnitus, and vertigo. Diagnosis is frequently delayed, and over time, orthostatic features may disappear and chronic daily headache may develop. Etiology is CSF leakage caused by spontaneous rupture of arachnoid membrane, most frequently localized to the thoracic or cervicothoracic spine, and rarely at the skull base. Some patients, particularly those with connective tissue disorders, may have meningeal diverticula or dilation of nerve root sleeves that predispose the leaks. Minor trauma, sexual intercourse, and Valsalva maneuvers may be inciting events. By definition, CSF pressure is low (less than 60 mm H_2O), although a spinal tap is not required and diagnosis can be made by imaging. MRI brain with contrast suggestive of diagnosis includes findings of subdural hematoma or hygroma, diffuse meningeal enhancement (including infratentorial and supratentorial pachymeninges, but not leptomeninges; there should be no abnormal enhancement in depth of cortical sulci), engorgement of venous structures, pituitary enlargement, and sagging of the brain. Spine MRI can help identify location of CSF leakage with extradural CSF extravasation or meningeal diverticula. If nondiagnostic, then CT radioisotope cisternography can be performed to confirm the diagnosis, and in some patients reveal the cite of the leak, or CT or MR myelography may be used to identify the leak cite.

TREATMENT

If prolonged bed rest and other conservative treatments including hydration and **caffeine** intake fail to relieve the symptoms, interventional approaches may be undertaken. Many patients will respond to an **epidural blood patch** at the level of the CSF leakage, although the procedure may need to be performed several times. Epidural fibrin glue is an alternative, and surgical repair may be required in some instances.

Giant Cell Arteritis

Also known as temporal arteritis, giant cell arteritis is a chronic vasculitis of large and medium-sized vessels that occurs almost exclusively in patients over 50 years of age. In addition to headache that may be temporal, occipital, or generalized and progressively worsening or waxing and waning, patients have systemic symptoms of weight loss, fevers, jaw claudication, and diffuse myalgias. The most feared complication is visual loss (see Chapter 12). The ESR is elevated in almost all patients, usually to high levels of over 50 mm/h.

TREATMENT

If the diagnosis is suspected, without visual loss, **prednisone may be started at a daily dose of 40 to 60 mg.** With visual loss, urgent IV pulse dose treatment with methylprednisolone 1000 mg daily can be given for 3 days followed by oral prednisone at 60 mg/day. Bilateral temporal artery biopsies with long sections should be performed within a few days to confirm the diagnosis. In most patients, headache and systemic symptoms improve over a few days after initiating therapy. Steroid therapy may be required over months to several years, but because the illness is self-limited, it usually can be gradually tapered off.

Neuromuscular Respiratory Failure

Generalized weakness is usually the primary complaint in patients with severe neuromuscular disease. The most common diseases presenting as acute paralysis and acute respiratory failure are **myasthenia gravis** and **Guillain-Barré syndrome (GBS)** (acute inflammatory demyelinating polyneuropathy). Patients may also present with acute respiratory failure as a presenting symptom of myasthenia gravis or GBS. Weakness of the bulbar or respiratory muscles could lead to life-threatening respiratory failure by two potential mechanisms: (1) lack of upper airway protection and (2) hypoventilation because of respiratory muscle weakness. Your management should be directed toward stabilizing the patient, assessing the need to intubate and ventilate, and establishing a diagnosis and starting definitive treatment expeditiously. The most important goals of monitoring patients with neuromuscular respiratory failure closely are preventing crash intubations and assessing response to definitive treatment.

PHONE CALL

Questions

1. **What are the vital signs?**
2. **Is the patient in respiratory distress or complaining of shortness of breath?**

Patients with acute neuromuscular respiratory failure might not appear in obvious respiratory distress caused by respiratory muscle weakness. Even a subjective complaint of shortness of breath should be evaluated diligently and followed up with bedside pulmonary function testing (PFT). *Rapid, shallow breathing and paradoxical breathing* could be danger signs of impending ventilatory failure. Patients with acute weakness who are in obvious respiratory distress should be intubated immediately.

3. **Over what time period has the weakness developed? Any preceding illnesses, vaccinations, or travel history?**

    Fluctuating weakness with diurnal variation that has been present for weeks or months is characteristic of myasthenia gravis. Progressive ascending paralysis over hours to days is suggestive of GBS. A history of diarrhea 1 to 2 weeks prior to the onset of weakness has been classically described for GBS.

4. **Has the patient had difficulty swallowing or change in voice?**

    Dysphagia (coughing or choking after swallowing), dysarthria, and drooling are symptoms of bulbar muscle weakness. Affected patients are at risk for aspiration and should undergo formal swallow assessments (Table 16.1).

Orders

1. **Administer oxygen.**

    Oxygen can be administered via nasal cannula, face mask, high-flow nasal cannula, 100% nonrebreather mask, or noninvasive positive pressure ventilation (NIPPV). Reassess oxygen requirements on arrival at the bedside. Patients with suspected or diagnosed myasthenia gravis could benefit from NIPPV such as bilevel positive airway pressure (BiPAP), but for patients with GBS, NIPPV is not recommended because they are likely to worsen and require intubation for a few days or weeks prior to any improvement in neuromuscular respiratory failure.

2. **Perform a focused clinical exam. Look for any signs of respiratory distress, hypotension, any arrhythmias.**

    On your systemic exam look for any signs of infection, auscultate the lungs for any signs of aspiration pneumonia/

TABLE 16.1	Respiratory Muscle Groups and Clinical Symptoms and Signs in Patients With Acute Neuromuscular Dysfunction
Muscle Group	**Clinical Symptoms and Signs**
Inspiratory	Dyspnea, tachypnea, hypoxia
Inspiratory muscles	Paradoxical breathing, neck flexion/neck extension weakness
Bulbar	Dysphagia, dysarthria, weak mastication, facial weakness, nasal speech, lingual weakness
Expiratory muscles	Ineffective cough
All	Hypoventilation, hypoxemia, hypercarbia
Accessory muscles	Unlike patients with other causes of respiratory failure, accessory muscles will be weak so flaring of nostrils, retractions of chest wall, etc. may not be that obvious

pneumonitis and skin for any rashes. On your neurologic exam, focus on eliciting muscle strength, cranial nerve deficits, and any sensory signs. Check a single breath count (ask the patient to take a deep breath and count as far as possible starting from one in a single breath), and check neck flexion and extension strength. The strength of the neck flexors and extensors that are innervated by nerve roots C3-C5 are a good surrogate for diaphragmatic strength.

3. **Perform bedside pulmonary function tests.**
   - *Vital capacity (VC)* is the maximal exhaled volume after full inspiration and is normally 60 mL/kg (approximately 4 L in a 70-kg person). Patients generally require intubation when VC falls below 40 mL/kg.
   - *Peak inspiratory pressure or negative inspiratory force (NIF)* (normally greater than -50 cm H_2O) measures the force of inhalation generated by contraction of the diaphragm and is an index of the ability to maintain lung expansion and avoid atelectasis.
   - *Peak expiratory pressure (PEF)* (normally greater than 60 cm H_2O) correlates with the strength of cough and the ability to clear secretions from the airway.

     A good guide for determining which patients are at risk of impending respiratory failure is NIF < -20 cm H_2O, PEF < 30 cm H_2O, and/or VC < 40 cc/kg. However, for patients with facial diplegia, these bedside PFTs may not be accurate because of the lack of a good seal. Trends in these numbers are more helpful than isolated values alone (Box 16.1).

4. **Measure arterial blood gas levels on room air.**
     Patients with neuromuscular respiratory failure will develop hypercarbia and hypoxia only late in the course of their

---

BOX 16.1	Signs of Impending Respiratory Failure

Clinical
1. Single Breath count <13 (out of 20)
2. Neck flexion/extension weakness
3. Use of accessory muscles of respiration
4. Hypoxemia (late sign)
5. Acute hypercarbia (late sign)

Pulmonary Function Testing
1. NIF < -20 cm H_2O
2. MEF < 30 cm H_2O
3. Forced vital capacity < 40 cc/kg

MEF, Maximum expiratory flow; *NIF,* negative inspiratory force.

respiratory failure. Worsening trends in PFTs, single breath count, neck flexion/extension, and subjective dyspnea will help identify patients with impending respiratory failure before the development of hypercarbia or hypoxia. *Hypercarbia* (P_{CO_2} greater than 45 mm Hg) results from alveolar hypoventilation. *Hypoxia* (P_{O_2} less than 60 mm Hg) is indicative of impaired ventilation-perfusion matching and in this setting is usually related to atelectasis or pneumonia.

5. **Obtain a chest radiograph and, if available, assess lungs with point-of-care ultrasonography (POCUS) if possible.**
6. **The patient should eat nothing by mouth (NPO).**
7. **Insert two peripheral intravenous (IV) lines.**

   IV access should be established in anticipation of acute deterioration.

ELEVATOR THOUGHTS

What can cause generalized weakness leading to respiratory failure?

An anatomic approach is the most useful way to classify causes of generalized weakness. Further discussion of many of the entities listed here can be found later in this chapter.

1. **Spinal cord lesion**
   - Cervical cord compression
   - Transverse myelitis
2. **Motor neuron lesion**
   - Amyotrophic lateral sclerosis
   - Polio
3. **Peripheral nerve lesion**
   - GBS (acute inflammatory polyneuropathy) and variants
   - Chronic inflammatory demyelinating polyneuropathy
   - Postdiphtheritic polyneuropathy
   - AIDS related
   - Demyelinating polyneuropathy
   - Toxic neuropathy (lead, arsenic, hexacarbons, dapsone, nitrofurantoin)
   - Lyme disease
   - Tick paralysis
   - Critical illness polyneuropathy
   - Acute intermittent porphyria
4. **Neuromuscular junction lesion**
   - Myasthenia gravis
   - Lambert-Eaton syndrome
   - Botulism
   - Organophosphate poisoning

5. **Muscle lesion**
   - Polymyositis or dermatomyositis
   - Critical illness myopathy
   - Hyperthyroid myopathy
   - Mitochondrial myopathy
   - Acid maltase deficiency (Pompe disease)
   - Periodic paralysis (hyperkalemic or hypokalemic)
   - Congenital myopathy (muscular dystrophy)

MAJOR THREAT TO LIFE

These patients should be monitored continuously on telemetry.
- **Hypoxia** ($Pao_2 < 60$ mm Hg)
- **Hypercarbic respiratory acidosis** with pH < 7.2.
- **Arrhythmias** caused by autonomic dysfunction.

BEDSIDE

Quick-Look Test

Does the patient look well (comfortable), sick (uncomfortable), or critical (about to die)?

Agitation, diaphoresis, difficulty finishing sentences, accessory respiratory muscle contraction, and rapid or labored breathing may signal impending respiratory failure.

Airway and Vital Signs

Is the upper airway clear?

Weakness of the tongue and oropharyngeal muscles can lead to upper airway obstruction, which increases resistance to airflow and the work of breathing. *Stridor* is indicative of potentially life-threatening upper airway obstruction.

Weakness of the laryngeal and glottic muscles can lead to impaired swallowing and aspiration of secretions. A *wet, gurgled voice* and *pooled oropharyngeal secretions* are the best clinical signs of significant dysphagia.

What is the respiratory rate?

Check for *paradoxical respirations* (Fig. 16.1) (inward movement of the abdomen on inspiration), which is indicative of diaphragmatic paralysis.

What is the heart rate and blood pressure (BP)?

Sinus tachycardia, hypertension, or BP lability can result from dysautonomia in GBS.

What is the temperature?

Fever or hypothermia can occur because of an obvious or occult source of infection.

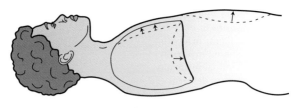

Normal inspiration

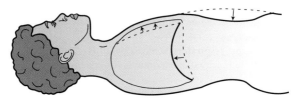

Paradoxical respiration

FIG. 16.1 Paradoxical respirations.

Selective History

To make the diagnosis, it is important to establish the time course and distribution of weakness (Table 16.2). Key questions to keep in mind when obtaining a history in patients with generalized weakness include the following: (1) Is a spinal cord lesion a possibility? (2) Is the process purely motor or is sensation involved? (3) Is the patient at risk for sudden respiratory failure?

1. **When did the weakness develop?**

    Early symptoms of weakness can be subtle. Ask about difficulty arising from a chair, climbing stairs, lifting packages, combing or brushing hair, or turning keys or doorknobs.

2. **Was there an antecedent illness?**

    Approximately 70% of cases of GBS are triggered by an antecedent viral illness or *Campylobacter jejuni* gastroenteritis. Respiratory crisis in myasthenia gravis is triggered by infection in approximately 40% of patients.

3. **Does the weakness fluctuate?**

    Fluctuating weakness (on an hourly basis) is almost pathognomonic for myasthenia gravis.

4. **Has there been any blurred or double vision?**

    Blurred vision occurs with botulism.

5. **Has there been any neck or back pain?**

    Neck pain should raise suspicion for a cervical cord lesion. Low backache occurs frequently with GBS.

TABLE 16.2	Key Aspects of History and Physical Exam in Neuromuscular Dysfunction

History and Physical	
History and collateral info	Etiology, risk factors
	Medication compliance, any follow-ups with other neurologists
	Bulbar function, autonomic dysfunction, visual symptoms
	Travel history, vaccination, sick contacts
	Any advanced directives
Timing and progression	Acute, subacute, chronic
	Progressive
	Ascending/descending
ABC's	Assess for stability
Systemic exam	Concomitant pulmonary diagnosis, for example: aspiration pneumonia or pneumonitis, OSA, COPD, etc.
	Previous signs of NM disease
	Signs of infection
	Skin: rash, insect bite, vaccination

ABC, Airway breathing and circulation; *COPD,* chronic obstructive pulmonary disease; *NM,* neuromuscular; *OSA,* obstructive sleep apnea.

6. **Has there been any numbness or tingling?**
   Distal paresthesias are common in GBS.
7. **Have there been any muscle aches, cramps, or tenderness?**
   Aching and tenderness generally occur with myopathy. Cramps can occur with motor neuron disease or with severe electrolyte derangements.
8. **Has there been any exposure to toxins or insecticides?**
   Organophosphate is the most common toxin that can lead to respiratory failure.

Selective Physical Examination

Once the patient has been stabilized, the goal is to identify signs of airway or respiratory compromise and to search for clues to the diagnosis.

General Physical Examination

- **Head, ears, eyes, nose, and throat (HEENT):**
Oropharynx: Check for *pooled secretions,* which are diagnostic of impaired swallowing and ability to handle secretions. *Exudative pharyngitis* occurs with diphtheria.
  - **Swallow test:** Give the patient a small amount (3 ounces) of water to drink. Coughing after swallowing is diagnostic of aspiration.

- **Speech:** Check for *dysphonia.* A nasal voice results from palatal paralysis. A soft, strangulated voice results from vocal cord paralysis. Evaluate *dysarthria* by checking the buccal (ma, ma), lingual (la, la), and pharyngeal (ga, ga) components of articulation.
- **Respiratory**

Lungs: Auscultate for wheezes, rales, rhonchi, or consolidation.

- **Diaphragm:** Palpate for normal, outward abdominal movement during inspiration.
- **Cough:** Check the strength of the patient's cough.
- **Ventilatory reserve:** Ask the patient to inhale fully and count from 1 to 20. A patient with adequate ventilatory reserve should be able to do this in a single breath.
- **Skin**

Rashes: Check for a rash (Lyme disease, dermatomyositis).

Neurologic Examination

- **Pupils:** Pupillary reactivity may be lost with botulism or in the Miller-Fisher variant of GBS (triad of ophthalmoplegia, ataxia, and areflexia).
- **Extraocular muscles:** *Ptosis and ocular muscle weakness* is characteristic of myasthenia gravis but can occur with the Miller-Fisher variant of GBS, botulism, diphtheria, polymyositis, Graves disease, mitochondrial myopathy, or critical illness myopathy.
- **Face, palate, tongue, and neck strength**
- **Limb strength**
- **Fasciculations:** Fasciculations are seen with motor neuron disease or organophosphate poisoning.
- **Reflexes:** *Areflexia* is **always** seen with GBS.
- **Coordination:** Ataxia occurs with the Miller-Fisher variant of GBS.
- **Sensation:** A cervical or upper thoracic *sensory level* associated with quadriparesis suggests a cervical cord lesion. Mild sensory loss in the distal extremities is common in GBS.

MANAGEMENT

Airway Management and Mechanical Ventilation

A plan should be verbalized because these patients often are managed by multidisciplinary teams. The threshold for intubation including the induction medications, whether paralytics should be used or not, and if all the equipment and medications needed should be readily available (Box 16.2). Whether a patient may benefit from a trial of NIPPV should be determined based on patient characteristics and the anticipated trajectory of recovery from acute neuromuscular dysfunction (Box 16.3).

BOX 16.2	Key Principles of Critical Care Management

1. Recognize: Pitfalls in identifying NM weakness
2. Monitor: Transfer patient to appropriate settings, neuro checks, PFTs
3. Determine thresholds: Intubation, extubation, tracheostomy, hospice/palliative care
4. Treat: Underlying disease, secondary neurologic complications like respiratory failure, systemic complications
5. Prognosticate: Review/address goals of care

NM, neuromuscular; *PFT*, pulmonary function testing.

BOX 16.3	Suggested Criteria for Noninvasive Ventilation

1. BiPAP can be used in patients who are awake, alert with minimal secretions
2. BiPAP can be used in patients with a known neuromuscular diagnosis such as myasthenia gravis or ALS
3. BiPAP should not be used in patients with undifferentiated neuromuscular respiratory failure or in GBS and its variants

ALS, Amyotrophic lateral sclerosis; *BiPAP*, bilevel positive airway pressure; *GBS*, Guillain-Barré syndrome.

Criteria for Intubation

A number of factors must be considered when deciding when to intubate and ventilate (Box 16.4). The most important factor, perhaps, is the overall comfort level and any a priori discussions about code status or goals of care. Preventing crash intubations is extremely important.

Remember that conservative, early intubation and institution of positive-pressure ventilation can minimize the development of atelectasis and pneumonia and may lead to earlier extubation. Crash intubations are associated with worse outcomes in GBS patients.

BOX 16.4	Suggested Absolute Criteria for Intubation

1. Hypercarbia pH < 7.3
2. O_2 saturation $< 92\%$
3. Usual indications for intubation
4. PFTs: NIF < -10 cm H_2O, VC < 20 cc/kg
5. Severe dyspnea (subjective) or excess work of breathing (objective)
6. Delirium or confusion
7. Severe oropharyngeal paresis with inability to protect the airway

NIF, Negative inspiratory force; *PFT*, pulmonary function testing; *VC*, vital capacity.

Initial Ventilator Management

The initial goals of ventilator management immediately after intubation are (1) to provide rest and (2) to promote lung expansion. These goals are best accomplished using IV sedation and *assist control volume control (ACVC)* at a rate of 12 to 14 breaths/min, using tidal volumes of about 8 mL/kg ideal body weight (IBW). *Positive end-expiratory pressure (PEEP)* aids in the expansion of collapsed alveoli and should be used in all patients at levels of 5 to 15 cm H_2O. Use of higher tidal volumes and generous application of PEEP is acceptable as long as peak airway pressures are <30 cm H_2O, and it may be beneficial for promoting lung expansion.

Patients with long-standing weakness and CO_2 retention should be intentionally hypoventilated (P_{CO_2} at or higher than 45 mm Hg). Normal or reduced P_{CO_2} levels will result in alkalosis and renal serum bicarbonate wasting, which in turn will make it more difficult to successfully wean the patient.

Bronchoscopy

Fiberoptic bronchoscopy for pulmonary toilet should be performed aggressively in patients with hypoxia, severe atelectasis, or lobar collapse because of mucus plugging.

Tracheostomy

After the patient has been on mechanical ventilation for approximately 7 days, tracheostomy should be discussed and performed (Box 16.4). Compared with prolonged endotracheal intubation, tracheostomy (1) is more comfortable, (2) poses less risk of permanent laryngeal or tracheal injury, (3) facilitates weaning from mechanical ventilation by reducing dead space and airway resistance, (4) makes it easier to clear airway secretions by cough or suctioning, and (5) promotes early mobilization. Early tracheostomy within the first week of intubation is reasonable in patients who have severe weakness and clear risk factors for a prolonged course of mechanical ventilation (Table 16.3).

Weaning to Extubation

For patients who were intubated primarily because of neuromuscular respiratory failure, after starting them on definitive treatment, it might be worthwhile to continue pressure support trials on pressure support of 8 to 15 cm H_2O to prevent respiratory muscle atrophy and ventilator-induced diaphragmatic dysfunction. Prior to initiating pressure support trails, confirm that the patient is not hemodynamically unstable, hypoxic, or hypercarbic.

TABLE 16.3	Risk Factors for Prolonged (>2 Weeks) Ventilator Dependence in Patients With Neuromuscular Respiratory Failure

- Age > 50 years
- Failure to tolerate >12 hours of CPAP with pressure support 5 cm H_2O
- Vital capacity fails to exceed 25 mL/kg within 6 days of intubation
- Preintubation serum bicarbonate ≥30 mg/dL (compensated chronic respiratory acidosis)
- Preexisting lung disease

Continuous positive airway pressure (CPAP) with pressure support is the preferred mode for weaning patients with respiratory muscle weakness. Each time the patient inhales, "pressure support" delivers additional inspiratory volume until a preset level of pressure is reached. The amount of inspiratory pressure support given (range, 5–15 cm H_2O) should be initially adjusted to attain tidal volumes of approximately 300 to 500 mL in an adult.

Extubation can be performed once the patient has demonstrated the ability to tolerate at least a few hours of CPAP with pressure support equal to 5 to 10 cm H_2O without fatigue. Fluctuating PFTs, excessive secretions, or concurrent medical problems (i.e., infection or cardiovascular instability) are relative contraindications to extubation. Consider extubation to NIPPV support, such as BiPAP or high-flow nasal canula, to provide additional support in the immediate periextubation period (Box 16.5).

General Care of the Patient With Neuromuscular Respiratory Failure

1. **Elevate the head of the bed**

   With diaphragmatic weakness, lung volumes become diminished and work of breathing increases in the supine

BOX 16.5	Suggested Criteria for Extubation and Tracheostomy

Suggested Criteria for Extubation
1. Clinical Improvement
2. Improvement in PFTs
3. Usual parameters for extubation met

Suggested Criteria for Tracheostomy
1. In line with patient's goals of care
2. Difficulty weaning from ventilator by 7–10 days
3. Based on underlying disease process and overall prognostication

PFT, Pulmonary function testing.

position. Head elevation also reduces the risk of ventilator-associated pneumonia.

2. **Chest physical therapy**

Chest percussion and airway suctioning are essential for preventing mucus plugs and aiding in the clearing of secretions. Prescribe *incentive spirometry* every 6 hours if the patient is not intubated.

3. **Serial measurements of VC**

VC should be checked every 4 to 6 hours in nonintubated patients and every 12 to 24 hours in intubated patients.

4. **Prophylaxis for deep vein thrombosis (DVT)**

In addition to dynamic compression stockings, order **enoxaparin 40 mg subcutaneously (SC) once daily** or **heparin 5000 U SC every 12 hours**.

5. **Nutrition**

Patients with bulbar weakness should be made NPO and fed via a *small-bore nasogastric tube.*

6. **Fluids and electrolytes**

Hypokalemia and *hypophosphatemia* can exacerbate muscle weakness and should be periodically checked for and treated.

7. **Bowel and bladder care**

Paralysis predisposes to constipation and can be prevented with **docusate sodium (Colace) 100 mg three times a day and milk of magnesia 30 mL every night.** Intermittent straight catheterization carries a lower risk of infection than an indwelling Foley catheter.

Specific Disorders

GUILLAIN-BARRÉ SYNDROME

GBS is a monophasic, acute inflammatory demyelinating polyneuropathy. The etiology is related to an autoimmune attack directed against surface antigens on peripheral nerves, resulting in focal segmental demyelination (Box 16.6).

ONSET

In approximately 70% of cases, the syndrome follows a respiratory or gastrointestinal infection by 5 days to 3 weeks. Viral upper respiratory infection and *C. jejuni* gastroenteritis are the most common precipitating infections. Other causes include HIV infection, immunization, pregnancy, Hodgkin disease, and surgery.

CLINICAL FEATURES

The syndrome usually begins with rapidly progressive ascending paralysis, associated with cranial nerve and respiratory muscle weakness, loss of deep tendon reflexes, and distal paresthesias and sensory loss. Unlike other neuropathies, proximal muscles are often

BOX 16.6	Checklist for the Management of Guillain-Barré Syndrome

1. *Diagnostic workup:* Lumbar puncture, electromyography/nerve conduction studies, hepatitis and Lyme disease serologies, CMV, EBV, HSV, and HIV titers, urine porphyrin levels, urine heavy metal screen, stool analysis for *Campylobacter*

2. *Pain management:* Pain can be severe and may result from meningeal inflammation or neuropathic mechanisms; NSAIDs (ketorolac 30 mg IM every 6 h), opioids (morphine 2–10 mg every 2–4 h as needed), or medications such as gabapentin (start with 100 mg via nasogastric tube or orally TID and increase as tolerated)

3. *Dysautonomia:* The most frequent cardiovascular manifestation of dysautonomia is sustained hypertension and tachycardia; treatment with beta-blockers (propranolol PO 10–40 mg every 6 h or labetalol infusion or calcium channel blocker infusion such as nicardipine or clevidipine) may be desirable in older patients with coronary artery disease

CMV, Cytomegalovirus; *EBV*, Epstein-Barr virus; *HSV*, herpes simplex virus; *IM*, intramuscularly; *NSAID*, nonsteroidal antiinflammatory drug; *PO*, by mouth; *TID*, three times a day.

affected more than distal muscles. The weakness progresses over 7 to 21 days; the median duration from onset to maximal weakness is 12 days. Respiratory failure requiring intubation occurs in 20% of patients. Papilledema, autonomic disturbances (e.g., hypertension, hypotension, urinary retention, sinus tachycardia, cardiac arrhythmias), and syndrome of inappropriate antidiuretic hormone (SIADH) are seen in some patients.

LABORATORY DATA

The cerebrospinal fluid (CSF) classically shows dissociation between albumin levels and cytologic findings, with elevated protein levels and normal white blood cell counts (5 cells/μL or fewer). The elevation in the protein level can sometimes take up to 2 weeks to develop. A mild lymphocytic or monocytic pleocytosis is sometimes seen (10–100 cells/mm^3) and should raise suspicion for an infectious polyradiculopathy (e.g., HIV, cytomegalovirus [CMV], West Nile virus, or Lyme disease) or poliomyelitis. Nerve conduction studies show loss of F waves and reduced conduction velocities. Reduced motor fiber amplitudes reflect secondary axonal damage and imply a worse prognosis for recovery.

TREATMENT

Patients with signs of respiratory muscle weakness should be admitted to an intensive care unit (ICU) for observation until it is clear that the illness has stabilized. **Plasmapheresis,** when initiated within

10 days of the onset of symptoms, can speed the onset of recovery. A total of five treatments are performed every 1 to 2 days, with a total of 2 to 4 L of plasma exchanged for 5% albumin during each treatment. High-dose **IV immunoglobulin (IVIG), 0.4 g/kg/day for 5 consecutive days,** has been shown to be as effective as plasmapheresis and may be slightly superior. Rebound deterioration after completing a course of IVIG can sometimes occur. The management of pain and dysautonomia is discussed in Box 16.7.

PROGNOSIS

Features shown to have a poor prognosis in GBS include (1) advanced age, (2) very low distal motor amplitudes, (3) rapidly progressive weakness occurring over the first week, (4) respiratory failure requiring intubation, and (5) axonal rather than demyelinating features on electromyography (EMG)/nerve conduction velocity (NCV) studies.

MYASTHENIA GRAVIS

Myasthenia gravis is caused by an antibody-mediated attack on nicotinic acetylcholine receptors, resulting in a defect in neuromuscular transmission. This phenomenon manifests clinically as *fluctuating weakness* and *muscle fatigability,* which are the hallmarks of myasthenia gravis.

CLINICAL FEATURES

Fluctuating weakness is typical of myasthenia gravis; it tends to involve the eyes (in 90% of patients); face, neck, and oropharynx (in 80% of patients); and limbs (in 60% of patients). The age distribution at onset is bimodal, with an early peak between ages 20 and 40 (primarily in women) and a later peak between ages 50 and 80 (in both sexes). The limbs are almost never affected in isolation. Sensation is always normal, and reflexes are preserved unless the muscle is plegic. Most patients reach the maximum severity of their disease within the first 1 to 2 years; thereafter, spontaneous remission is common (in approximately 30% of patients), and the disease process tends to become less severe. *Malignant thymoma* is present in approximately 15% of patients with myasthenia and is associated with more severe disease.

Myasthenic crisis is defined by respiratory failure requiring intubation and mechanical ventilation (Box 16.7). Crisis is most often provoked by infection (in 40% of patients) but can also occur spontaneously (in 30% of patients) or result from aspiration, surgery, pregnancy, medications, or emotional upset. Approximately 25% of patients can be extubated within 1 week, 50% within 2 weeks,

BOX 16.7	Checklist for the Management of Myasthenic Crisis

1. Eliminate and avoid all contraindicated medications (see Table 16.4).
2. *Diagnostic workup:* Edrophonium test, acetylcholine receptor antibody level, repetitive nerve stimulation, single-fiber EMG, thyroid function tests, chest CT scan.
3. *Treatment:* Anticholinesterase medications should be *discontinued* while patients are mechanically ventilated because they lead to excessive secretions (see Table 16.5). A course of plasmapheresis or IVIG is indicated in all patients.

CT, Computed tomography; *EMG*, electromyography, *IVIG*, intravenous immunoglobulin.

TABLE 16.4	Drugs That Can Exacerbate Weakness in Myasthenia Gravis

Antibiotics	Neuromuscular junction blockers
Aminoglycosides (gentamicin, streptomycin, others)	(vecuronium, rocuronium, succinylcholine)
Peptide antibodies (polymyxin B, colistin)	Quinine
Tetracyclines (tetracycline, doxycycline, others)	Steroids
Erythromycin	Lithium
Clindamycin	Magnesium toxicity
Ciprofloxacin	Verapamil
Ampicillin	Thyroid hormones (thyroxine, levothyroxine, others)
Antiarrhythmics	Beta-blockers (propranolol, timolol, others)
Quinidine	Chloroquine
Procainamide	Phenytoin
Lidocaine	Penicillamine (induces autoimmune myasthenia gravis)

and 75% within 1 month. One-third of patients intubated for crisis will proceed to experience a second crisis. Although a crisis is by definition is life-threatening, with modern ICU management, death (approximately 5% mortality rate) results only from overwhelming medical complications (e.g., myocardial infarction, sepsis).

LABORATORY DATA

The diagnosis of myasthenia gravis can be established with the following tests:

1. *Edrophonium (Tensilon) testing* reveals transient improvement in patients with ocular and facial weakness. **Edrophonium**

10 mg is used in adults; infuse 2 mg initially and observe for severe cholinergic muscarinic effects such as nausea, bradycardia, and hypotension. **Atropine 0.4 mg** should be kept at the bedside and can be used to reverse these symptoms. If there are no severe effects, inject the remaining 8 mg of edrophonium and observe for improvement, which generally occurs within 2 to 10 minutes.

2. *Repetitive nerve stimulation* at 2 to 3 Hz characteristically produces a greater than 10% decrement in amplitude between the first and fifth compound muscle action potential. Sensitivity and specificity are 90% when weak, proximal muscles are tested; however, sensitivity falls to less than 50% in myasthenic patients without limb weakness.

3. *Single-fiber EMG* reveals "jitter," which is variation in the time interval between firing of muscle fibers in the same motor unit. Single-fiber EMG is highly sensitive (sensitivity greater than 95%) for myasthenia gravis but is not specific.

4. *Acetylcholine receptor antibodies* are present in approximately 80% of patients with generalized myasthenia but in only 50% of patients with ocular myasthenia. Titers do not correlate with the severity of illness.

5. *Anti-MuSK (muscle-specific tyrosine kinase) antibodies* are present in half of patients who lack acetylcholine-receptor antibodies. Anti-MuSK–positive patients tend to be female, with predominant neck and oropharyngeal weakness. They respond variably to acetylcholinesterase inhibitors and do not tend to respond to thymectomy, but they usually improve after plasmapheresis.

TREATMENT

Therapeutic options for treating myasthenia gravis can be divided into three categories: *symptomatic therapy* (with acetylcholinesterase inhibitors), *short-term disease suppression* (with plasmapheresis and IVIG), and *long-term immunosuppression* (with thymectomy, steroids, or chemotherapy).

Symptomatic therapy: Acetylcholinesterase inhibitors (Table 16.5) improve myasthenic weakness by allowing acetylcholine to accumulate at the neuromuscular junction. **Pyridostigmine (Mestinon) is started at 30 mg by mouth (PO) three times a day, increased to 60 to 120 mg every 4 to 6 hours as a maintenance dose, and increased to 120 mg every 3 hours as a maximal dose.** A long-acting 180-mg tablet (Mestinon Timespan) can be given at bedtime for patients with nocturnal or morning weakness. Excessive muscarinic side effects (e.g., pulmonary secretions, diarrhea) can be controlled by concurrently giving an antimuscarinic agent such as **glycopyrrolate**

TABLE 16.5	Anticholinesterase Drugs Used for Myasthenia Gravis				
	Route	Equivalent Dosage	Onset	Maximal Response	Dosage Range
Pyridostigmine bromide (Mestinon)	PO[a]	60 mg	30–60 min	1–2 h	30–120 mg every 3–8 h
Pyridostigmine long-acting	IM, IV[b]	2 mg	5–10 mins	20–30 min	—
Mestinon Timespan	PO	—	3–5 h	3–5 h	180 mg/day at night
Neostigmine bromide (Prostigmin)	PO	15 mg	30 min	1 h	15–30 mg every 2–3 h
Neostigmine methylsulfate (Prostigmin injectable)	IV[b]	0.5 mg	1–2 min	20 min	0.5–1 mg every 2 h
	IM	1.5 mg	30 min	1 h	1.5–3 mg every 2–3 h

[a]Can be given as a tablet or as a liquid.
[b]Equivalent intravenous dose of pyridostigmine or neostigmine is $\frac{1}{30}$ of the oral dose.
IM, Intramuscularly; *IV*, intravenously; *PO*, by mouth

(Robinul) 1 to 2 mg PO three times a day or **propantheline bromide (Pro-Banthine) 15 mg PO four times a day.**

Short-term disease suppression: This is indicated to hasten clinical improvement in hospitalized patients. **Plasmapheresis (five exchanges of 2–4 L every 1–2 days)** can lead to improvement within days, but the effect is short-lived, lasting only 2 to 4 weeks. Similar benefits have been reported in 70% of patients treated with **IVIG (0.4 g/kg daily for 5 days),** but experience with this therapy remains limited.

Long-term immunosuppression: This treatment is indicated when weakness is inadequately controlled with anticholinesterase medications. **Prednisone** is most commonly prescribed; to use the lowest dose possible, start with **15 to 20 mg/day** and gradually increase to **40 to 100 mg/day over 4 to 8 weeks** until an adequate response is achieved. Temporary worsening of symptoms within the first 2 weeks of starting steroids can be expected in up to 40% of patients. **Azathioprine 1 to 2 mg/kg PO per day** can also be used for long-term immunosuppression in patients who cannot tolerate the side effects of steroids. **Thymectomy** leads to disease remission in 40% of patients and clinical improvement in another 40%, but these benefits can take months or years to occur. Thymectomy is indicated in any patient between the ages of 15 and 60 with thymoma or with generalized myasthenia.

UNCOMMON CAUSES OF PARALYSIS AND RESPIRATORY FAILURE

Botulism

Botulism is caused by an exotoxin produced by *Clostridium botulinum,* which is an anaerobic, gram-positive, spore-forming rod that contaminates food. Weakness occurs because the toxin is a potent inhibitor of presynaptic acetylcholine release. Clinical symptoms begin within 12 to 24 hours of ingestion and are characterized by gastrointestinal complaints, dilated and nonreactive pupils, blurred vision, and weakness that begins with the extraocular and oropharyngeal muscles before becoming generalized. Urinary retention, dry mouth, and anhidrosis may also occur. **Botulism trivalent antitoxin** (Table 16.5) (one vial IV and one vial intramuscularly [IM] every 2–4 hours) should be given as soon as possible. Guanidine hydrochloride (40 mg PO every 4 hours) is an acetylcholine agonist that can counteract the presynaptic blockade caused by the toxin. The Centers for Disease Control and Prevention(CDC) has guidance on sample testing and treatment for botulism (see https://www.cdc.gov/botulism/botulism-specimen.html).

Poliomyelitis

Poliovirus is an enterovirus that can cause selective destruction of motor neurons in the spinal cord and brain stem, resulting in *flaccid, areflexic paralysis.* Modern vaccination has made the disease a clinical rarity. Acute paralysis from poliomyelitis is differentiated from that caused by GBS by the presence of headache, high fever, mental status changes, asymmetric weakness, and neutrophils in the CSF.

Acute Flaccid Myelitis

The CDC has been investigating AFM cases since October 2014. None of these cases tested positive for the polio virus. The CDC has detected coxsackievirus A16, Enterovirus EV-A71, and EV-D68 in the CSF of 4 of 558 confirmed cases of AFM since 2014. For all other patients, no pathogen (germ) has been detected in their spinal fluid to confirm a cause. Most AFM cases are children (over 90%) and have occurred in 48 states and Washington, DC. For more information, see https://www.cdc.gov/acute-flaccid-myelitis/afm-surveillance.html.

Tetanus

Tetanus results from an exotoxin produced by *C. tetani,* which is an anaerobic gram-positive coccus that can infect soft-tissue wounds. The toxin results in neuronal hyperexcitability, which can cause seizures, autonomic instability, and sustained "tetanic" muscle contractions involving the jaw ("lockjaw"), neck, back, and respiratory muscles. Treatment is directed toward (1) airway management and ventilation and administration of neuromuscular blocking agents, (2) neutralizing the toxin with intramuscular or intrathecal **tetanus immunoglobulin 250 U (single dose),** and (3) eradicating the soft-tissue infection with **procaine penicillin 1.2 million U every 6 hours for 10 days.**

Syncope

Syncope is brief loss of consciousness caused by a sudden reduction of cerebral blood flow. Patients will often use the words "fainting" or "passing out" to describe a syncopal event. *Presyncope* refers to the sensation of impending loss of consciousness, but the patient does not actually pass out. Presyncope and syncope represent varying degrees of the same disorder and should be addressed as manifestations of the same underlying problem. Your task is to confirm that the event was syncope and to discover the cause of the syncopal attack.

PHONE CALL

Questions

1. **Did the patient actually lose consciousness?**
   Ask if the patient was unresponsive and whether the patient remembers the event.
2. **Is the patient still unconscious?**
   If so, this is coma (see Chapter 5) until proven otherwise.
3. What **are the vital signs?**
   Bradycardia suggests a vasovagal event.
4. Was **the patient standing, sitting, or lying down when the attack occurred?**
   Syncope in the recumbent position is almost always cardiac in origin. Syncope that occurs immediately after standing up suggests orthostatic hypotension.
5. **Was there any witnessed shaking or stiffness?**
   Brief involuntary movement such as shaking or stiffness lasting 5 to 10 seconds can be seen in syncope (also known as "convulsive syncope"), but involuntary movements lasting longer than 30 seconds are more suggestive of seizure.
6. **Did the patient sustain any injury from the fall?**
   Serious injury is more characteristic of cardiac syncope or seizure (Fig. 17.1).

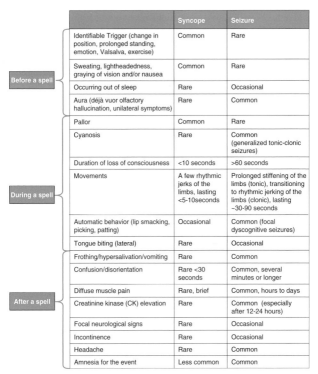

	Syncope	Seizure
Before a spell		
Identifiable Trigger (change in position, prolonged standing, emotion, Valsalva, exercise)	Common	Rare
Sweating, lightheadedness, graying of vision and/or nausea	Common	Rare
Occurring out of sleep	Rare	Occasional
Aura (déjà vuor olfactory hallucination, unilateral symptoms)	Rare	Common
During a spell		
Pallor	Common	Rare
Cyanosis	Rare	Common (generalized tonic-clonic seizures)
Duration of loss of consciousness	<10 seconds	>60 seconds
Movements	A few rhythmic jerks of the limbs, lasting <5-10seconds	Prolonged stiffening of the limbs (tonic), transitioning to rhythmic jerking of the limbs (clonic), lasting ~30-90 seconds
Automatic behavior (lip smacking, picking, patting)	Occasional	Common (focal dyscognitive seizures)
Tongue biting (lateral)	Rare	Occasional
After a spell		
Frothing/hypersalivation/vomiting	Rare	Common
Confusion/disorientation	Rare <30 seconds	Common, several minutes or longer
Diffuse muscle pain	Rare, brief	Common, hours to days
Creatinine kinase (CK) elevation	Rare	Common (especially after 12-24 hours)
Focal neurological signs	Rare	Occasional
Incontinence	Rare	Occasional
Headache	Rare	Common
Amnesia for the event	Less common	Common

FIG. 17.1 **Clinical features distinguishing syncope from seizure.**

Orders

If the patient is still unconscious, give the following orders:

1. Administer intravenous (IV) D5W to keep the vein open (KVO) if IV is not already in place.
2. Turn the patient onto the left side (this maneuver minimizes the risk of upper airway obstruction and aspiration).
3. Order a stat 12-lead electrocardiogram (ECG) and rhythm strip.
4. Obtain a finger-stick glucose level.

If the patient has regained consciousness, if there is no evidence of head or neck injury, and if the vital signs are stable, do the following:

1. Instruct the registered nurse (RN) to keep the patient supine for at least 10 to 15 minutes, until the patient feels comfortable and is fully aware and oriented. To return the patient to bed, slowly

raise the patient to the sitting position, and then to a standing position.
2. Have the RN check orthostatic vital signs (blood pressure [BP] and heart rate with the patient lying down and standing).
3. Order an ECG and rhythm strip.
4. Have vital signs taken every 15 minutes until you arrive at the bedside. Instruct the RN to call you back immediately if the patient becomes unstable before you are able to perform your assessment.

ELEVATOR THOUGHTS

Is this syncope?

The main differential diagnosis is seizure versus syncope, the proverbial "fit" versus "faint." Accordingly, your initial evaluation should first focus on determining if this event was syncopal in nature. See Table 17.1 for features distinguishing seizure from syncope.

What causes syncope?

A comprehensive list of the causes of syncope and the approximate relative frequency of each of the main categories in an emergency room (ER) population are given here. In the majority of patients (90%), syncope results from a transient drop in systemic BP and can be explained on the basis of vasovagal syncope (most common cause of syncope in young people), cardiac disease, orthostatic hypotension, or medications.

1. **Reflex vasodilation (60% of ER patients)**
   A. Vasovagal or neurocardiogenic syncope
   B. Situational syncope (micturition, defecation, cough)
   C. Carotid sinus syncope

TABLE 17.1	Symptoms Suggestive of a Specific Cause of Syncope
Symptom or Precipitating Factor	**Diagnosis to Be Considered**
Triggered by unpleasant stimulus (blood draw, sight of blood), preceded by lightheadedness, graying of vision	Vasovagal syncope
Occurs with micturition, defecation, or coughing	Situational syncope
Occurs with head turning/tight collar	Carotid sinus syncope
Occurs on standing	Orthostatic hypotension
Sudden loss of consciousness without prodrome	Cardiac arrythmia

Adapted from Kapoor WN. Syncope. *N Engl J Med.* 2000;343:1856.

2. **Cardiac causes (25% of ER patients)**
   A. Cardiac arrhythmias
      (1) Tachyarrhythmias (ventricular tachycardia, fibrillation)
      (2) Bradyarrhythmias (heart block, sick sinus syndrome)
   B. Cardiac outflow failure
      (1) Obstruction to left ventricular outflow (aortic stenosis, hypertrophic cardiomyopathy)
      (2) Obstruction to pulmonary outflow (pulmonary embolus)
      (3) Pump failure (myocardial infarction, tamponade)
3. **Orthostatic (postural) hypotension (10% of ER patients)**
   A. Volume depletion (anemia, dehydration)
   B. Drug induced (Table 17.2)
   C. Autonomic dysfunction
4. **Rare neurological causes (less than 5% of ER patients)**
   A. Vertebrobasilar stenosis/occlusion
   B. Subclavian steal syndrome
   C. Bilateral hemispheric ischemia from carotid artery stenosis or occlusion
   D. Increased intracranial pressure (subarachnoid hemorrhage, space-occupying lesion)

TABLE 17.2	Drugs and Medications That Can Cause Syncope

Antihypertensive Agents
Calcium channel blockers
Diuretics
Angiotensin-converting enzyme inhibitors
Beta-blockers
Others (hydralazine, prazosin)

Antiarrhythmic Agents (Long QT Syndrome, Torsades de Pointes)
Quinidine, procainamide, disopyramide
Sotalol
Dofetilide, ibutilide
Amiodarone
Flecainide, propafenone

Other Medications or Drugs
Tricyclic and tetracyclic antidepressants
Monoamine oxidase inhibitors
Phenothiazines (haloperidol, thioridazine)
Antineoplastic agents
Antianginal agents (ranolazine, ivabradine, nitrates)
HIV antiretrovirals (efavirenz, lopinavir, saquinavir)
Antifungal (fluconazole, itraconazole, ketoconazole)
Macrolide antibiotics (azithromycin, erythromycin, clarithromycin)
Levodopa
Digoxin
Ethanol
Marijuana
Methadone

5. **Psychiatric causes (less than 1% of ER patients)**
   A. Hyperventilation
   B. Conversion disorder (technically not syncope but mimics syncope)

MAJOR THREAT TO LIFE

- *Aspiration* is the main threat if the patient is still unconscious.
     Remember that syncope generally lasts only a few minutes. If the patient remains persistently unconscious (longer than 5 minutes), the diagnosis is coma, and your evaluation should proceed as outlined in Chapter 5.
- *Cardiac syncope* (*fatal cardiac arrhythmia or structural heart disease*) is potentially life-threatening, and it is imperative to consider this diagnosis in all cases of syncope.
     If a cardiac rhythm disturbance is suspected, then the patient should be attached to an ECG monitor, and consideration should be given to observing the patient in an intensive care unit (ICU). Other potentially life-threatening illnesses that can present with syncope include gastrointestinal (GI) bleeding, pulmonary embolism, aortic dissection, and myocardial infarction.

BEDSIDE

Quick-Look Test

Does the patient look well (comfortable), sick (uncomfortable), or critical (about to die)?

Most cases of syncope are brief (loss of consciousness less than 5 minutes), and most patients look well shortly after regaining consciousness. Others may appear mildly nauseated, pallid, and diaphoretic; these signs represent the systemic autonomic response to hypotension and should resolve rapidly.

Are there any external signs of head or neck trauma?

Significant head injury is unusual after syncope but should be checked for. In most cases, a period of presyncope warns the patient that something is amiss and allows him or her to avoid a hard fall. *Cardiac syncope often occurs without warning and is more likely to lead to traumatic injury.*

Airway and Vital Signs

Abnormal vital signs can help make your diagnosis of the specific cause of syncope much easier (Fig. 17.2).

Is the airway clear?

If the patient is still unconscious, ensure that he or she is lying on the left side and that respirations and oxygen saturation are adequate; treat this as coma until proven otherwise.

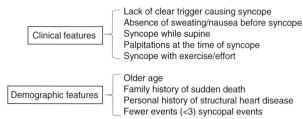

FIG. 17.2 **"Red flags" showing when to consider a diagnosis of cardiac syncope.**

What is the heart rate?

Supraventricular or ventricular tachycardia should be documented on ECG tracings. If the patient is hypotensive, call for a cardiac arrest team and treat immediately with electrical cardioversion.

Sinus bradycardia suggests vagally mediated vasodepressor syncope. In this case, both the heart rate and the BP should normalize quickly as the patient remains supine, and the patient should regain consciousness quickly.

What is the BP?

Persistently low BP or significant orthostatic hypotension combined with normal sinus rhythm or sinus tachycardia implicates volume depletion. Begin IV volume resuscitation with D5 normal saline (NS) and order a stat hematocrit. Rule out GI bleeding, ruptured aortic aneurysm, and sepsis, which rarely present with syncope.

Hypertension, if found in association with headache, stiff neck, or altered level of consciousness, may indicate subarachnoid hemorrhage.

What is the temperature?

Patients with syncope are rarely febrile. If fever is present, it is usually caused by a concomitant illness not related to the syncopal attack. If the attack was unwitnessed and the patient is febrile, consider meningitis or encephalitis associated with a seizure.

Selective History

Taking the history is probably the most important part of the bedside evaluation; interview the patient and the witnesses. Focus on signs and symptoms immediately preceding and after the attack.

1. **Has this ever happened before?**

    If it has, ask the patient if a diagnosis was made after the previous attack.

2. **What do the patient or witnesses recall from the period immediately before the syncope? (See Table 17.2 for symptoms commonly associated with specific causes of syncope.)**

   - Syncope occurring while changing from the supine or the sitting position to the standing position suggests *orthostatic hypotension.*
   - Palpitations or the complete absence of prodromal symptoms suggest *cardiac arrhythmia.*
   - A prodrome of dizziness, lightheadedness, pallor, diaphoresis, and graying of vision and muffling of ambient sounds (i.e., presyncope) is highly characteristic of *vasovagal syncope.*
   - Syncope during or immediately after Valsalva maneuver (coughing, micturition, defecation) can result from mechanical disruption of venous return and is termed *situational syncope, which is a form of reflex syncope.*
   - One or more episodes of vertigo, diplopia, dysarthria, numbness, weakness, or ataxia preceding the attack, alone or in combination, are suggestive of *vertebrobasilar insufficiency.*
   - An event occurring in the setting of pain or venipuncture is suggestive of reflex/vasovagal syncope.

3. **How does the patient feel on waking from the syncopal attack?**

   Headache is unusual in true syncope and suggests subarachnoid hemorrhage. Persistent lethargy and confusion are atypical for true syncope and suggest an unwitnessed seizure or subarachnoid hemorrhage.

4. **Were any shaking movements observed?**

   Brief shaking movements (at most a few seconds) that *follow a loss of consciousness* can be seen in syncope, but shaking movements *lasting more than 30 seconds with a loss of consciousness* is much more likely caused by a seizure.

5. **Was the patient incontinent of stool or urine?**

   If the attack was unwitnessed, incontinence is highly suggestive of a seizure. Be aware that incontinence can also occur with true syncope.

6. **What are the medications?**

   Refer to Table 17.2 for a list of medications that can cause syncope.

7. **Is there a history of cardiac disease?**

Selective Physical Examination

Your physical examination is directed toward finding a cause for the syncope. However, a search for evidence of injuries sustained by a fall is equally important at this time.

General Physical Examination

Vital signs	Repeat now, including *orthostatic* tests if not performed yet
	Tongue lacerations, especially at lateral borders (seizure)
	Ecchymoses, abrasions, lacerations
Neck	Neck stiffness (SAH)
Cardiac	Heart murmur (mitral, pulmonic, or aortic stenosis)
	Pericardial rub (cardiac tamponade)
GU	Urinary incontinence (seizure)
Extremities	Palpate for evidence of fracture

GU, Genitourinary; *SAH,* subarachnoid hemorrhage.

MANAGEMENT

Apart from an ECG, there are no laboratory tests that are routinely indicated for the evaluation of syncope. In approximately 50% of cases, a careful history, brief targeted examination (including orthostatic BP), and ECG are all that are needed to establish a diagnosis, especially in cases of vasovagal syncope. For patients with likely vasovagal syncope and orthostatic intolerance, non-pharmacologic management strategies are the most effective. Patients benefit greatly from education about the condition, identification, and then avoidance of potential triggers and learning how to perform maneuvers to abort an episode (supine posture; physical counterpressure maneuvers consist of leg crossing, arm tensing, or hand grip).

If the cause of syncope is unexplained, further workup should be directed toward ruling out a cardiac cause of syncope. Because of the high morbidity associated with cardiac syncope, it is imperative to consider this diagnosis when evaluating an individual with syncope. The clinical features most predictive of cardiac syncope include age >60 years, male gender, known structural heart disease, fewer events (less than three events by history), syncope while supine, and syncope during effort/exercise.

Tests to evaluate a cardiac cause of syncope may include the following:

A. Echocardiography
B. Cardiac telemetry
C. Holter monitoring or event monitoring
D. Tilt table testing
E. Cardiac electrophysiologic studies
F. Cardiac stress testing
G. Coronary angiography

Pain Syndromes

Pain is the chief complaint in many patients. Although pain may arise from a variety of nonneurologic causes, this chapter will cover the diagnosis and management of six pain syndromes that are uniquely neurologic. Headache is covered in Chapter 15. Treatment of pain, independent of the underlying cause, is usually possible with appropriate therapeutic agents, but rational management decisions can be made only after identification of the site of the pain-producing lesion and recognition of the pathophysiology of the particular pain syndrome. Pain can be either acute or chronic in which nociceptor and spinothalamic sensitization may contribute to the development of chronic pain. Fig. 18.1 outlines the possible sites and mechanisms of pain. This chapter will address the following pain syndromes:

- Complex regional pain syndrome (CRPS; reflex sympathetic dystrophy, causalgia, sympathetically maintained pain [SMP])
- Facial pain (trigeminal neuralgia)
- Postherpetic neuralgia
- Peripheral neuropathy
- Cervical or lumbar radiculopathy
- Brachial plexopathy/neuritis

PHONE CALL

Questions

Questions to be asked at the time of initial contact depend on the pain syndrome. Localization will determine the subsequent path of questioning, but certain questions are pertinent to all pain syndromes. The first three questions can be asked over the phone to prepare for the history taking and examination.

1. **Where is the pain?**

   Is the pain localized or diffuse? Does it correspond to a particular anatomic pattern or dermatomal distribution? Does it radiate?

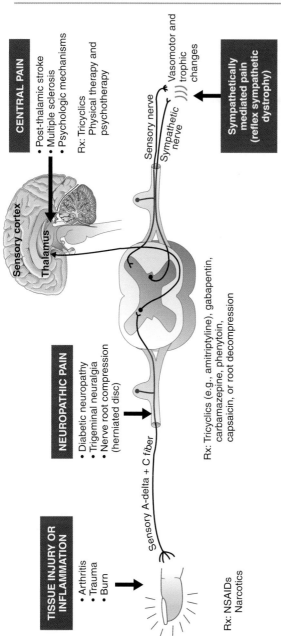

FIG. 18.1 Sites of origin of pain within the nociceptive pathway. *NSAID,* Nonsteroidal antiinflammatory drugs.

2. **When did it begin?**

    Did it come on suddenly or worsen over time?

3. **Is there a history of injury, underlying neurologic disease, or other chronic medical condition?**

    Acute injury from lifting or from a mechanical task is common for radicular pain. Traumatic injury to a limb may precede CRPS. A variety of underlying medical conditions predispose to painful peripheral neuropathies, including diabetes mellitus, alcoholism, and a variety of medications.

4. **Are there red flags?**

    Is there acute and significant weakness or sensory loss? Is there a change in normal bowel or bladder function? Does the patient have a fever or unintentional weight loss? Is there a known history of cancer or other immunocompromised condition?

Orders

No orders should be given over the phone. Although analgesia may be required to obtain an adequate history and perform an adequate physical examination, it is best to evaluate the patient yourself first.

Inform RN

"Will arrive at the bedside as soon as possible."

ELEVATOR THOUGHTS

What is the differential diagnosis based on the location of pain?

Face: trigeminal neuralgia (tic douloureux), herpes zoster (ophthalmicus or oticus), temporomandibular joint disease, atypical facial pain, carotid artery dissection, cavernous sinus thrombosis

Neck: rheumatoid arthritis, osteoarthritis/spondylosis, discogenic pain, meningitis, subarachnoid hemorrhage, vertebral artery dissection, carotid artery dissection, tumor/mass, tension headache, myofascial pain

Low back: herniated nucleus pulposus, epidural abscess, vertebral metastasis, osteomyelitis, osteoarthritis/spondylosis, discitis, herpes zoster, musculoligamentous strain, ankylosing spondylitis, retroperitoneal disease (referred pain from neoplasm, pancreatitis, ulcer, aortic aneurysm, etc.), kidney stone, pyelonephritis, compression fracture, sacroiliac (SI) joint

Arms/shoulders: cervical radiculopathy, brachial plexitis, ischemic heart disease, entrapment syndromes (suprascapular syndrome, radial nerve entrapment, interosseous syndrome) musculoskeletal pain (intraarticular pathology, bursitis, tendinosis, fracture), CRPS

Legs/hips: osteoarthritis, diabetic amyotrophy, lumbar radiculopathy, polyradiculopathy (cytomegalovirus [CMV], neoplastic), spinal stenosis, lumbar plexopathy, musculoskeletal pain (intraarticular pathology, bursitis, tendinosis, fracture)

Hands/feet (e.g., painful peripheral neuropathies): acquired peripheral neuropathy (diabetes mellitus, alcoholism, HIV/AIDS, paraproteinemia/myeloma toxin exposure, amyloidosis, paraneoplastic), mononeuritis multiplex, carpal tunnel syndrome, inherited neuropathies (Fabry disease, Tangier disease, dominantly inherited sensory neuropathy), CRPS, musculoskeletal pain (intraarticular pathology, bursitis, tendinosis, fracture), erythromelalgia

MAJOR THREAT TO LIFE

Neck pain is one category in which a missed early diagnosis could lead to significant disability or death. Etiology of pain syndromes in this category includes carotid artery dissection, meningitis, and subarachnoid hemorrhage.

Low back pain can also be a harbinger of a more threatening diagnosis, which may lead to permanent disability such as an epidural abscess, hematoma, or mass lesion.

BEDSIDE

Quick-Look Test
Does the patient appear acutely ill?

Tachypnea, diaphoresis, or a decreased level of alertness suggests that the medical illness should be attended to before the pain syndrome is addressed.

How severe does the pain appear to be?

Pain is very subjective, and tolerance can vary; one should ask about severity and observe the patient's pain behaviors.

Vital Signs

Fever suggests infection. Tachypnea may mean an underling medical condition or hyperventilation in response to pain. Tachycardia and elevated blood pressure often accompany acute pain.

Selective History and Chart Review

1. **Define the character of the pain.**

    The questions posed during the phone call should be asked directly (Where is the pain? When did the pain begin?). One strategy is to differentiate between neuropathic and somatic pain. Neuropathic pain is often described as burning, sharp, or shooting. Neuropathic pain may be induced by normally innocuous stimuli such as the touch of a shirt or spray from a shower (dysesthesia, allodynia). Somatic pain is oftentimes described as dull or achy. You should also ask about the presence of radiating pain.

2. **What makes the pain better or worse?**

    Ask if certain positions lessen or worsen pain. For example, an acute herniated lumbar disk is often worse with lumbar flexion, whereas peripheral neuropathy can be most bothersome at rest.

3. **What is the patient's medical history?**

    Ask about specific conditions (such as diabetes) and exposures to neurotoxic substances (such as chemotherapy or alcohol) when considering a diagnosis of peripheral neuropathy. Any history of trauma may lead to a diagnosis of nerve or root compression or CRPS. Malignancy may produce neural pain either by compression from a mass or by neural infiltration. A previous stroke, particularly in the thalamus, the lateral medulla, or the parietal lobe, may produce a central pain syndrome.

4. **What medications has the patient tried already?**

Selective Physical Examination I
General Physical Examination

Musculoskeletal: If there is pain in or around a joint, look for signs of inflammation, palpate for tenderness, and test the joint for active and passive range of motion. Be sure to percuss the spine to check for osseous lesions such as fractures, infection, or neoplastic disease. A straight leg raise test should be done when there is low back or leg pain (Fig. 18.2).

Skin: Rash may accompany an infection or a drug reaction. Vesicles of herpes zoster may precede or follow the associated neuralgia. Peripheral neuropathy and CRPS can cause hair loss and trophic changes.

Abdomen: Hepatomegaly may suggest chronic alcohol abuse. Abdominal or pelvic masses may produce pain that is referred to the back or the legs.

Neurologic Examination

Focus on the motor and sensory examinations in the location of the pain. Look for muscular atrophy in the distribution of the pain to suggest chronic sensorimotor neuropathy or local nerve entrapment or compression. Sensory loss will often map to the same territory as the pain. Hyporeflexia usually accompanies peripheral neuropathy and radiculopathy. Check for allodynia because this might suggest the presence of CRPS.

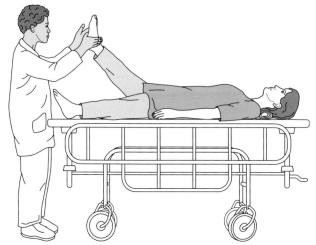

FIG. 18.2 Straight leg raise test. The physician raises each of the patient's legs, in turn, while the patient is supine. A positive test occurs when the pain is reproduced as a result of stretch on a nerve root. Pain of muscle stretch in the posterior thigh does not constitute a positive test.

MANAGEMENT

Management of individual pain syndromes is discussed later. There are, however, some general principles of pain management that apply in any symptomatic treatment of pain. Tailor the therapy to the type, location, and duration of pain. Specific pharmacologic therapy remains the cornerstone of treatment, but nonpharmacologic treatment such as transcutaneous electric nerve stimulation (TENS), local or regional anesthetic blocks, or physical therapy may be useful in specific instances. Psychologic support is especially important in management of chronic pain.

Selected Pain Syndromes

COMPLEX REGIONAL PAIN SYNDROME TYPES 1 AND 2 (TYPE 1: AKA REFLEX SYMPATHETIC DYSTROPHY, TYPE 2: AKA CAUSALGIA)

Clinical Presentation

This syndrome occurs after trauma, most frequently to a limb. The diagnosis of type II is given when there is a demonstrable peripheral nerve injury. The typical presentation is pain disproportional to the inciting injury and lasting beyond normal time to resolve. There is often allodynia, skin changes such as sweating, with red, glossy skin and abnormalities of the hair and nails. Long-term consequences may be fixed joints and osteoporosis.

Diagnosis

This syndrome is diagnosed clinically. A triple phase bone scan can be a helpful image but is rarely ordered in an emergency setting.

Treatment

Acutely, nonsteroidal antiinflammatory drugs (NSAIDs) (i.e., ibuprofen 400–800 mg three times a day [TID]), corticosteroids (e.g., prednisone 30–80 mg/day in divided doses), anticonvulsants (e.g., gabapentin up to 1800 mg daily in divided doses), antidepressants (e.g., amitriptyline up to 150 mg per day), and opioids can be considered, although there is no clear consensus on treatment and little data. Physical and occupational therapy need to be started on an outpatient basis. Referral to pain management for sympathetic blockade or spinal cord stimulation can also be considered.

TRIGEMINAL NEURALGIA (TIC DOULOUREUX)

This disorder of the sensory division of the trigeminal nerve usually occurs in the middle and late stages of life but can also present earlier. The cause is unknown, but important underlying diagnoses to rule out include multiple sclerosis and mass lesions. Degenerative or fibrotic changes in the gasserian ganglion have been reported. In some cases, the trigeminal nerve may be compressed by a tumor or a blood vessel.

Clinical Presentation

Paroxysmal unilateral lightning-like jabs of pain occur in one or more divisions of the trigeminal nerve, most commonly in the second or third division (V2 or V3). Paroxysms can last seconds to minutes and can be followed by a refractory period up to minutes. There may also be mild ipsilateral parasympathetic symptoms such as lacrimation and conjunctival injection. The frequency of pain ranges from several times daily to once or twice a month. Typically, patients describe a trigger that induces the paroxysm, for example, chewing, facial movements, or light touch. Patients may avoid eating/chewing or conversation in a desperate attempt to avoid triggering an attack. There is generally no objective sensory loss or weakness in the distribution of the pain, although patients may refuse to be examined for fear of inducing a paroxysm.

Diagnosis

Because of an absence of signs, the diagnosis of trigeminal neuralgia is made on the basis of history and observation. The differential diagnosis includes dental and sinus pain, other cranial neuralgias, and herpes zoster. Herpes (and postherpetic neuralgia) most commonly involves the first division, however. The appearance of vesicles verifies the diagnosis of active herpes infection.

Treatment

Carbamazepine 200–400 mg two times a day is the first-line treatment, and it induces remissions in a high percentage of patients. **Phenytoin, oxcarbazepine, gabapentin,** or **lamotrigine** may be a medical alternative. Radiosurgery of the trigeminal ganglion may be successful in refractory cases.

HERPETIC NEURALGIA (SHINGLES), POSTHERPETIC NEURALGIA

Clinical Presentation

Herpes zoster infection causes a painful neuropathy in a unilateral dermatomal distribution, thought to result from the reactivation of a latent infection of the virus in sensory ganglion cells (i.e., from childhood chickenpox). It occurs during the lifetime of 10% to 20% of the general population, but this incidence is mostly in the elderly and in those who are immunocompromised. The associated pain is described as sharp and radiating. A thoracic dermatome is the most common site of occurrence, followed by the cervical and then the lumbosacral dermatome. Herpes zoster ophthalmicus results from infection in the first division of the trigeminal ganglion, producing a painful vesicular eruption over the upper face and the eye (which, if untreated, may lead to blindness). The rash of herpes zoster appears 1 to 4 days after a prodrome of fever, malaise, and dysesthesias. The vesicular eruption becomes pustular in 3 to 4 days and then crusts over by 7 to 10 days. In the normal host, the lesions resolve without sequelae in 2 to 3 weeks. In immunocompromised hosts, however, the infection may linger.

Postherpetic neuralgia is the persistence of pain 4 to 6 weeks after the resolution of the rash. This occurs in 10% to 20% of patients with herpes zoster, with the bulk of occurrences in the elderly and the immunocompromised. Fifty percent of patients with postherpetic neuralgia will have a resolution of the pain in 2 months, and 70% of patients are better in 1 year. In some patients, however, the neuralgia may persist for many years.

Diagnosis

You can make the clinical diagnosis on the basis of the typical unilateral dermatomal rash. Pain, hypesthesia, and mild sensory loss should follow the same dermatomal distribution. For confirmatory diagnosis, consultation from the infectious disease or dermatology service may be helpful. Vesicles may contain polymorphonuclear leukocytes. A scrape biopsy may show giant cells and intranuclear inclusions. Varicella-zoster virus antibody titers may increase fourfold. Postherpetic neuralgia after the resolution of rash is diagnosed on a clinical basis and also follows a dermatomal distribution.

Treatment

1. **Acute herpes zoster infection**

    Acyclovir 800 mg by mouth (PO) q4h for 7 to 10 days in immunocompetent patients, and 10 mg/kg intravenously (IV) (infuse over 1 hour) three times a day for 7 days in immunocompromised patients will shorten the period of acute dermatomal pain and accelerate healing of the rash but will not reduce the incidence or severity of postherpetic neuralgia. Famciclovir and valacyclovir may also be used. **Prednisone 60 mg PO per day for 7 days followed by a taper** may reduce acute pain and potentially reduce the incidence of postherpetic neuralgia. Beware of using prednisone in immunocompromised hosts.

2. **Postherpetic neuralgia**

    This condition is notoriously difficult to treat, and a variety of anticonvulsants and antidepressants have been tried. Amitriptyline 50 to 150 mg PO per day, gabapentin 300 to 900 mg PO three times a day, and oxycodone/acetaminophen (Percocet) 1 to 2 tablets every 6 hours may reduce the burning pain. Lidoderm (5% lidocaine) patch has been shown to be an effective topical treatment. Intrathecal treatment with methylprednisolone (60 mg) plus 3% lidocaine (3 mL) has been shown to be effective in patients with refractory pain.

PERIPHERAL NEUROPATHY

Clinical Presentation

Peripheral neuropathy describes a disease caused by diffuse lesions of peripheral nerves. Systemic disease affecting the peripheral nervous system produces symptoms in the longest nerves first. Dysesthesias and sensory loss in a symmetric, stocking-glove distribution are typical for early peripheral neuropathy. The patient may describe the pain as burning, stinging, or pressure like. There may be hypersensitivity to touch, which typically affects the feet before the hands. There may be gait disturbance from pain and/or from sensory loss affecting joint position sense.

During the examination, look for wasting of the very distal muscles, sensory loss (vibratory sense may be the first to be lost), distal weakness, and hyporeflexia particularly at the ankles.

Diagnosis

The clinical diagnosis may often be made from the history and physical examination. Be sure to ask about diabetes mellitus, alcohol use, and medication history. Occupational history may reveal exposure to toxins.

Electromyography (EMG) and nerve conduction studies can confirm a diagnosis of peripheral neuropathy and distinguish between demyelinating and axonal pathology. Laboratory tests to order should include a hemoglobin A1c and full chemistry panel including liver and thyroid function tests, rheumatologic screen (erythrocyte sedimentation rate [ESR], antinuclear antibody [ANA], and rheumatoid factor [RF]), serum protein electrophoresis (SPEP) (screen for multiple myeloma), complete blood count (CBC), and serum vitamin B_{12}, B6, and B1 levels. Antibodies associated with celiac disease may also be checked because this is another possible cause.

Treatment

1. Treat any underlying metabolic/systemic disorder or malignancy or remove any offending neurotoxins.
2. Symptomatic treatment of painful peripheral neuropathy typically consists of anticonvulsants, antidepressants, and/or topical agents. One may begin with **gabapentin 100 mg three times a day** (lower dosage for elderly patients) and taper up to 1800 to 3600 mg per day divided into three doses. **Pregabalin 50 to 300 mg twice a day (BID)** also may be used. Antidepressants such as amitriptyline 25 to 100 mg daily and Cymbalta 30 to 60 mg per day are alternatives.
3. For topical treatment, use **Lidoderm (5% lidocaine) gel or capsaicin (0.075% to 0.25%) ointment.**
4. Nonpharmacologic therapies such as TENS and acupuncture can supplement the treatment regimen.

CERVICAL OR LUMBOSACRAL ROOT COMPRESSION

Clinical Presentation

Axial low back or neck pain with radiating pain down a limb is often caused by nerve root compression. In the acute setting, this is often caused by a herniated nucleus pulposus and may be precipitated by a specific physical event such as lifting a heavy weight or twisting. In the chronic setting in the absence of acute injury, this may be caused by spondylitic changes resulting in neural foraminal narrowing. One must also consider a compressive mass, hematoma, or abscess causing nerve root compression in the appropriate context. The differential diagnosis includes neck or back muscle strain or ligamentous sprain without neural injury, as well as plexopathy and discogenic pain (i.e., annular fissure). Radicular pain usually presents as shooting pain into an arm or leg, typically in the distribution of a nerve root. There is often associated myofascial pain at the level of compression. With disk herniation, the pain is often increased by coughing or sneezing. Lumbar disks tend to herniate posterolaterally, and cervical disks tend to herniate centrally.

Diagnosis

The typical symptom of lumbar radiculopathy is radiation of pain from the back into the leg, often in a dermatomal distribution. In the acute setting, this is often exacerbated by lumbar flexion. The most commonly affected roots are L5 (produced by herniation of the L4-L5 disk) and S1 (produced by herniation of the L5-S1 disk). Upper lumbar root compressions are less common. In the cervical region, C5, C6, and C7 are the roots most commonly affected. Higher cervical involvement or thoracic radiculopathies warrant further investigation for neoplastic disease or neurofibromatosis. Table 18.1 lists the pain, sensory, and reflex changes for common cervical and lumbosacral radicular syndromes. Also, see the **dermatome and myotome charts** in Appendix section. Clinical diagnosis can usually be made from the history and examination. Be sure to check motor, sensory, and reflex function in the distribution of the pain and the affected nerve root. When considering the diagnosis of lumbosacral radiculopathy, a dural stretch test such as the straight leg raise should be performed as part of the physical examination, which will reproduce radicular pain in the affected limb (see Fig. 18.2). *Cervical or lumbosacral spinal magnetic resonance imaging (MRI)* is the diagnostic test of choice to visualize the spinal cord, the vertebrae, the disks, and the nerve roots. If there is any suspicion of a neoplastic or infectious lesion, a contrast-enhanced MRI should be obtained.

Treatment

1. **Conservative management** usually suffices to achieve good recovery. This can be accomplished with a short course of anti-inflammatories (NSAIDs, i.e., **naproxen 500 mg PO every 12 hours** or Medrol Dosepak) and physical therapy, focusing

TABLE 18.1 | **Clinical Features of Cervical and Lumbosacral Root Compression Syndromes**

Root	Area of Pain	Sensory Loss	Motor Loss	Reflex
C5	Lateral upper arm	Lateral upper arm	Shoulder abduction, internal and external rotation, and elbow flexion	Biceps reflex
C6	Lateral forearm, thumb, and index finger	Lateral forearm and thumb	Elbow supination	Brachioradialis reflex
C7	Over the triceps, midforearm, and middle finger	Middle fingers	Elbow extension and wrist extension	Triceps reflex
C8	Medial forearm and little finger	Medial forearm and little finger	Finger adduction and abduction	—
L4	Knee to medial malleolus	Medial knee and leg	Knee extension	Patellar reflex
L5	Back of thigh, lateral calf, and dorsum of foot	Dorsum of foot	Foot and toe dorsiflexion	None
S1	Back of thigh, back of calf, and lateral foot	Behind lateral malleolus, sole of foot	Foot plantar flexion	Achilles reflex

on core strengthening. If there is associated myofascial pain, a short course of muscle relaxants may be prescribed (i.e., **cyclobenzaprine 5mg PO every 8 hours as needed**).

2. **Epidural steroid injection** can be considered if the patient's pain prohibits participation in physical therapy, or if there is persistent pain despite 6 weeks of conservative therapy

3. **Surgical intervention** should be reserved for three indications: (1) evidence of cauda equina syndrome (i.e., bowel/bladder involvement); (2) severe neurologic deficit, such as a complete foot drop; and (3) failure to control pain or reverse a neurologic deficit with medical management.

BRACHIAL NEURITIS (IDIOPATHIC BRACHIAL PLEXOPATHY, NEURALGIC AMYOTROPHY, BRACHIAL NEURALGIA, PARSONAGE-TURNER SYNDROME)

Clinical Presentation

This rare syndrome typically begins with pain in the axilla, shoulder, and arm. Pain in the shoulder may have an aching quality that radiates into the arm. Some patients have mild sensory loss in the distribution of the affected nerves. The acute phase of pain may last hours to weeks, and within a few days the shoulder girdle musculature becomes weak and atrophic, affecting primarily the C5 and C6 myotomes (although any nerve may be affected). The disease is idiopathic and sporadic, affecting men more than twice as frequently as women. Most cases occur after the third decade. The syndrome may occur after trauma, exertion, surgery, infection, or vaccination and is usually unilateral and rarely bilateral. It is thought to be the result of an immune-mediated process. Guarding of the shoulder may lead to a frozen shoulder.

Diagnosis

The clinical pattern of relatively rapid onset of pain followed by weakness is typical for brachial neuritis. The differential diagnosis at the early stage in which pain is the only complaint includes inflammatory and orthopedic involvement, as well as cervical radiculopathy and root compression from a rudimentary cervical rib. **EMG/nerve conduction studies usually show evidence of denervation in the affected myotomes and decreased amplitude of sensory nerve action potentials.** Subtle signs may also be present on the unaffected side in up to 25% of patients.

Treatment

Because the cause of brachial neuritis is unknown, there is no specific therapy. Gentle physical therapy with **passive range-of-motion exercises** should be used to avoid a frozen shoulder and aid with recovery of muscle strength. **Ibuprofen 600 mg every 4 to 6 hours** may be used as the first therapy for analgesia. A tapering course of steroids, beginning with **prednisone 60 mg PO per day,** also may be used early in the disease course. The prognosis is good, with 90% of patients making a good recovery. The prognosis is poor if the EMG shows no voluntary motor units.

Brain Death

The Uniform Determination of Death Act (UDDA) of 1981 defined death in two ways: (1) there is the traditional definition of death involving the irreversible cessation of circulatory and respiratory function; and (2) there is the irreversible cessation of all function of the entire brain including the brain stem, which defines brain death. The concept of brain death did not exist before the era of modern medicine, critical care, and the advent of ventilators. Brain death has the same legal standing as cardiac death, and it allows for many lives to be saved by organ transplantation.

CLINICAL SIGNIFICANCE OF BRAIN DEATH

Brain death determination should be made accurately and expeditiously to:
1. Avoid prolonged suffering of loved ones,
2. Avoid wasting resources on nonrecoverable patients, and
3. Enable patients to become an organ donor.

Brain death determination should be made using accepted medical standards. Each state has different laws, and every hospital has different policies regarding brain death. All brain death determination procedures must include the following:

1. There must be radiographic evidence or historical evidence that is consistent with the diagnosis of brain death.
2. Adequate time must be given to ensure that the state is irreversible.
3. All confounding factors, including drug effects and metabolic derangement, must be mitigated.
4. A provider must do and detail neurological examinations that evaluate cerebral and brain stem function.
5. Apnea test provision must be made to document lack of respiratory effort.
6. There must be provisions for the confirmatory tests that may be done if unable to adequately perform specific portions of the brain death determination procedure.

Clinical Guidance

Patients with severe facial trauma or those who have preexisting pupillary abnormalities, those who have toxic drug levels, and those with chronic CO_2 retention may limit the ability to perform the brain death determination procedures. Providers should wait at least five times the half-life of any central nervous system (CNS) depressant if there is no ability to measure levels. In the case of alcohol, the legal limit of intoxication is a good reference. A patient who has received neuromuscular blockade should have a train of four performed to confirm intact muscle contraction to electrical stimulation before undergoing the brain death determination procedure. One neurological examination should be sufficient to pronounce brain death, but this should be compliant with local laws.

CRITERIA FOR THE CLINICAL DIAGNOSIS OF BRAIN DEATH

1. **Absent Cerebral Function**

   The patient must be in a deep coma. There must be no reflexes or responses that are mediated by structures in the brain. Decorticate or decerebrate posturing is not consistent with brain death. Localization or withdrawal are not consistent with brain death. Reflexes and responses including triple flexion, deep tendon reflexes, and extensor plantar response are consistent with brain death.

2. **Absent Brain Stem Function**

   a. **Pupils**

   In brain death, pupils may be midrange to large, round, or irregular and must be nonreactive to light via the direct and consensual response bilaterally.

   b. **Eye movements**

   After ensuring that the cervical spine is clear, the head should gently be turned from side to side and flexed and extended taking care not to dislodge and medical devices. In brain death, turning the head does not produce movement of the eyes. It is as if the eyes are painted on the head like old-fashioned "doll's eyes"; this is the absence of the "oculocephalic reflex."

   After checking for intact tympanic membranes, 50 to 60 mL of cold saline should be used to irrigate both tympanic membranes independently. In brain death, there should be no movement of the eyes. This is the absence of the "oculovestibular reflex." Before doing this maneuver, place the bed at 45 degrees. This orients the semilunar canals to allow for lateral eye movement if a response is to occur. The cold saline simulates a brain stem lesion ipsilateral to the side of the irrigation. In a comatose patient with intact brain stem function, irrigation of cold saline should provoke smooth eye movements toward the side of irrigation. Time should be given between both sides of the test to allow for the endolymph in the semilunar canals to warm up.

c. **Facial sensation and motor response**

The "corneal reflex" should be tested by taking a wisp of a cotton swab and touching the corneas in both eyes. There should be no response to the movement (i.e., blinking, grimacing, etc.). Similarly, there should be no response to applying supraorbital pressure on both sides.

d. **Pharyngeal and tracheal reflexes**

A tongue depressor or suction catheter should be used to gently stimulate the back of the throat. In brain death, there should be no response to this action, such as a gag. Also, using an in-line suction tube down the endotracheal tube should not produce a cough if there is brain death.

3. **Apnea**

In brain death, there should be no spontaneous respiration. Patients without remaining intrinsic respiratory drive can often appear to be breathing over the set rate on a control-mode ventilator setting. This "overbreathing" may be a result of some extraneous movement in the intensive care unit (ICU) environment that is picked up by the pressure or flow trigger within the ventilator as respiratory effort. An apnea test (Table 19.1) is

TABLE 19.1	**Apnea Test Procedure**
Apnea Test	
Prerequisite	Core temperature > 36.0°C
	SBP > 90 mm Hg
	Euvolemia (positive fluid balance in the previous 6 h)
	Normal P_{CO_2} (arterial P_{CO_2} > 40 mm Hg)
	Normal P_{O_2} (preoxygenate to a P_{O_2} > 200 mm Hg)
Testing procedure	Make sure patient is connected to a pulse oximetry
	Disconnect from the ventilator
	Deliver 100% oxygen into the trachea
	Monitor for respiratory movements
	Measure P_{CO_2} at around 7–10 min and reconnect to the ventilator
Testing results	If respiratory movements are noted the test is negative
	Take arterial sample and abort the test if SBP < 90 mm Hg or patient develops an arrhythmia or significant desaturations
	Test is consistent with brain death if P_{CO_2} is > 60 mm Hg and no respiratory movements are observed

SBP, Systolic blood pressure.

done to formally test a patient's respiratory drive. This test is done after cerebral and brain stem function testing. Before doing an apnea test, the patient should be at least 36°C and should be deemed able to tolerate removal from the ventilator for several minutes from a hemodynamic and oxygenation standpoint. These patients are often on pressor medication drips and often may need these medications to be adjusted during the test. Before doing an apnea test, a baseline arterial blood gas (ABG) should be obtained. If necessary, the ventilator setting should be adjusted to obtain P_{CO_2} in the normal range before the test. Preoxygenation before performing the test helps to ensure that the patient does not become hypoxic during the procedure.

To perform the test, the patient is disconnected from the ventilator. A nasal cannula with the nasal prongs cut off can be placed down the endotracheal tube to allow for passive oxygenation. The provider observes for any chest wall motion indicative of respiratory effort. The patient should remain off the ventilator for at least 7 minutes, then a follow-up ABG should be performed and the patient placed back on the ventilator. The P_{CO_2} should rise approximately 3 mm Hg for every minute a person is disconnected from the ventilator and not breathing. The test should be aborted if patient becomes hemodynamically unstable (systolic blood pressure [BP] < 90 mm Hg) or hypoxic (pulse oximetry < 90). No spontaneous respiratory movement while the patient is disconnected from the ventilator and a P_{CO_2} of ≥60 mm Hg is consistent with brain death. A patient with chronic obstructive pulmonary disease (COPD)/emphysema with chronic elevation of the P_{CO_2} at baseline complicates the interpretation of these ABGs. They often may require further confirmatory testing.

CONFIRMATORY TESTING

A perfect confirmatory test would have no "false positives"; it would not be susceptible to drugs or metabolic disturbances. The test would be safe and readily available and be standardized and sufficient on its own to establish brain death. No such test exists. Next is a list of possible confirmatory tests. Brain death is a clinical diagnosis. Confirmatory tests such as electroencephalography (EEG) are not essential to the declaration of brain death but may be required according to state laws or institutional policy. In circumstances in which the clinical diagnosis of brain death cannot be made with certainty, a confirmatory test may be needed (Fig. 19.1).

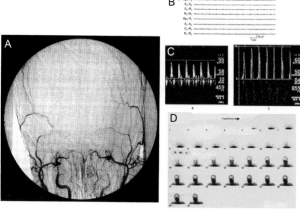

FIG. 19.1 Diagnostic tests for the confirmation of brain death. (A) Anteroposterior view of a cerebral angiogram demonstrating complete intracranial circulatory arrest at the level of the petrous internal carotid arteries. Note the persistence of external carotid artery flow. (B) Flat electrocerebral silence electroencephalography demonstrating artifactual electrocardiographic activity generated by the heart. (C) Transcranial Doppler sonography of the middle cerebral arteries demonstrating isolated systolic spikes with reversed *(left panel)* or absent *(right panel)* diastolic flow. (D) Radionuclide cerebral perfusion scan demonstrating the complete absence of blood flow to the brain.

- **Angiography, i.e., formal cerebral angiogram, computed tomographic angiography (CTA), magnetic angiography (MRA):** Complete absence of intracranial blood flow in a four-vessel angiogram confirms the diagnosis of brain death.
- **Transcranial Doppler (TCD):** A velocity profile showing systolic spikes with absent or reversed diastolic flow is consistent with the cessation of cerebral blood flow and brain death.
- **Nuclear medical tests:** The complete absence of cerebral perfusion also can be established using radionuclide angiography or single-photon emission computed tomography (SPECT).
- **EEG:** Confirmation of neocortical death can be documented by at least 30 minutes of electrocerebral silence by using a 16-channel instrument with increased gain settings, according to guidelines developed by the American Electroencephalographic Society. If any brain wave is present, then the diagnosis of brain death cannot be made. EEG confirmation of brain death also is not valid in patients exposed to sedatives or toxins because they can directly suppress the brain electrical activity.

- **Somatosensory evoked potentials (SSEPs) and brain stem auditory evoked potentials (SSEPs and BEARs):** Loss of median SSEPs and all BEARs are seen in brain death.

PSYCHOSOCIAL ISSUES

The emotional and psychosocial effect of death is always stressful for those who survive the patient; this can be even more difficult in the setting of brain death. Communication of the concept and meaning of brain death to the patient's family is paramount. This communication, however painful, should be initiated as early as possible to give those involved time to adjust to the situation. Although family permission is generally *not* required to discontinue life support once a patient is declared legally brain dead, their consent and understanding are extremely important. Misunderstanding, bereavement, emotional upset, and religious or moral beliefs may lead family members to object to "pulling the plug" in some cases. In these instances, third-party mediation by a medical ethics consultant or member of the clergy may be desirable.

INTENSIVE CARE UNIT MANAGEMENT OF POTENTIAL ORGAN DONORS

Brain death eventually leads to severe homeostatic derangements and cardiac arrest despite mechanical ventilation and aggressive life-support measures. This inexorable progression toward multisystem organ failure creates a challenge in managing the potential organ donor in whom the goal is to maintain and optimize organ viability for transplantation.

Most patients become hypotensive because sudden loss of resting sympathetic tone and require intravenous (IV) pressors at the time brain death occurs, and soon thereafter they develop diabetes insipidus (DI) (because antidiuretic hormone secretion ceases). Adrenergic vasopressors, such as dopamine or arginine vasopressin, both of which cause peripheral vasoconstriction in this setting, are considered the first-line interventions for hypotension. In some cases, continued hypotension will respond to thyroid and glucocorticoid hormone replacement, indicating a relative deficiency of these hormones.

The situation usually deteriorates when brain dead patients are maintained on a ventilator for a prolonged period of time. Hypothermia, refractory hypoxia, disseminated intravascular coagulation, metabolic acidosis, renal failure, and adult respiratory distress syndrome may all occur. The key to management is to be ready for these complications.

Protocol for Management of the Potential Organ Donor in the Intensive Care Unit

1. Insert a central venous catheter or two large-bore peripheral IV lines.
2. Insert an arterial line for continuous BP monitoring.
   a. Maintain systolic BP at or higher than 100 mm Hg with step-wise intervention:
      (1) **500 mL 0.9% saline fluid bolus (two times at 10-minute intervals)**
      (2) **Dopamine 800 mg/500 mL normal saline (NS) (start at 13 mL/h, 5 mg/kg/min), titrated to maintain systolic BP at or higher than 100 mm Hg**
      (3) If refractory hypotension (systolic BP less than 90 mm Hg) or tachyarrhythmia occurs with dopamine treatment, **start vasopressin (Pitressin) 4 U/h.**
      (4) If hypotension is refractory to dopamine and/or IV Pitressin, perform thyroxine (T_4) replacement protocol:
         a. Administer as IV boluses:
            i. **Dextrose 50% (1 amp)**
            ii. **Methylprednisolone 1 g**
            iii. **Regular insulin 10 U**
            iv. **Levothyroxine 20 mg**
         b. If the BP responds to these boluses, start **levothroxine 5 mg/h as a continuous infusion (200 mg/500 mL NS at 12.5 mL/h)** and titrate to maintain the SBP > 100 mm Hg. Note that T_4 can precipitate cardiac arrhythmias, particularly in younger, hypokalemic patients.
3. Start baseline IV flow: **0.9% saline at 150 to 200 mL/h.**
   a. Check serum sodium levels every 6 hours:
      (1) If sodium level is 150 to 159 mmol/L, change baseline IV to 0.45% saline.
      (2) If sodium level is >160 mmol/L, change baseline IV to 0.25% saline.
4. Transfuse if hematocrit is lower than 24%.
5. Adjust fraction of inspired oxygen and positive end-expiratory pressure to maintain Pa_{O_2} > 100 mm Hg and oxygen saturation higher than 92%.
6. Insert a Foley catheter. Measure fluid input and urine output (UO) and monitor urine specific gravity every 2 hours.
   a. If the UO over 2 hours is greater than 500 mL with specific gravity of 1.005 or lower, begin treatment for DI:
      (1) Administer **aqueous vasopressin 6 to 10 U IV push (IVP).**

(2) Start **IV vasopressin 2 to 4 U/h titrated to maintain systolic blood pressure (SBP) > 100 mm Hg and UO < 200 mL/h.**

(3) Replace hourly UO milliliter for milliliter with D5W.

7. Check the finger-stick glucose level every 4 hours.

c. If finger-stick glucose level is higher than 140 mg/dL, begin **insulin drip (100 U regular insulin in 1000 mL 0.9% saline) starting at 20 mL/h (2 U/h), titrated to maintain blood glucose between 80 and 120 mg/dL.**

Selected Neurologic Disorders

Nerve and Muscle Diseases

Patients with neuromuscular disease generally present with weakness, sensory loss, or both of these conditions. Your approach should initially focus on localizing the problem to a specific component of the peripheral nervous system that is involved (e.g., neuropathy or myopathy) and then be directed toward identifying a specific disease process. The major anatomic components of the peripheral nervous system are listed in Table 20.1.

Approach to the Patient With Suspected Neuromuscular Disease

HISTORY

1. **Clarify the pattern of weakness.** Proximal weakness suggests myopathy; distal weakness suggests neuropathy.
2. **Characterize any sensory symptoms.** Have the patient identify the exact regions involved and symptom character (sensory loss or unpleasant sensation).
3. **Ask about cramps and muscle twitches (fasciculations).** These symptoms point to disease of the motor neuron (amyotrophic lateral sclerosis [ALS]) or muscle (myopathy).
4. **Ask about pain.** Pain may be related to a musculoskeletal structure (e.g., herniated disk), or it may be neuropathic or muscular.
5. **Is there any autonomic involvement?** Ask about orthostatic dizziness, anhidrosis, visual blurring, urinary hesitancy or incontinence, constipation, and impotence. These symptoms can result from autonomic neuropathy.

EXAMINATION

1. **Determine whether the patient has true weakness.** Decreased strength needs to be differentiated from limitation arising from

TABLE 20.1	Basic Anatomic Subtypes of Neuromuscular Disease	
Anatomic Site	**Typical Pattern of Motor and Sensory Deficit**	**Examples**
Motor neuron disease	Weakness, wasting, fasciculations; no sensory deficits; hyperreflexia with ALS	ALS, spinal muscular atrophy, polio
Monoradiculopathy	Distribution of a single nerve root (dermatomal pattern)	L5 or S1 root compression herniated disk form
Polyradiculopathy	Distribution of multiple nerve roots	Cauda equine syndrome; carcinomatous meningitis
Plexopathy	Distribution of a nerve plexus	Acute brachial neuritis
Mononeuropathy	Distribution of a single peripheral nerve	Carpal tunnel syndrome
Mononeuropathy multiplex	Multifocal process affecting several discrete peripheral nerves	Vasculitis, leprosy
Polyneuropathy	Diffuse, symmetric, distal stocking-glove pattern; distal hyporeflexia	Diabetic polyneuropathy
Neuromuscular junction disease	Fluctuating weakness with fatigability; no sensory deficits; reflexes preserved	Myasthenia gravis
Myopathy	Diffuse proximal muscle weakness; no sensory deficits; preserved reflexes until late	Polymyositis; muscular dystrophy

ALS, Amyotrophic lateral sclerosis.

pain, and from submaximal effort. Effort-limited weakness is inconsistent and tends to "give way" suddenly.

2. **Map out any sensory deficits.** Think in terms of identifying *diffuse, distal sensory loss* (stocking-glove pattern), as seen in polyneuropathy; *focal sensory loss* restricted to a single root dermatome or peripheral nerve; or *multifocal sensory loss*, which suggests mononeuropathy multiplex or a plexus lesion (Fig. 20.1).

3. **Test the reflexes.** Loss of deep tendon reflexes suggests peripheral nerve involvement.

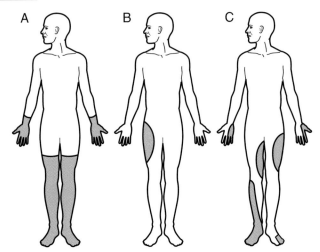

FIG. 20.1 Patterns of sensory loss in patients with neuropathy. (A) Polyneuropathy. Diffuse stocking-glove pattern. (B) Mononeuropathy. Focal involvement corresponding to a single peripheral nerve. (C) Mononeuritis multiplex. Pattern of multiple, asymmetric regions of sensory loss, corresponding to multiple peripheral nerves.

4. **Undress the patient to check for wasting and fasciculations** (irregular individual muscle twitches). These findings indicate lower motor neuron disease.

MOTOR NEURON DISEASE

The clinical hallmarks of anterior horn cell disease are the lower motor neuron signs of **weakness, wasting (atrophy), and fasciculations.** These signs may be seen alone or in combination with upper motor neuron signs (hyperreflexia, upgoing toes) as in the case of ALS. Sensory disturbances are absent. There are several distinct forms of motor neuron disease:

AMYOTROPHIC LATERAL SCLEROSIS (ALS)

Also known as Lou Gehrig disease, ALS is the most common form of motor neuron disease. It is easily recognized on the basis of progressive weakness, wasting, fasciculations, and upper motor neuron signs. It is familial in 10% of cases. The presence of bulbar involvement (dysarthria, dysphagia, dyspnea) carries a worse prognosis. Median survival after diagnosis is 3 years. ALS is a clinical diagnosis that is supported by exclusion of other causes and evidence of denervation in at least three regions on electromyography (EMG).

SPINAL MUSCULAR ATROPHY

This condition resembles ALS but is limited to pure lower motor neuron degeneration (e.g., no upper motor neuron signs are seen). Spinal muscular atrophy typically has infantile or childhood onset, but adult forms also occur. Adult-onset progression is slower than ALS and is more often hereditary. Testing for the survival motor neuron 1 (SMN1) copy number is available. Nusinersen (Spiranza ®), an antisense oligonucleotide that increases SMN copy number, was approved by the Food and Drug Administration (FDA) in 2016.

MULTIFOCAL MOTOR NEUROPATHY

This condition is an immune-mediated motor neuropathy, differentiated by the presence of **conduction block** on nerve conduction studies (NCSs). The course is protracted over many years, and the weakness is asymmetric; patients progress without treatment. Up to 50% of patients have anti-GM1 antibodies. Treatment with frequent intravenous immunoglobulin (IVIG) is the mainstay of treatment; IVIG is approved by the FDA for this condition.

OTHER MOTOR NEURON DISEASES

These diseases include poliomyelitis (West Nile causes a polio-like condition), hereditary neurodegenerative diseases, and metabolic systemic storage disorders.

Diagnosis

Diagnostic testing for suspected motor neuron disease should include the following: EMG/NCS, serum electrophoresis, serum immunofixation electrophoresis, quantitative immunoglobulins, and anti-GM1 antibody levels. Cervical spine magnetic resonance imaging (MRI) and lumbar puncture (LP) should be considered. In patients with a paraprotein, bone marrow biopsy may be indicated.

Treatment

ALS is incurable, but **riluzole 50 mg by mouth (PO) twice per day,** a glutamate antagonist, may slow the progression of the disease. Clinical trials of additional agents are ongoing. Patients with multifocal motor neuropathy may improve with treatment with **IVIG 0.5 to 1.0 g/kg given every 2 to 4 weeks.**

MONORADICULOPATHY AND POLYRADICULOPATHY

Monoradiculopathies typically result from disk herniation and nerve root compression. They present with a radicular distribution of pain and are discussed in Chapter 18. *Polyradiculopathy* involving multiple lumbosacral nerve roots (cauda equina syndrome) presents with low back pain, urinary disturbances, and gait failure.

PLEXOPATHY

Diseases that cause diffuse injury to either the brachial or the lumbosacral plexus lead to **regional motor, sensory, and reflex disturbances in one limb.** The key to identifying the syndrome is to find a pattern of deficits that cannot be explained by involvement of one nerve root or a single peripheral nerve. EMG and NCS are helpful in confirming and defining the syndrome; weakness is typically more severe in plexopathy than compressive radiculopathy. See Appendix for the anatomy of the brachial and lumbosacral plexus.

Brachial Plexopathy

Upper brachial plexus injury (arising from C5-C7) results in weakness and atrophy of the shoulder and upper arm muscles (Erb palsy). Lower brachial plexus injury (arising from C8 and T1) leads to weakness, atrophy, and sensory deficits in the forearm and hand (Klumpke palsy). The main causes of brachial plexopathy include the following:

1. **Trauma**
2. **Idiopathic brachial neuritis (Parsonage-Turner syndrome)**
   This under recognized syndrome presents with the sudden onset of pain in the shoulder and arm; as the pain resolves over 2 to 4 weeks, weakness and muscle wasting become evident.
3. **Tumor infiltration**
   Metastatic disease and neurofibroma are most common.
4. **Radiation plexopathy**
   High-dose irradiation for lymphoma or breast cancer can lead to painless progressive brachial plexopathy 1 to 5 years later. *Myokymia* (irregular wormlike muscle movement) may be a distinguishing feature.
5. **Cervical rib or bands (thoracic outlet syndrome)**
   This rare condition is caused by compression of the lower trunk of the brachial plexus as it passes over an abnormal first cervical rib or rudimentary first rib. Patients complain of pain and paresthesias in the C8-T1 distribution of the hand and medial forearm when carrying heavy objects or when raising the arm above shoulder level. Surgical decompression may be helpful in rare cases.

Lumbosacral Plexopathy

Unilateral lumbosacral plexopathy is rare. The main diagnostic considerations include idiopathic neuritis, diabetic infarction, and compression from a retroperitoneal abscess, hemorrhage, or neoplasm.

Diagnosis

In many cases, the cause of brachial or lumbosacral plexopathy is readily apparent (e.g., trauma or radiation). If not, chest and cervical spine radiographs, LP, and MRI, or computed tomography (CT) of the plexus should be considered.

Treatment

Physical therapy can help speed recovery, minimize muscle wasting, and prevent contractures.

MONONEUROPATHIES

Mononeuropathies result from injury, compression, or entrapment of a single nerve, usually at a specific site. There are multiple different syndromes.

Carpal Tunnel Syndrome

Carpal tunnel syndrome is by far the most common cause of mononeuropathy; it results from compression of the median nerve at the wrist and usually presents with wrist pain and tingling of the first three digits. The pain may radiate proximally to the elbow and is almost always worse at night. Examination may reveal a *Tinel sign* (radiation of pain into the first three digits when the wrist is tapped with a hammer). Thenar muscle wasting and persistent sensory deficits in the distal median nerve distribution are advanced findings (Fig. 20.2). Risk factors include repetitive "overuse" injury, thyroid disease, pregnancy, acromegaly, diabetes, and amyloidosis.

Diagnosis

EMG and NCS show focal sensory and/or motor slowing across the wrist in the median nerve. Nerve ultrasound is a complimentary diagnostic test. Check thyroid function tests (TFTs) and fasting glucose level to screen for hypothyroidism and diabetes.

Treatment

Mild disease can be treated with a neutral position to 20-degree extension wrist splint; more severe disease requires surgical decompression. Repetitive stress to the wrist can be minimized with special occupational devices.

Facial Palsy (Bell Palsy)

Facial palsy (Bell palsy) is the most common cranial mononeuropathy. Patients present with acute unilateral facial paralysis, with equal involvement of the forehead and lower half of the face. The disorder is thought to result from inflammation of cranial

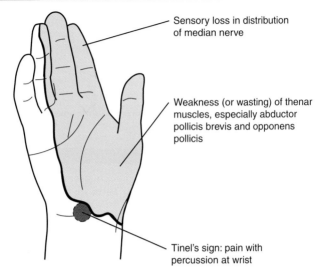

Sensory loss in distribution of median nerve

Weakness (or wasting) of thenar muscles, especially abductor pollicis brevis and opponens pollicis

Tinel's sign: pain with percussion at wrist

FIG 20.2 Sensory and motor involvement in proximal median neuropathy; note that carpal tunnel syndrome spares sensation over thenar muscles.

nerve 7 within the facial canal. In some patients, an antecedent viral infection is identified, and approximately 25% of cases are associated with pain in the ipsilateral ear. If the injury to the facial nerve is proximal to the chorda tympani in the facial canal, loss of taste occurs on the anterior two-thirds of the tongue ipsilaterally. Complete or near-complete recovery occurs in 85% of cases.

Diagnosis

The majority of cases are idiopathic (Bell palsy). Examination should focus on searching for signs of other treatable diseases that can present with facial paralysis:

- Decreased hearing or a decreased afferent corneal reflex is suggestive of a cerebellopontine angle tumor (e.g., acoustic neuroma), which should be excluded by MRI with gadolinium.
- Vesicles in the external auditory canal are indicative of the Ramsay Hunt syndrome, which results from herpes zoster infection of the ipsilateral geniculate ganglion.
- An antecedent annular rash or tick bite is suggestive of Lyme disease. Serum Lyme antibody titers and LP with testing for

cerebrospinal fluid (CSF) Lyme antibodies are required to establish the diagnosis.
- Interstitial lung disease with hilar adenopathy, uveitis, or parotitis may be a clue to neurosarcoidosis. CSF examination may reveal a lymphocytic pleocytosis; biopsy of involved tissue is required to establish the diagnosis.

Treatment

Recovery from idiopathic Bell palsy can be accelerated by treatment with **prednisone 80 mg PO daily for 5 days,** followed by a 7-day taper. Ramsay Hunt syndrome is treated with **acyclovir 800 mg PO five times daily for 7 days** in addition to prednisone. The likelihood of complete recovery is increased when treatment is started within 7 days of onset. Treatment for Lyme disease (see Chapter 22) and neurosarcoidosis (see Chapter 21) is discussed elsewhere. Patients with incomplete eye closure should use an ophthalmic ointment (e.g., Lacri-Lube) and a protective eye shield at night to prevent corneal abrasions.

Other Common Nerve Entrapment Syndromes

The nerves implicated in additional selected entrapment syndromes include the following:
- Ulnar nerve at the elbow (cubital tunnel syndrome, tardy ulnar palsy)
- Median nerve at the pronator teres (pronator syndrome)
- Radial nerve at the spiral groove of the humerus (Saturday night palsy)
- Obturator nerve at the obturator foramen (childbirth)
- Fibular nerve at the fibular head (leg crossers, total hip replacement, and surgical malpositioning)
- Lateral femoral cutaneous nerve (meralgia paresthetica)
- Posterior tibial nerve at the tarsal tunnel (tarsal tunnel syndrome).
- Accessory nerve in the posterior triangle (surgical neck dissection).

MONONEUROPATHY MULTIPLEX

Diseases that affect multiple peripheral nerves at different sites result in the syndrome of *mononeuropathy multiplex.* The presence of **asymmetric and multifocal motor, sensory, and reflex deficits** is the key to identifying the syndrome. The patient's history may reveal a subacute, stepwise progression of deficits. The differential diagnosis of mononeuropathy multiplex includes the following:

- *Vasculitis*

  Polyarteritis nodosa is the most common vasculitis associated with this condition. Systemic lupus erythematosus, rheumatoid arthritis, and cryoglobulinemia may occasionally produce the condition.
- *Diabetes mellitus*
- *Leprosy*
- *Sarcoidosis*
- *HIV infection*
- *Lymphoma*
- *Lyme disease*
- *Hereditary liability to pressure palsies*
- *Multifocal motor neuropathy (pure motor)*
- *Chronic inflammatory demyelinating polyneuropathy (CIDP)*

Diagnosis

Initial blood tests should include fasting glucose level with Chem-20 screen, complete blood count (CBC), erythrocyte sedimentation rate (ESR), antinuclear antibody (ANA), rheumatoid factor (RF), antineutrophil cytoplasmic antibody (ANCA), HIV testing, hepatitis serologies, cryoglobulins, and serum angiotensin-converting enzyme (ACE) activity. LP should be considered to rule out inflammatory conditions (e.g., CIDP, neurosarcoidosis) and carcinomatous meningitis. A comprehensive EMG and NCS examination is often needed to prove multifocal involvement. Muscle or nerve biopsy is sometimes necessary to rule out vasculitis, sarcoidosis, leprosy, and lymphoma. Vasculitic neuropathy may indicate an underlying malignancy if no rheumatological condition is present.

Treatment

Therapy is directed toward treating the underlying disease.

POLYNEUROPATHY

The prototypical polyneuropathy patient presents with gradual **distal, symmetric sensorimotor deficits, and hyporeflexia.** Typically, the longest nerves in the body are affected first, resulting in a stocking-glove distribution of symptoms and signs (see Fig. 20.1). Dysesthetic sensory changes are often the first symptom; weakness develops later or not at all.

The number of entities that can cause peripheral neuropathy is vast (Table 20.2), and pinpointing a precise cause can be difficult. An organized and stepwise approach is essential. **Consideration of the following points can help narrow the possibilities and allow screening for the most common and important (i.e., treatable) causes.**

TABLE 20.2	Causes of Peripheral Polyneuropathy

Metabolic and Endocrine Diseases
Diabetes mellitus[a]
Renal failure[a]
Hepatic failure
Porphyria
Hypothyroidism
Critical illness polyneuropathy[a]

Vitamin Deficiency States
Beriberi (thiamine deficiency)
Vitamin B_6 (pyridoxine) deficiency
Vitamin B_{12} deficiency
Vitamin B complex deficiency
Pellagra (niacin deficiency)
Vitamin E deficiency
Copper deficiency (also causes myelopathy)

Toxins and Poisons
Alcohol
Heavy metals: arsenic, lead, mercury, thallium
Organic and industrial solvents: carbon disulfide, n-hexane, acrylamide,
     methyl-N-butyl ketone
Pyridoxine (vitamin B_6) overdose
Nitrous oxide (also causes myelopathy)
Medications
Antibiotics: dapsone, nitrofurantoin, isoniazid, ethambutol, metronidazole, HIV
     nucleoside analogs, linezolid, fluoroquinolones (controversial)
Antiarrhythmics: amiodarone, propafenone
Chemotherapeutic agents[a]: vinca alkaloids, platins, taxoids, ixabepilone,
     bortezomib, eribulin mesylate, thalidomide, cetuximab, arsenic trioxide
Chloroquine (also causes myopathy)
Colchicine (also causes myopathy)
D-Penicillamine
Disulfiram
Gold salts
Leflunomide, teriflunomide
Lithium
Podophyllin
Pyridoxine
Phenytoin
Statins
Tacrolimus

Immunologic or Paraprotein-Mediated Diseases
Acute inflammatory polyneuropathy (Guillain-Barré syndrome)[a]
Chronic inflammatory polyneuropathy (chronic inflammatory demyelinating
     polyneuropathy)[a]
Paraneoplastic disease (sensorimotor or pure sensory)[a]
Multiple myeloma
Antimyelin-associated glycoprotein antibody-mediated disease
Amyloidosis

TABLE 20.2	Causes of Peripheral Polyneuropathy—cont'd

Lymphoma with paraprotein
Monoclonal gammopathy
Cryoglobulinemia
Collagen vascular disease (systemic lupus erythematosus, rheumatoid
　arthritis, etc.)
Sarcoidosis
Waldenström macroglobulinemia
Celiac disease

Genetic/Hereditary Diseases
Charcot-Marie-Tooth disease[a]
Refsum disease
Storage diseases (metachromatic leukodystrophy, adrenomyeloneuropathy, etc.)
Inherited metabolic enzyme defects

Infectious Diseases
HIV infection*
Cytomegalovirus infection
Leprosy
Lyme disease
West Nile virus
Zika virus

[a]Common.

Clinical Approach to the Patient with Polyneuropathy
Diagnosis

1. **History**
   - **Is the neuropathy acute or chronic?** Acute polyneuropathy (Guillain-Barré syndrome) is discussed in Chapter 16.
   - **Ask a carefully directed set of questions to identify an obvious cause.** Ask about diabetes, renal disease, HIV infection, current medications, alcohol use, potential exposure to toxins, and family history. *The majority of polyneuropathies are complications of previously evident medical disorders, medications, or alcohol.*
   - **Do the symptoms fluctuate?** Fluctuations suggest a relapsing demyelinating neuropathy (CIDP) or repeated exposures to toxins.
2. **Examination**
   - **Determine the predominant systems involved.** Most neuropathies are sensorimotor, with the sensory component predominant. Identifying a predominantly motor, pure sensory, or particularly painful neuropathy helps to limit the differential diagnosis considerably (Table 20.3).

TABLE 20.3	Features Helpful in Narrowing the Cause of Peripheral Neuropathy: Syndromes Other Than Distal Axonal Neuropathies
Pure (or predominantly) motor neuropathy	Lymphoma, multifocal motor neuropathy (with or without anti-GM 1 antibodies) *Toxic:* dapsone, lead, organophosphates Porphyria Guillain-Barré syndrome Tick paralysis Diphtheria
Pure (or predominantly) sensory neuropathy[a]	Acute idiopathic sensory neuropathy Primary biliary cirrhosis Sjögren syndrome Diabetes mellitus Human immunodeficiency virus infection Leprosy Hereditary sensory and autonomic neuropathies Uremia Paraneoplastic sensory ganglioneuritis (anti-Hu, ANNA-1 antibodies) *Toxic:* thallium, pyridoxine (vitamin B_6) intoxication, copper deficiency
Palpably enlarged nerves	*Genetic:* Charcot-Marie-Tooth disease, Dejerine-Sottas disease, Refsum disease, neurofibromatosis, hereditary liability to pressure palsies Leprosy Chronic inflammatory demyelinating polyneuropathy
Demyelinating neuropathies	*Immunologic:* Guillain-Barré syndrome, chronic inflammatory demyelinating polyneuropathy, paraproteinemia, anti-MAG antibodies *Toxic:* diphtheria, buckthorn toxin, amiodarone, perhexiline *Genetic:* Charcot-Marie-Tooth type I disease, storage diseases, hereditary liability to pressure palsies *Paraneoplastic:* osteosclerotic multiple myeloma

[a]Usually small-fiber sensory loss (pain, temperature) with prominent autonomic dysfunction.
MAG, Myelin-associated glycoprotein.

- **Determine whether the findings are asymmetric.** Patchy and asymmetric motor, sensory, and reflex deficits suggest *mononeuropathy multiplex* or *polyradiculopathy* (see earlier discussion).
- **Check for palpably enlarged nerves.** Although it is unusual, a finding of enlarged nerves can help pinpoint the diagnosis (see Table 20.3).

3. **Electrodiagnostic studies: EMG and NCS**
   - **Determine whether the neuropathy is axonal or demyelinating.** Electrodiagnosis is critical for making this distinction, which can help to narrow your differential diagnosis. *Distal axonal sensorimotor neuropathies* are the most common. *Demyelinating neuropathies* have a much smaller differential diagnosis (see Table 20.3).

Management

LABORATORY TESTING FOR EVALUATION OF POLYNEUROPATHY

1. If an obvious cause for the neuropathy exists (e.g., post–vincristine chemotherapy), no further workup may be needed; otherwise, proceed with the next steps.
2. The following initial laboratory tests should be performed: fasting glucose with full chemistry panel including liver function tests (LFTs), CBC, TFTs, initial rheumatologic screen (ESR, ANA, Sjögren antibodies, RF), serum protein electrophoresis, and vitamin B_{12} level.
3. Other tests to consider include LP, testing of urine for paraproteins, serum immunofixation electrophoresis, quantitative immunoglobulins, testing urine for heavy metals, tests for HIV, cytomegalovirus (CMV), Lyme antibody, gliadin and tissue transglutaminase, other vitamin levels (vitamins B_6 and E), ANCA, ACE level, homocysteine/methionine levels (vitamin B_{12} deficiency), genetic testing (Charcot-Marie-Tooth disease), special antibody assays (anti-Hu, anti-GM1, anti-MAG, and anti-sulfatide), and bone marrow biopsy.
4. A nerve and muscle biopsy is occasionally helpful for confirming several specific diagnoses (Table 20.4), but it is most useful in evaluating *mononeuropathy multiplex* and is not routinely performed.

TABLE 20.4	**Causes of Peripheral Neuropathy That Can Be Diagnosed by Nerve Biopsy**

- Vasculitis
- Leprosy
- Lymphoma
- Cytomegalovirus (causes polyradiculopathy or mononeuropathy multiplex)
- Storage diseases (MLD, AMN, Krabbe disease)
- Amyloidosis
- Immune-mediated diseases (IgM and complement deposition)

AMN, Adrenomyeloneuropathy; *IgM,* immunoglobulin M; *MLD,* metachromatic leukodystrophy.

Selected Causes of Neuropathy

- **Diabetes mellitus**

  Diabetes is the most common cause of neuropathy worldwide. Several different forms of neuropathy may occur, and an individual may have more than one type.

  1. **Distal axonal sensorimotor neuropathy** is most common. Sensory symptoms (small fiber) usually predominate, including painful dysesthesias.
  2. **Autonomic neuropathy** is commonly seen in combination with axonal small-fiber sensory neuropathy. Symptoms may include anhidrosis, orthostatic hypotension, impotence, gastroparesis, and bowel and bladder disturbances.
  3. **Mononeuropathy** may occur from either nerve infarction or entrapment (e.g., carpal tunnel syndrome).
  4. **Mononeuropathy multiplex**
  5. **Diabetic amyotrophy (radiculoplexus neuropathy)** presents with dull, aching proximal pain, followed by asymmetric proximal leg weakness and wasting not limited to a root, plexus, or nerve territory. Underlying distal diabetic neuropathy is often minimal in these patients.

- **Ethanol**

  Chronic ethanol is a common cause of axonal sensorimotor neuropathy with prominent distal paresthesias and numbness; superimposed thiamine deficiency produces subacute progression weakness and imbalance. Vitamin B complex supplements and alcohol cessation can lead to improvement.

- **Uremia**

  Renal failure often leads to a distal, axonal, sensorimotor neuropathy with prominent cramps and unpleasant dysesthesias. Improvement may occur with dialysis or kidney transplantation.

- **Chronic Inflammatory Demyelinating Polyneuropathy (CIDP)**

  CIDP presents as a chronic relapsing sensorimotor polyneuropathy or, rarely, as mononeuropathy multiplex. The diagnosis is confirmed by *elevated CSF protein* and *a demyelinating pattern on EMG/NCS*. Proximal and distal weakness is typically present. In some cases, a plasma cell dyscrasia or paraprotein may be identified. **IVIG (2.0 g/kg for initiation then 1.0 g/kg every 2–4 weeks) is the mainstay of treatment; this approach is approved by the FDA. Prednisone, starting at 60 mg/day,** is a secondary alternative treatment. **Plasmapheresis, azathioprine 150 mg/day, and rituximab** are other secondary treatment options.

- **Paraprotein-associated neuropathy**

  These neuropathies can result in a demyelinating or axonal sensorimotor neuropathy. CSF protein is elevated in 80% of demyelinating cases. The protein can be identified by either serum or urine protein electrophoresis or immunofixation electrophoresis. IgM forms are less common but much more likely to produce neuropathy. IgA and IgG forms are less commonly associated with neuropathy; POEMS syndrome and amyloidosis are possible associations. Bone marrow biopsy may be helpful in the two-thirds of cases with plasma cell dyscrasia; in the remaining patients, multiple myeloma (in 12%), amyloidosis (in 9%), lymphoma (in 5%), leukemia (in 3%), or Waldenström macroglobulinemia (in 2%) may be identified. **Prednisone 40 to 100 mg/day** or **azathioprine 150 mg/day** may benefit some patients; **plasmapheresis, rituximab**, and **IVIG** are other treatment options. If severe sensory ataxia and imbalance are present, an IgM monoclonal gammopathy that includes antibodies against myelin-associated glycoprotein (anti-MAG), rituximab is the primary treatment option.

- **Critical illness polyneuropathy**

  This polyneuropathy is associated with sepsis and multisystem organ failure. It often presents as failure to wean from mechanical ventilation. EMG/NCS is consistent with severe sensorimotor axonal neuropathy. There is no specific treatment, but if the patient survives, recovery is possible.

- **Paraneoplastic neuropathy**

  Paraneoplastic neuropathy most often manifests as an axonal sensorimotor neuropathy, but it also can take the form of a large-fiber pure sensory neuropathy, a demyelinating sensorimotor neuropathy, or a pure motor neuronopathy (usually seen with lymphoma). These and other paraneoplastic syndromes (see Chapter 23) are mediated by autoimmune responses against peripheral nerve.

- **Genetic (hereditary) neuropathies**

  These neuropathies are unusual except for **Charcot-Marie-Tooth disease,** which comes in two forms: type I (demyelinating) and the less common type II (axonal). The disease is most commonly autosomal dominant, with variable expression from one generation to the next. Patients present with insidious distal lower extremity weakness and wasting ("stork leg deformity"), high arches, pes cavus, and minimal sensory symptoms. Multiple gene defects are known.

General Care of the Patient with Neuropathy

1. *Remove any potential neurotoxic medications,* even if these are not the primary cause (see Table 20.2 for a list).
2. *Treat neuropathic pain* with **gabapentin (300–3600 mg daily),** tricyclic antidepressants **(nortriptyline 10–25 mg daily), pregabalin (50–100 mg three times a day [TID]),** or the selective serotonin reuptake inhibitors **duloxetine (20–60 mg every day [QD]), or the atypical pain agent, tramadol (50 mg QD to 100 mg four times a day [QID]); narcotics are typically avoided except in refractory cases.**
3. *Initiate occupational and physical therapy* in patients with moderate to severe disability for gait and balance training, prevention of contractures, orthoses, and assistive devices.
4. *Skin care* is important in patients with severe sensory neuropathy to prevent trophic ulcers, infections, and neuropathic (Charcot) joints.
5. *Autonomic neuropathy* may require treatment for orthostatic hypotension **(fludrocortisone 0.1–0.3 mg a day or midodrine 2.5–10 mg two to three times a day, or droxidopa 100–600 mg three times a day)** or gastroparesis (treat with **metoclopramide 5–10 mg three times a day).**

NEUROMUSCULAR JUNCTION DISEASE

Myasthenia gravis and **botulism,** both of which can lead to respiratory failure, are discussed in Chapter 16.

Lambert-Eaton myasthenic syndrome (LEMS) is an autoimmune disease caused by antibodies directed against voltage-gated calcium channels of the presynaptic nerve terminals, causing impaired neuromuscular transmission. Many cases are paraneoplastic and are mostly small-cell lung carcinoma. The disease is initially identified with proximal limb weakness. Lower extremity areflexia, myalgias, dry mouth, and impotence may also occur, but diplopia, dysphagia, and dyspnea do not occur. The disease is diagnosed by the presence of an incremental response on repetitive nerve stimulation (10 Hz) and supporting antibody titers. **3,4-Diaminopyridine 20 mg TID (amifampridine) improves strength and fatigue, and**, is the only FDA approved treatment. Pyridostigmine, plasmapheresis, and IVIG may also be tried.

MYOPATHY

Diseases of muscle typically lead to **proximal, symmetric weakness** without sensory deficits or bowel or bladder symptoms. The patient may complain of difficulty reaching above the head, getting out of a chair, or climbing stairs.

Questions to Ask the Patient with Suspected Myopathic Disease

1. Does the patient have muscle aches or tenderness, suggestive of muscle inflammation or necrosis?
2. Has the patient noticed darkened, cola-colored urine (*myoglobinuria*)?
3. Does the weakness fluctuate or worsen with exercise, suggestive of myasthenia gravis or periodic paralysis?
4. Are there any sensory or bowel or bladder symptoms? (Such symptoms would make a myopathic disease unlikely.)
5. Have there been any new cardiac symptoms? (Many entities affect both skeletal and cardiac muscle.)

Examination

1. Map out the pattern of weakness (proximal versus distal). Most myopathies cause proximal weakness; exceptions include myotonic dystrophy, inclusion body myositis, and rare genetic causes.
2. Check for *myotonia* (prolonged muscle contraction after voluntary contraction or percussion), which can be tested by handgrip, forced eye closure, or muscle percussion.
3. Palpate for muscle tenderness.
4. Undress the patient to evaluate for a pattern of muscle wasting.

Management

Diagnostic Testing

1. **Initial laboratory tests:** creatine kinase (CK) level, Chem-20 screen, TFTs, sedimentation rate, electrocardiogram (ECG).
2. **EMG/NCS:** needle EMG in patients with myopathy shows abnormal, short-duration, low-amplitude, polyphasic motor unit potentials and overly rapid recruitment of motor units with an excessively low-amplitude interference pattern (see Chapter 3).
3. **Muscle biopsy** may be needed to establish a diagnosis.
4. **Other tests to consider** include ACE level, serum cortisol level, serum and CSF lactate (mitochondrial myopathy), genetic testing (for muscular and myotonic dystrophy), and toxicology screen.

Causes of Myopathy

Causes of myopathy can be categorized into five main groups: **inflammatory, endocrine, toxic, hereditary, and infectious.**

1. **Inflammatory myopathies**
   a. *Polymyositis*
      This inflammatory autoimmune muscle disease is characterized by chronic and relapsing proximal limb weakness. Although the eyes and face are almost never affected, pharyngeal and neck weakness is common (in approximately 50% of

patients). Cardiomyopathy, interstitial lung disease, and other systemic autoimmune diseases (e.g., systemic lupus erythematosus, Crohn disease) are also found in a significant proportion of patients. Isolated polymyositis is highly atypical.

(1) *Diagnosis:* CK levels are elevated in almost all cases, and EMG shows myopathic findings with denervation secondary to segmental muscle necrosis. Muscle biopsy reveals endomysial lymphocytic infiltrates, necrotic and atrophic muscle fibers, and connective tissue deposition.

(2) *Treatment:* Prednisone 60 to 100 mg daily leads to improvement in most patients within 2 to 3 months and is most effective early in the disease course. Azathioprine 1 to 3 mg/kg per day or methotrexate 25 to 50 mg per week can be used for disease suppression in steroid nonresponders.

b. *Dermatomyositis*

Dermatomyositis is similar to polymyositis but is accompanied by a characteristic rash that precedes or accompanies muscle weakness. Skin manifestations include a heliotrope (bluish) rash on the upper eyelids, erythematous rash on the face and trunk, violaceous scaly eruptions on the knuckles (Gottron papules), and subcutaneous calcifications.

(1) *Diagnosis:* Muscle biopsy findings differ from polymyositis in showing perivascular inflammation and *perifascicular atrophy.* A malignancy screen is prudent with a later age of onset.

(2) *Treatment:* Treatment is the same as for polymyositis.

c. *Inclusion body myositis*

This entity differs from polymyositis in that it tends to produce distal and asymmetric weakness, it occurs primarily at an older age, and it responds poorly to steroids. Muscle biopsy reveals rimmed vacuoles and eosinophilic cytoplasmic inclusions with amyloid. Finger flexor and quadriceps weakness is a hallmark. No effective treatment is known.

d. *Sarcoidosis*

Patients with sarcoidosis can develop focal or generalized myopathy. Biopsy shows noncaseating granulomas. Steroids usually produce clinical improvement.

2. **Endocrine myopathies**

Patients with endocrine myopathy usually show systemic signs of endocrine disease before the onset of weakness, but in some instances, myopathy is the presenting feature. CK levels are usually normal or only mildly elevated. In all cases, weakness is reversed by treating the underlying endocrinopathy, which includes thyroid disease, Cushing disease (hyperadrenalism), or parathyroid disease.

3. **Toxic myopathies**
    a. *Medications*

    Drugs and medications produce subacute, generalized proximal muscle weakness through a variety of mechanisms. Table 20.5 lists some medications and toxins commonly associated with myopathy.

    b. *Critical illness myopathy*

    This myopathy presents as a failure to wean from mechanical ventilation in intensive care unit (ICU) patients treated with steroids and nondepolarizing paralyzing agents (e.g., vecuronium); however, neither precipitant is necessary for disease development. Muscle biopsy shows selective loss of thick myosin filaments. This condition is much more common than typically diagnosed. There is no treatment, but recovery over weeks to months is the rule. This condition is much more common than critical illness neuropathy.

    c. *Neuroleptic malignant syndrome*

    Dopamine blockers (e.g., haloperidol, chlorpromazine [Thorazine]) can produce this rare, idiosyncratic response characterized by generalized muscle rigidity with rhabdomyolysis, fever, altered mental status, tremor, and autonomic instability (especially hypertension). CK levels are always elevated, and white blood cell counts are usually increased. Treatment includes discontinuation of the offending agent, surface cooling, dantrolene 1 to 10 mg/kg per day intravenously (IV) (every 4–6 hours as needed to attain muscle relaxation), and bromocriptine 2.5 to 5 mg three times a day.

    d. *Malignant hyperthermia*

    This autosomal dominant condition predisposes to severe muscle rigidity, rhabdomyolysis, fever, and metabolic acidosis following exposure to inhalation anesthetics or

TABLE 20.5	Drugs That Can Cause Myopathy	
Rhabdomyolysis	**Hypokalemic Myopathy**	**Myopathy (Weakness and Myalgia)**
Amphotericin B	Diuretics	Colchicine
ε-Aminocaproic acid	Azathioprine	Zidovicine
Fenfluramine	Myositis	Steroids
Heroin	(inflammatory)	Clofibrate
Phencyclidine	Penicillamine	Chloroquine
Alcohol	Procainamide	Emetine
Barbiturates	Cimetidine	Labetalol
Cocaine		Statin class anticholesterol

succinylcholine. Treatment is with dantrolene 2.5 to 10 mg/kg IV in repeated doses.

4. **Hereditary myopathies**
   a. *Muscular dystrophy*

   Muscular dystrophy is a progressively degenerative genetic myopathy. Weakness is usually present in early life, gets worse over time, and often leads to early death.

   (1) **Duchenne muscular dystrophy (X-linked).** The onset is by age 5 with inability to walk occurring by age 10 and with eventual respiratory failure. Features include calf pseudohypertrophy, cardiomyopathy, and occasional mental impairment. *Becker muscular dystrophy* is a later-onset form of the disease with less severe manifestations. **Prednisone 20 to 40 mg per day** can increase strength and function, but it does not alter the overall course. Genetic testing of the dystrophin gene is the primary mode of testing. Genetic-based treatments are in advanced stages of testing.

   (2) **Myotonic dystrophy (autosomal dominant).** This most common form of muscular dystrophy leads to progressive *distal* myopathy. The disease occurs earlier and is more severe with successive generations (genetic anticipation). Along with myotonia, features include distinctive facies with ptosis and frontal balding, cataracts, cardiac conduction defects, gonadal atrophy, and mental impairment. **Mexiletine 150 to 200 mg 3 times daily, phenytoin 300 mg per day PO, and procainamide 20 to 50 mg/kg per day three times a day** are occasionally necessary to treat the myotonia, but most patients do not require treatment. ECGs performed at least yearly are prudent to assess for evolving heart block. Definitive genetic triple repeat analysis is available for diagnosis confirmation.

   (3) **Other hereditary myopathies.** These entities include facioscapulohumeral (autosomal dominant), limb girdle (autosomal recessive and dominant, multiple genes), oculopharyngeal (autosomal recessive), and Emery-Dreifuss (X-linked) myopathies. Many of these myopathies now have precise genetic diagnoses. Discerning a clinical pattern of involvement may narrow genetic testing required for diagnosis.

   b. *Metabolic myopathies*

   Seen mostly in the pediatric population, these diseases result from deficiencies of specific enzymes involved in the utilization of glucose or lipid (the two main sources of skeletal muscle energy). Along with muscle weakness, patients with metabolic myopathies often experience *rhabdomyolysis* and *myoglobinuria.* Muscle biopsy is necessary to establish the diagnosis. The most common metabolic myopathy is McArdle disease, which is an autosomal recessive disorder resulting from myophosphorylase deficiency. It presents in childhood with painful muscle cramps and myoglobinuria after intense exercise. A lack of increase in lactate levels with ischemic forearm testing is characteristic. Laboratory confirmation of urinary or serum myoglobin in an acute phase is key.

c. *Periodic paralysis*

These rare disorders are caused by genetic abnormalities of membrane ion channels. The majority are inherited in autosomal dominant fashion. Patients are usually normal between attacks of severe weakness. Hypokalemic and hyperkalemic forms have been described.

d. *Congenital myopathies*

This group of rare disorders presents mostly at birth with floppy infant syndrome, and the disorders are usually nonprogressive or very slowly progressive. Examples include nemaline (rod) body myopathy, myotubular (centronuclear) myopathy, and central core disease. Adult-onset cases may be seen.

e. *Mitochondrial myopathy*

These diseases result from defects in the mitochondrial genome and hence are maternally inherited. Muscle biopsy shows "ragged red fibers." Suspicious signs for mitochondrial diseases include ptosis, ophthalmoparesis, and high serum lactate levels. Variants include myoclonic epilepsy with ragged red fibers, which is known as mitochondrial encephalomyopathy, encephalopathy, lactic acidosis, and strokelike episodes (*MELAS*), and *Kearns-Sayre syndrome* (pigmentary retinopathy, cardiac conduction defects, high CSF protein). Genetic analysis is available for many types of mitochondrial myopathies.

5. **Infectious myopathies**

Muscle infiltration with the organisms that cause *trichinosis, toxoplasmosis,* and *cysticercosis* can lead to a widespread or a localized inflammatory myopathy. Acute rhabdomyolysis and myoglobinuria can occur as a result of infection with influenza virus, rubella virus, coxsackievirus, echoviruses, and mycoplasma. HIV myopathy has declined in incidence but is a consideration.

Demyelinating and Inflammatory Disorders of the Central Nervous System

Demyelinating and inflammatory diseases of the central nervous system (CNS) are varied and often enigmatic. *Multiple sclerosis (MS),* the prototypical inflammatory demyelinating disease, is a chronic autoimmune disorder characterized by loss of myelin and relative preservation of axons. *Acute disseminated encephalomyelitis (ADEM)* is a monophasic illness that is pathologically similar to MS but is typically triggered by an antecedent viral infection. *Central pontine myelinolysis (CPM)* refers to osmotic demyelination in the setting of rapid correction of hyponatremia. *Sarcoidosis* and *Behçet disease* are idiopathic systemic inflammatory diseases that may involve the CNS. Dysmyelinating diseases, such as Alexander and Canavan diseases, are genetic disorders in which there is an intrinsic abnormality of myelin; they present in childhood and will not be discussed in this chapter.

MULTIPLE SCLEROSIS

The hallmark of MS is episodic or progressive multifocal deficits affecting the CNS in otherwise healthy young adults. The most common initial clinical manifestations of MS are sensory disturbances, visual loss, and weakness. Diagnosis relies on recognition of the clinical patterns of disease and is supported by magnetic resonance imaging (MRI) studies of the brain and spinal cord, and analysis of cerebrospinal fluid (CSF; in those with a progressive onset). Systemic illnesses that can mimic the symptoms of MS must be excluded.

General Considerations

Next to trauma, MS is the most common cause of disability in young adults. MS affects approximately 350,000 to 500,000 Americans and more than 1 million individuals worldwide. The cause of MS is unknown, and because there is no single diagnostic test, accurate diagnosis relies on clinical recognition of the disease. The hallmarks of MS are multifocal waxing and waning, or progressive neurologic deficits, that localize to the CNS. *The signs and symptoms of MS are separated in space (multiple areas of the CNS) and evolve over time (during the life of the patient).* MS affects only the CNS and spares the peripheral nerves.

MS has a distinct pathology characterized by focal demyelination within the brain and spinal cord. MS is considered an autoimmune disease because inflammatory infiltrates are present within the damaged myelin. However, it is not known whether the immune response is a primary process or is triggered by infectious, toxic, or metabolic etiologies. There is no cure for MS, and current treatments are only partially effective, although tremendous progress has been made, particularly in relapsing forms of the illness.

Epidemiology

MS affects women two to three times as often as men. MS is rare in the pediatric population, but its risk increases steadily from adolescence up to the age of 35, then gradually decreases, and is rarely diagnosed after the age of 65. MS is uncommon in equatorial climates, and its prevalence increases with northern distance from the equator.

Genetics

The risk of MS is much higher in populations of Northern European ancestry than in other ethnic groups residing at the same latitudes. Twin studies demonstrate concordance rates of approximately 30% in identical twins and 5% in fraternal twins. The rate for first-degree relatives of MS patients also is 5%. Genome-wide association studies have identified over 100 risk alleles for MS. These alleles provide clues to pathophysiology and potential therapeutic targets.

Pathology

The term *multiple sclerosis* refers to discrete hard or rubbery plaques within the white matter of the brain and spinal cord. These lesions are composed of areas of myelin and oligodendrocyte loss accompanied by infiltrates of macrophages and lymphocytes.

The focal loss of myelin indicates a highly specific demyelinating process and distinguishes MS from leukodystrophies. In addition, preserved axons and neurons discern MS from other destructive processes. Although axons in MS plaques are relatively spared, axonal transection occurs, is irreversible, and presumably leads to neuronal death by Wallerian degeneration.

Clinical Features
Symptomatic Onset

The initial focal manifestations may be acute or insidious and can vary in severity. Acute neurologic deficits caused by MS are called *relapses* and are known as flares, attacks, or exacerbations. The most common initial symptoms are sensory disturbances, visual loss, and weakness, although abnormal gait, loss of dexterity, diplopia, ataxia, vertigo, or sphincter disturbances can occur. Nonspecific symptoms such as malaise or fatigue often precede the initial focal disturbance.

Sensory Disturbance

The most common presenting symptom of MS is paresthesia (tingling, pins and needles), dysesthesia (burning, gritty, sandy, electrical, or wet sensations), or hypesthesia (loss of sensation or procaine-like numbness). Some patients describe a squeezing sensation as if a limb or the trunk were tightly wrapped. These symptoms can be intermittent or constant and can spread from one location to adjoining areas. Spinal cord involvement is implied by ascending numbness with a sensory level. A Lhermitte symptom, an electrical or shocklike paresthesia that radiates down the spine and into one or more limbs after neck flexion, localizes the lesion to the cervical spine. Sensory disturbances associated with MS flares usually resolve spontaneously but sometimes evolve into chronic neuropathic pain. Trigeminal neuralgia also occurs in MS, perhaps caused by demyelination in the root entry zone of the trigeminal nerve.

Optic Neuritis

The next most common presenting manifestation of MS is optic neuritis, which causes loss of vision affecting usually one eye evolving over hours or days. Bilateral simultaneous optic neuritis is much less frequent and should raise the possibility of an alternate diagnosis such as neuromyelitis optica spectrum disorder (NMOSD). Loss of vision can be complete or partial; patients will often report a scotoma, which is an area of diminished or blurred vision in the monocular field. Optic neuritis is often associated with periorbital pain elicited by eye movements. Loss of vision can be subtle and affect only color vision. Red desaturation, or the inability to distinguish shades of red, can be quantified using Ishihara color plates. Demyelination of the optic nerve close to the retina causes optic disc pallor. The differential diagnosis of acute visual loss is shown in Table 21.1.

Motor Symptoms

Motor symptoms are as common as optic neuritis as initial manifestations of MS and include limb weakness, loss of dexterity, and

TABLE 21.1	Differential Diagnosis for Acute Visual Loss
V	**Vascular:** nonarteritic anterior ischemic optic neuropathy, giant cell arteritis, diabetic retinopathies, Susac syndrome (microangiopathy of the brain, retina, and inner ear), acute posterior multifocal placoid pigment epitheliopathy, Eales disease (noninflammatory occlusive disease of the retinal vasculature), Cogan syndrome (interstitial keratitis, vestibular dysfunction, and deafness), amaurosis fugax, central retinal vein occlusion, aneurysms and arteriovenous malformations, systemic hypercoagulable states including anticardiolipin syndrome
I	**Infectious:** rarely cause such rapid visual loss without other symptoms and can be local (retinitis, periostitis, meningitis) or systemic (syphilis, toxoplasmosis, typhoid fever, leptospirosis)
T	**Trauma:** rare
A	**Autoimmune:** sarcoidosis, optic neuritis
M	**Metabolic /toxic:** vitamin B_{12} deficiency, toxins (e.g., ethyl alcohol, ethambutol, methanol, amiodarone, clioquinol, chemotherapeutic agents, benzene), tropical ataxic neuropathy (cassava diet, tobacco use associated with a defect in cyanide detoxification), radiation-induced optic neuropathy
I	**Idiopathic/hereditary:** Leber hereditary optic neuropathy, Kearns-Sayre syndrome, MELAS, NARP, Friedreich ataxia
N	**Neoplastic/paraneoplastic/infiltrative:** infiltrating neoplasms (e.g., lymphoma, leukemia, myeloma, carcinomatous meningitis), optic nerve glioma, optic nerve glioblastoma, optic sheath meningioma, CAR, CACD, MAR, DUMP, PCGN, Langerhans cell disorders
S	**Psychiatric:** conversion reaction
Others:	central serous chorioretinopathy, optic disc drusen, ophthalmic migraine, big blind spot syndromes (acute zonal occult outer retinopathy, acute macular neuroretinopathy, multiple evanescent white dot syndrome, acute idiopathic blind spot enlargement syndrome)

CACD, Cancer-associated cone dysfunction; *CAR,* cancer-associated retinopathy; *DUMP,* diffuse uveal melanocytic proliferation; *MAR,* melanoma-associated retinopathy; *PCGN,* paraneoplastic ganglion cell neuronopathy; *MELAS,* mitochondrial encephalopathy with lactic acidosis and strokes; *NARP,* neuropathy, ataxia, and retinitis pigmentosa syndrome.

gait disturbance. Symptoms typically evolve over hours or days; sometimes patients will awaken with a motor deficit. Weakness can affect a single limb or cause hemiparesis or paraparesis. The hemiparesis of MS usually spares the face. Sometimes weakness becomes apparent only during exertion. Weakness is usually accompanied by spasticity and hyperreflexia.

Diplopia

Dysconjugate eye movements resulting in diplopia are common in MS. Intranuclear ophthalmoplegia (INO) is caused by demyelinating plaques within the medial longitudinal fasciculus (MLF). Lesions in the MLF typically occur ipsilateral to the affected third nucleus and result in impaired ipsilateral adduction with compensatory nystagmus of the abducting eye. MS also can cause vertical diplopia and isolated impairments of the sixth, third, and fourth nerves.

Ataxia and Tremor

Dyscoordinated movements of the limbs or trunk are common in MS because of plaques affecting the cerebellar afferent or efferent pathways and range in severity from subtle to disabling. Tremor and dysmetria, an error in measurement of movement, are often observed on finger-nose-finger and heel-knee-shin tests. Dysrhythmia can be demonstrated by finger or toe tapping. *Romberg sign,* truncal swaying on standing with the feet together and eyes closed, can be caused by impaired proprioception from spinal cord dorsal column lesions.

Neuropsychiatric Dysfunction

Cognitive impairments are present in 40% to 65% of MS patients and can result in loss of vocation and impairment of activities of daily living. Patients often report difficulties with short-term memory, attention, information processing, problem-solving, multitasking, and language function. Cognitive deficits may not be detected by the Mini-Mental Status Examination and often require neuropsychiatric testing. Emotional lability is common; up to 60% of MS patients suffer from depression.

Bladder and Bowel Dysfunction

Patients often complain of urinary urgency, frequency, hesitancy, and incontinence. Incontinence can occur in the setting of a spastic bladder that is incapable of filling completely or with a distended (denervated) bladder that overflows. It is often not possible to determine the nature of bladder dysfunction by history. Measurement of the volume of postvoid residual urine, by catheterization, ultrasound, or urodynamic studies, is essential for distinguishing between a spastic and denervated bladder. Bladder dyssynergia, an impairment of sphincter and detrusor coordination, also is a cause of hesitancy and incomplete voiding. Patients with urinary retention are susceptible to urinary tract infections, and such infections may trigger MS relapses by stimulating the immune system.

Bowel dysfunction is common in MS and is presumably caused by spinal cord plaques. Chronic constipation can worsen spasticity. Incontinence occurs either as a consequence of sphincter dysfunction or from bowel spasticity and fecal urgency.

Vertigo

Vertigo caused by MS is sometimes associated with other signs or symptoms of brain stem pathology such as facial sensory loss or diplopia. Vertigo can be fleeting or last for days or even weeks. Although uncommon, unilateral hearing loss occurs in MS, sometimes in conjunction with vertigo. Vertigo caused by labyrinthine pathology identified by the Dix-Hallpike maneuver (see Chapter 14) is not caused by MS.

Dysarthria

Impairments of speech are common in MS and can be caused by tongue weakness from lower brain stem dysfunction, spastic dysarthria from corticobulbar injury, or scanning dysarthria from cerebellar dysfunction.

Dysphagia

Impairment of swallowing occurs in MS, particularly later in the course of the disease. Choking on thin liquids is consistent with neurologic injury as opposed to solid food dysphagia, which is typically caused by a pharyngeal structural abnormality. Barium swallow and fiberscope endoscopic evaluation of swallowing are helpful in assessing aspiration risk.

Facial Weakness

Lower motor neuron facial weakness, similar to Bell palsy, can occur when MS plaques affect intraparenchymal emerging fibers of the seventh cranial nerve. Ipsilateral loss of taste, hyperacusis, retroauricular pain, and synkinesis are hallmarks of peripheral facial neuropathy and do not occur with central facial weakness. Facial myokymia is a chronic flickering contraction of the orbicularis oculi or other muscles of facial expression caused by injury to the facial nerve or corticobulbar tracts within the brain stem.

Fatigue

Fatigue is the most common symptom of MS and contends with cognitive impairment as the major cause of loss of vocation. Fatigue can occur as a consequence of exertion (neuromuscular weakness), as a manifestation of depression, as a consequence of insomnia (daytime drowsiness), or as a generalized lassitude. Fatigue is often worse in the afternoon but can be present on awakening and persist throughout the day.

Paroxysmal Symptoms

Virtually all symptoms of MS, including the Lhermitte symptom, sensory disturbances, weakness, ataxia, vertigo, and diplopia, can occur as transient paroxysms lasting for seconds to minutes, sometimes in clusters. *Flexor spasms* are brief tonic spasms of a limb or the face and often occur at night and in clusters. Flexor spasms are frequently preceded by paresthesias and can be elicited by movements, hyperventilation, or other precipitating factors.

Disease Course

Relapsing-Remitting Multiple Sclerosis

Because there is no specific test for MS, diagnosis of the disease relies on the clinical history. Patients experience relapses when an acute plaque develops in an eloquent area, such as the optic nerves, spinal cord, brain stem, and cerebellum. However, many plaques evolve in clinically silent areas such as the corpus callosum and the periventricular white matter. Often patients gradually recover after resolution of the acute inflammation, possibly through myelin repair and reorganization. These periods of recovery of neurologic function are termed *remissions*, and the term *relapsing-remitting multiple sclerosis* (RRMS) describes this pattern of episodic attacks and recoveries with intervening stability. Approximately 85% of patients will initially follow this disease course (Fig. 21.1). Although complete recovery of neurologic function may follow acute attacks, patients may suffer sustained neurologic deficits.

Secondary Progressive Multiple Sclerosis

If untreated, approximately 85% of subjects with RRMS will develop secondary progressive MS (SPMS), which is the insidiously progressive accumulation of neurologic impairments that lead to physical and cognitive disability. The median time from disease onset to SPMS is 10 years. Relapses can still occur in SPMS; however, the frequency of relapses declines, and eventually most patients stop experiencing attacks. Although some patients with SPMS plateau

Natural History of MS

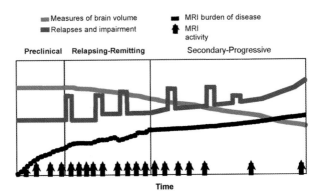

FIG. 21.1 The natural history of multiple sclerosis (MS). Approximately 85% of MS patients follow a similar disease course. Brain magnetic resonance imaging *(MRI)* scans show that MS begins prior to the onset of the first focal neurologic deficit of which the patient is aware. Relapses occur during the relapsing-remitting phase of the disease, and each relapse is followed by varying degrees of neurologic recovery. The secondary progressive phase of the disease is characterized by progressive neurologic deterioration independent of relapses. Relapses occur during the secondary progressive phase of the disease but are less frequent and eventually stop. MRI activity, measured by new, contrast-enhancing lesions, decreases during the secondary progressive phase of MS. The MRI burden of disease and the extent of brain atrophy increases during the course of the disease.

with stable deficits, disability relentlessly continues in other cases. It is difficult to quantify the effect of disease-modifying therapies on the transition to SPMS, which is a challenge for prognosticating outcomes in MS patients.

Primary Progressive Multiple Sclerosis

Fifteen percent of MS patients have primary progressive MS (PPMS). This is a disease course that is progressive from onset without relapses or remissions. PPMS typically presents with insidious onset of asymmetric leg weakness; however, sensory, brain stem/cerebellar, or sphincter dysfunction can be initial manifestations. In contrast to RRMS and SPMS patients, men are affected about as often as women, and the mean age of onset is 40 years compared with 30 years for RRMS. PPMS patients develop ambulatory disability similar to that of the progressive phase of SPMS. The pathology of PPMS lesions is identical to that of RRMS and SPMS. On brain MRI, PPMS patients tend to have fewer plaques compared with RRMS and SPMS, and these rarely enhance on MRI.

Diagnosis

MS is said to evolve over space and time because it afflicts multiple areas of the CNS during an affected individual's life span. The recognition of this pattern accompanied by corresponding physical findings forms the basis of the diagnostic criteria used to define the disease (Table 21.2).

TABLE 21.2 | Multiple Sclerosis Diagnostic Criteria

Diagnosis of MS requires that one of five sets of criteria be fulfilled and that other etiologies be excluded.

1. Two or more clinical attacks and two or more objective lesions
2. Two or more clinical attacks and one objective lesion *and* dissemination in space by MRI[a] *or* reasonable historical evidence of a prior attack
3. One clinical attack and two or more objective lesions *and* dissemination in time by MRI[b] *or* second clinical attack
4. One clinical attack and one objective lesion (clinically isolated syndrome) *and* dissemination in space by MRI[a] *and* dissemination in time by MRI[b] *or* second clinical attack
5. Progression from onset for at least 1 year and at least two of three of the following criteria:
   - Positive CSF: positive oligoclonal bands or elevated IgG index
   - Dissemination in space by MRI[a] brain
   - Dissemination in space by MRI spinal cord ($\geq$2 T2 lesions)

N.B.: An attack is an episode of neurologic disturbance of the kind typically seen in multiple sclerosis, lasting at least 24 hours. The time between attacks must be separated by 30 days. There must be *no better explanation* for the attacks or abnormalities identified by physical examination and by ancillary studies (magnetic resonance imaging [MRI], cerebrospinal fluid [CSF], and visual evoked potentials [VEPs]).

[a]Dissemination in space by magnetic resonance imaging; $\geq$1 T2 lesion in at least two of four areas of the central nervous system: periventricular, juxtacortical, infratentorial, spinal cord (a symptomatic brain stem or spinal cord lesion is excluded from lesion count).

[b]Dissemination in time by magnetic resonance imaging: a new T2 of gadolinium-enhancing lesion on any follow scan regardless of timing from baseline *or* simultaneous presence of asymptomatic enhancing and nonenhancing lesions.

CSF, Cerebrospinal fluid; *IgG,* immunoglobulin G; *MRI,* magnetic resonance imaging; *MS,* multiple sclerosis.

Adapted from Polman CH, et al. Diagnostic criteria for multiple sclerosis: 2010 revisions of the McDonald criteria. *Ann Neurol.* 2011;69:292–302.

Magnetic Resonance Imaging

MRI is particularly helpful in confirming the suspected diagnosis. The brain MRI is abnormal in 95% to 99% of cases of RRMS. Although sensitive, the specificity of the brain MRI is 50% to 65% because other disease states can present with a similar pattern (Table 21.3). Typically, there are multiple areas of increased signal intensity on T2-weighted brain MRI (T2, proton density, and fluid attenuation inversion recovery sequences) that often have a round or ovoid appearance and are characteristically located within the corpus callosum and the periventricular and subcortical white matter (Fig. 21.2). On sagittal views, these plaques appear as linear or flamelike streaks oriented perpendicular to the lateral ventricles; they are called Dawson fingers after the British pathologist who described similar findings at autopsy. The white matter of the brain stem and cerebellum also are often affected. Less often gray matter structures such as the thalamus and basal ganglia are affected. Although cortical plaques occur, they are not well visualized by standard field strength MRI. On T1-weighted imaging, areas of relative hypointensity can be identified that correspond to some of the areas of increased T2 signal. These so-called T1 "black holes" correspond to chronic MS plaques and are associated with axonal loss. Acute plaques show contrast uptake on gadolinium-enhanced

TABLE 21.3	Differential Diagnosis for Multifocal White Matter Changes on Magnetic Resonance Imaging
V	**Vascular:** microvascular ischemic leukoaraiosis, CADASIL, primary angiitis of the central nervous system, migraine
I	**Infectious:** Lyme disease, syphilis, progressive multifocal leukoencephalopathy
T	**Trauma:** perinatal trauma or hypoxia
A	**Autoimmune:** systemic lupus erythematosus, Sjögren syndrome, Behçet disease, sarcoidosis
M	**Metabolic/toxic:** central pontine myelinolysis, delayed post-hypoxic demyelination (Grinker myelinopathy), hexachlorophene poisoning, Marchiafava-Bignami disease, subacute combined degeneration (vitamin B_{12} deficiency), radiation
I	**Idiopathic/genetic:** adrenoleukodystrophy and adrenomyeloneuropathy, metachromatic leukodystrophy, eukaryotic initiation factor leukodystrophies, Krabbe disease, Lafora body disease, globoid leukodystrophy
N	**Neoplastic:** CNS lymphoma, glioma, paraneoplastic encephalomyelitis

CADASIL, Cerebral autosomal dominant arteriopathy with subcortical infarcts and leukoencephalopathy; *CNS,* central nervous system.

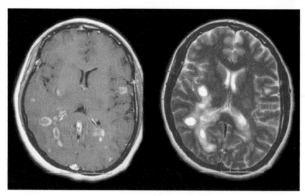

FIG. 21.2 Magnetic resonance imaging findings in a 36-year-old woman with acute fulminant relapsing-remitting multiple sclerosis. The T1-weighted image on the left shows multiple scattered ovoid foci of demyelination with ring enhancement. The T2-weighted image on the right shows high-intensity (white) signal changes associated with these lesions and diffuse edema affecting the deep white matter of the right parietooccipital regions.

T1-weighted imaging. The pattern of enhancement can be homogenous or ring, and it typically persists for 2 to 6 weeks, and then it subsides. The presence of new lesions on a follow-up brain MRI can help confirm the diagnosis of MS in patients who have suffered from only one clinical attack (see Table 21.2). Brain MRI also is useful for evaluating a patient's response to treatment.

Although not as sensitive as brain MRI, plaques within the parenchyma of the spinal cord can be seen on T2-weighted imaging or on T1-weighted imaging after administration of gadolinium and are highly specific for MS. Typically, these plaques are oriented longitudinally along the cord, often with a dorsal location, spanning one or two vertebral cord segments.

Cerebrospinal Fluid

In cases in which the MRI is normal or shows a pattern that is consistent with other disease processes such as microvascular ischemia, CSF analysis is indicated. The CSF is abnormal in 85% to 90% of MS patients. Typically, there is intrathecal synthesis of gamma globulins (increased total immunoglobulin [Ig]G, IgG/total protein ratio, or IgG synthesis rate) or the presence of two or more oligoclonal bands in the CSF that are not present in a simultaneously drawn serum sample. Intrathecal synthesis of gamma globulins also occurs in the setting of infections such as acute bacterial meningitis, chronic meningitis (Lyme disease, syphilis), viral encephalitis, and autoimmune disorders such as CNS vasculitis. A lymphocytic pleocytosis with cell counts >5 cells/μL is present in approximately 25% of MS patients and is usually less than 20 cells/μL. The total protein is usually normal or mildly elevated. Cell counts higher than 50 cells/μL, polymorphonuclear cells, or protein elevation >100 mg/dL should raise suspicion for alternate diagnoses such as infection, collagen vascular diseases, or neoplasm.

Evoked Potentials

Although no longer appearing in the diagnostic criteria for MS, electrophysiologic studies of the visual and somatosensory pathways can be useful when imaging studies or physical findings do not support the clinical impression. Delay or conduction block of the P100 visual evoked potential is found in 85% of MS patients. Delays or block of the N-20 potential on somatosensory evoked potentials of the median or tibial nerve are present in approximately 75% of MS patients. Evoked potential abnormalities are not specific for MS, which limits their diagnostic utility.

Rating Scales

The most commonly used measure of neurologic impairment in MS is the expanded disability status scale (EDSS; Fig. 21.3). The EDSS takes into account the extent of ambulatory disability and limitations in self-care and quantifies the neurologic examination as functional scale scores that quantify vision, brain stem, corticospinal, sensory, cerebellar, cognitive, and bowel and bladder functions.

Differential Diagnosis of MS

Because MS may affect any function of the CNS, the differential diagnosis potentially is broad. MS is difficult to distinguish from other disorders in several settings.

Progressive Myelopathy

Although PPMS can present as an asymmetric insidiously progressive myelopathy, several other diagnoses should be considered, including neoplasm, dural arteriovenous malformation (AVM), subacute combined degeneration (B$_{12}$ deficiency), sarcoidosis, Sjögren syndrome, hereditary spastic paraplegias (HSPs), adrenomyeloneuropathy (in women), syphilis, HIV, and human T-cell lymphotrophic virus I and II myelitis. MRI of the spinal cord is usually diagnostic of neoplasm and AVM. Blood tests help diagnose subacute combined degeneration (vitamin B$_{12}$, methylmalonic acid, and homocysteine), systemic sarcoidosis (angiotensin-converting enzyme [ACE]), Sjögren syndrome (anti-SSA and

Expanded Disability Status Scale (EDSS)

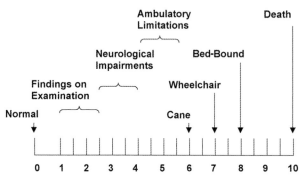

FIG. 21.3 Expanded disability status scale (EDSS). This is a non-linear rating scale with point intervals from 0 to 10. An EDSS score of 0 is normal. Scores of 1 to 2 reflect physical findings on examination. Scores of 2.5 to 3.5 correspond to impairments such as hemiparesis, paraparesis, cerebellar dystaxia, or substantial sensory loss. Scores from 4 to 5.5 usually reflect limitations in the distance a patient can walk without assistance. Scores of 6 and higher are based on the extent of ambulatory disability ability and the ability to perform activities of daily living. A score of 10 is death caused by multiple sclerosis. (From Kurtzke, JF. Rating neurologic impairment in multiple sclerosis: An expanded disability status scale (EDSS). *Neurology.* 1983;33:1444–1452. With permission.)

anti-SSB autoantibodies, rheumatoid factor, antinuclear antibody), adrenomyeloneuropathy (very long chain fatty acids), and infectious etiologies (Venereal Disease Research Laboratory [VDRL] and fluorescent treponemal antibody absorption test [FTA-ABS], HIV, and HTLV I/II serologies). In cases with minimal sensory involvement, normal bladder function, and relatively symmetric presentations of leg weakness and spasticity, primary lateral sclerosis (PLS) and HSP are possibilities. Genetic testing is available for some HSP mutations. PLS is a diagnosis of exclusion.

Progressive Cognitive Impairment With Symmetric White Matter Disease

Although leukodystrophies typically present in childhood, some have adult-onset variants that present with progressive cognitive impairment. White matter lesions similar to MS can be seen on brain MRI; however, MRI changes in the leukodystrophies usually have a symmetric and confluent appearance. Differential diagnoses include adrenoleukodystrophy, metachromatic leukodystrophy, eukaryotic initiation factor mutations, Krabbe disease, methylene-tetrahydrofolate reductase deficiency, biotinidase deficiency, cerebral autosomal dominant arteriopathy with subcortical infarcts and leukoencephalopathy (CADASIL), and polyglucosan storage disease.

Cranial Neuropathies

In addition to MS, Behçet disease and Sjögren syndrome can cause multiple cranial neuropathies. Behçet disease should be suspected in patients with cranial neuropathies and oral ulceration (aphthous sores). Genital ulcerations, dermatographia, and an elevated erythrocyte sedimentation rate (ESR) are other features of the disease. Sjögren syndrome is associated with xerostomia and xerophthalmia (dry mouth and eyes); the diagnosis is confirmed through biopsy of a minor salivary or lacrimal gland. **Glucocorticoids** and **immune suppressants** (i.e., cyclophosphamide) are used to treat Behçet disease and Sjögren syndrome. Lyme disease and sarcoidosis may cause bilateral facial paresis. Sarcoidosis also causes optic neuropathy, which may be poorly responsive to glucocorticoids.

Disease-Modifying Therapies

Treatment for MS is divided into two categories: disease-modifying therapies and symptomatic management. Although there is no cure for MS, currently there are 13 drugs approved by the US Food and Drug Administration (FDA) that alter the course of the disease (Table 21.4).

Interferons

Interferons are cytokines secreted by immune cells that inhibit viral replication. Interferon (IFN)-β has potent regulatory and antiinflammatory functions on the immune system and reduces disease activity in MS. **IFN-β1b** subcutaneously (SC) every other day reduces the relapse rate and slows accumulation of new lesions on brain MR in RRMS. **IFN-β1a** in its various preparations (intramuscular weekly, SC thrice weekly [TIW], pegylated SC every 14 days) also decreases the relapse rate, slows accumulation of new lesions on brain MRI, and lessens the accumulation of neurologic impairments. Patients treated with IFN-β are at risk for liver function abnormalities, leukopenia, thyroid disease, and depression. Liver functions (aspartate and alanine aminotransferase) and white cell count with differential should be monitored after initiation of treatment and periodically thereafter. Most patients do

Medication	Dosage Range	Serious Adverse Reactions	Common Adverse Reactions	Laboratory Monitoring
Amitriptyline (Elavil)	50–150 mg/day	Seizures, myocardial infarction, stroke, bone marrow suppression	Dry mouth, drowsiness, dizziness, constipation, urinary retention, confusion	CBC
Carbamazepine (Tegretol)	200–1200 mg/day	Hypersensitivity, cardiac arrhythmias, bone marrow suppression, cutaneous eruptions, hyponatremia	Dizziness, drowsiness, ataxia, blurred vision, allergic rash	CBC, Na
Gabapentin (Neurontin)	900–3600 mg/day	Leucopenia	Drowsiness, lightheadedness, ataxia, fatigue, weight gain	—
Lamotrigine (Lamictal)	50–200 mg/day	Cutaneous eruptions, bone marrow suppression, hepatic failure	Fatigue, dizziness, headache, rash, cognitive dysfunction	CBC, LFTs
Oxcarbazepine (Trileptal)	600–2400 mg/day	Angioedema, bone marrow suppression, cutaneous eruptions, hyponatremia	Dizziness, drowsiness, diplopia, fatigue, acne, alopecia, elevated LFTs	CBC, Na, LFTs
Topiramate (Topamax)	50–200 mg/day	Metabolic acidosis, nephrolithiasis, bone loss, angle closure glaucoma, bone marrow suppression, cutaneous eruptions	Metabolic acidosis, dizziness, somnolence, cognitive disturbance, visual disturbance, weight loss, agitation	CBC
Tramadol (Ultram)	50–400 mg/day	Seizures, respiratory depression, angioedema, cutaneous eruptions, serotonin syndrome, orthostatic hypotension, hallucinations, withdrawal symptoms	Dizziness, nausea, constipation, headache, somnolence, psychiatric disturbance, urinary retention	—
Zonisamide (Zonegran)	100–600 mg/day	Cutaneous eruptions, bone marrow suppression, heat stroke, nephrolithiasis, pancreatitis, psychiatric disturbance, withdrawal seizures	Somnolence, dizziness, psychiatric constipation	CBC

Medications used to treat neuropathic pain are listed with typical dosage range, adverse event, and laboratory studies for monitoring adverse reactions. See the manufacturer's package inserts for complete information. Not all known adverse events are listed.

CBC, Complete blood count; LFTs, liver function tests; Na, serum sodium.

not experience significant transaminitis requiring treatment discontinuation. A flulike reaction occurs in 60% of patients after IFN-β injection. With repeated treatments, the flulike reactions gradually subside over time. The flulike symptoms are reduced by coadministration with acetaminophen or a nonsteroidal antiinflammatory drug. Erythematous skin site reactions can occur with the SC injected preparations. Long-term follow-up studies show that IFN-β is safe and well tolerated for at least 10 years.

Glatiramer Acetate

Glatiramer acetate (GA) is a synthesized copolymer composed of L-*g*lutamic acid, L-*l*ysine, L-*a*lanine, and L-*t*yrosine in random order and is injected 20 mg SC daily or 40 mg SC TIW. GA resembles myelin basic protein and is thought to alter T-cell immune function, inducing "bystander suppression," so that T cells inhibit autoreactive T cells. GA reduces the attack rate in RRMS and reduces accumulation of contrast-enhanced lesions on brain MRI. Ten-year follow-up data demonstrate that many patients treated with GA are able to safely continue treatment. The typical flulike reaction characteristic of IFN-β does not occur with GA; however, approximately 15% of GA-treated patients will experience an immediate, self-limited, postinjection systemic reaction characterized by chest tightness, flushing, anxiety, dyspnea, and palpitations.

Mitoxantrone

Mitoxantrone is a cytotoxic agent that intercalates into DNA and inhibits topoisomerase II activity. It is a potent immune suppressor because of its cytopathic effects on replicating cells. In a study of RRMS and SPMS patients with incomplete recovery after attacks, mitoxantrone reduced the accumulation of neurologic impairment and number of relapses compared with placebo. Mitoxantrone has cardiotoxic properties that limit its total lifetime cumulative dose to 140 mg/m^2, and there is a risk of acute promyelocytic leukemia of approximately 0.25%. These toxicities limit the use of mitoxantrone in MS patients, particularly in light of highly effective alternative infusion-based agents.

Natalizumab

Natalizumab is a monoclonal antibody that binds a-4 integrin on monocytes and blocks the interaction between a-4 integrin and VCAM-1, which is an integrin expressed on the surface of vascular endothelial cells. The interaction between VLA4 and VCAM-1 is necessary for lymphocyte adherence to vascular endothelia and subsequent transmigration of lymphocytes into body tissues. Natalizumab was shown to reduce the number of MS flares, slow accumulation of neurologic disability, and reduce the accumulation of lesions on brain MRI. Natalizumab is dosed at 300 mg and is intravenously administered every 4 weeks. There is known risk of progressive multifocal leukoencephalopathy (PML), which can be estimated with John Cunningham Virus (JCV) antibody status and infusion number, as well as prior exposure to immunosuppressive agents.

Fingolimod

Fingolimod is a once-daily oral sphingosine phosphate receptor functional antagonist that limits lymphocyte egress from peripheral lymph nodes. It has been shown to reduce frequency of MS exacerbations by over 50% compared with placebo and is well tolerated. Benefit also was shown in reduction of brain atrophy rates and development of new and enlarging T2 lesions. Potential side effects include bradycardia at the time of first dose, macular edema, and lymphopenia. First-dose observation is undertaken to mitigate potential cardiovascular complications, and those with cardiac risk factors may avoid the medication.

Teriflunomide

Teriflunomide is a pyrimidine synthesis inhibitor dosed orally, once daily, that slows rapid expansion of lymphocytes by forcing cells to use the pyrimidine salvage pathway. Annualized relapse rate reduction of 31% was demonstrated, with a 30% reduction in 12-week sustained disability progression versus placebo. Potential adverse events include elevated liver enzymes, hair thinning, and gastrointestinal side effects such as nausea and diarrhea. Liver enzymes are monitored monthly for 6 months when starting teriflunomide. An accelerated elimination can be accomplished with activated charcoal or cholestyramine if necessary.

Dimethyl Fumarate

A fumaric acid ester related to a compound used for psoriasis, **dimethyl fumarate** is a twice-daily pill shown to reduce annualized relapse rate by about 50% in relapsing MS. It is thought to reduce oxidative stress through Nrf2 and NF-κB pathways. Side effects include flushing, gastrointestinal complaints, and lymphopenia.

Alemtuzumab

Alemtuzumab is an infused anti-CD52 monoclonal antibody that profoundly depletes circulating B and T lymphocytes. Infused on 5 consecutive days in year 1 and 3 consecutive days in year 2, alemtuzumab decreases relapse rate by 49% to 74% compared to IFN-β 1a given three times weekly. Patients may be retreated in the setting of active disease, but many patients have not required retreatment over a 5-year observation period. Potential risks include approximately 30% risk of development of secondary autoimmune conditions such as autoimmune thyroid disease.

Ocrelizumab

Ocrelizumab is a fully humanized monoclonal antibody directed against the CD20 receptor, causing selective reduction of memory B cells. Reduction of relapse rate versus IFN-β1a three times weekly was 46%, and there was a 94% reduction in gadolinium-enhancing lesions on ocrelizumab versus IFN-β1a. Most common side effects were infusion-related reactions. There is a slight increase in upper respiratory infections and herpes reactivations in ocrelizumab-treated patients. Reactivation of other dormant viruses may occur, and it is advised to screen for latent viral hepatitis prior to starting ocrelizumab. Ocrelizumab was approved for primary progressive and relapsing forms of MS, a first-ever approval for a disease-modifying treatment in the primary progressive form of the disease.

Glucocorticoids

Glucocorticoids are the mainstay of therapy for treatment of acute MS relapses. Intravenously administered **methylprednisolone (Solumedrol) dosed at** 1g/day administered over 3 to 5 days reduces the symptoms of flares and shortens the recovery time. A rebound in disease activity can occur after discontinuation of glucocorticoid treatment, and some clinicians follow intravenous treatment with a prednisone taper, gradually reducing the dose from 60 mg to off over 8 to 12 days. Monitoring of bone densitometry is recommended for patients treated with frequent pulsed doses of glucocorticoids. Short-term risks of glucocorticoids include fluid retention, hypokalemia, flushing, acne, insomnia, psychiatric disturbance, dyspepsia, and increased appetite. Patients with preexisting psychiatric illness may experience psychotic symptoms from glucocorticoids.

Plasma Exchange

Small trials showed that plasma exchange may help resolve acute flares of severe demyelinating disease that are not responsive to glucocorticoids. Plasma exchange was shown not to be beneficial in treatment of SPMS.

Treatments for SPMS

IFN-β1b appears to reduce the relapse rate and disability in patients who recently transitioned from RRMS into SPMS and are still experiencing relapses. IFN-β1b is probably of no benefit to SPMS patients who experience disease progression without relapses. Mitoxantrone is approved for rapidly worsening disease in SPMS patients who experience relapses, but it is rarely used because of potential cardiac side effects and leukemia risk. Ocrelizumab is approved for relapsing forms of MS, which could include SPMS with relapses. A study of natalizumab in patients with SPMS did not show benefit in slowing disease progression.

Off-Label Immunomodulatory Agents

Many other medications with immune-modulating or -suppressing properties are used to treat MS either alone or in combination with treatments approved by the FDA and include azathioprine, methotrexate, mycophenolate mofetil, cladribine, cyclophosphamide, and rituximab. Use of these agents is best left to experienced clinicians.

Symptomatic Therapies

Because MS affects multiple functions of the nervous system, the symptomatic treatment of MS patients can be complex, especially for patients with SPMS.

Spasticity

Spasticity is a velocity-dependent change in tone and occurs in MS as a consequence of reorganization within the spinal cord or higher centers after injury to the motor pathways. Physical therapy and daily stretching exercises are essential to prevent contracture formation. Antispasmodic treatments should start at low doses and escalate upward until symptomatic relief is obtained or until intolerable side effects occur (usually drowsiness). **Baclofen (10 mg three times daily)** and **tizanidine (2 mg three times daily)** should be the first agents prescribed. **Gabapentin started at 300 mg three times daily and rapidly escalated** also is an effective antispasmodic agent; doses of 3600 mg/day or higher are typical. **Diazepam started at 2 mg three times daily** can be titrated up to 20 mg three times daily. In patients with spasticity who experience excessive side effects or limited relief with oral medications, **intrathecal baclofen** can be administered by an indwelling pump.

Fatigue

MS patients may suffer from neuromuscular fatigue (weakness), fatigue associated with depression, daytime drowsiness secondary to insomnia, generalized lassitude, or deconditioning. MS patients are at high risk for depression, and if it is present, it should be adequately treated. Sleep disturbance also is common in MS, and patients should be educated about sleep hygiene. Some patients may require treatment with hypnotics for sleep. The lassitude associated with MS may respond to **amantadine 100 mg twice**

daily. Other stimulants include **modafinil (Provigil) 100 to 200 mg twice a day** and **methylphenidate (Ritalin) 10 to 20 mg twice a day.** All CNS stimulants can cause insomnia, which can further exacerbate fatigue, and caution must be exercised in patients who are treated with a hypnotic medication for insomnia and a stimulant for fatigue. Physical therapy and regular exercise are essential for MS patients. For patients who experience neuromuscular fatigue associated with increases in body temperature, aquatic exercise is recommended. **Dalfampridine** 10 mg twice daily may be used to improve walking in MS patients. This potassium channel blocker improves conduction along damaged axons and improves walking speed and endurance in MS patients. Those with a history of seizure should avoid the medication because of risk of enhancing aberrant conduction and precipitating a recurrent seizure.

Pain

Acute or chronic neuropathic pain is a frequent complication of MS and usually does not respond to treatment with nonsteroidal antiinflammatory medications. **Gabapentin** is often beneficial but usually requires doses of **1800 mg/day or higher** (see Table 21.4 for dosage ranges and side effects of commonly used medications). **Carbamazepine (Tegretol)** or **oxcarbazepine (Trileptal)** are particularly useful for the "squeezing" or "bandlike" dysesthesias and for trigeminal neuralgia. **Topiramate (Topamax), lamotrigine (Lamictal), and zonisamide (Zonegran)** also are useful in the treatment of neuropathic pain. Low-potency opiate analgesics may be used in combination with nonnarcotic analgesics. A continuous-release opiate preparation such as the fentanyl transdermal patch (Duragesic patch 25 to 75 μg/h) may be necessary for pain refractory to nonnarcotic medications.

Paroxysmal Symptoms

The Lhermitte symptom and tonic spasms respond to treatment with carbamazepine, oxcarbazepine, gabapentin, and acetazolamide (Diamox) 125 to 250 mg two to three times daily. Acetazolamide and ondansetron (Zofran), 4 to 8 mg twice a day, can be useful for intermittent central vertigo. Meclizine (Antivert) is rarely of benefit in central vertigo. Nocturnal flexor spasms respond well to antispasmodic agents such as baclofen or tizanidine.

Bladder Dysfunction

Bladder spasticity is treated with anticholinergic agents such as **oxybutynin (Ditropan) 5 mg three or four times daily** or **tolterodine (Detrol) 2 mg twice daily.** Long-acting formulations and an oxybutynin transdermal patch applied twice weekly are available. The denervated bladder is treated by intermittent self-catheterization, and patients should be taught this technique as soon as urinary retention is diagnosed. Sphincter dyssynergia can be treated with **terazosin (Hytrin) 1 to 5 mg at** night in combination with an anticholinergic and, in some cases, intermittent catheterization.

Bowel Dysfunction

Bowel dysfunction is often undertreated in MS. Constipation can be treated with a combination of fiber (e.g., **Metamucil, 1 teaspoon three times a day with meals),** a stool softener **(docusate sodium, 100 mg three times daily with meals),** and a stimulant **(e.g., senna, two tablets at night).** Enemas, suppositories, and digital stimulation may be necessary. Urge incontinence can be treated with a bowel regimen to trigger voiding at a convenient time each day.

Sexual Dysfunction

Male erectile dysfunction can be treated with **sildenafil (Viagra) 50 to 100 mg, vardenafil (Levitra) 5 to 20 mg,** or **tadalafil (Cialis) 5 to 20 mg before intercourse.** Alprostadil (Edex) 2.5 to 40 μg injected intracavernously is used for nonresponders to oral preparations. Diminished vaginal lubrication causes dyspareunia and can be treated with water-based lubrication. Vaginismus may respond to antispasmodic medications.

ACUTE TRANSVERSE MYELITIS

Acute transverse myelitis (ATM) is inflammation of the spinal cord that results in bilateral lower extremity weakness, a sensory level, and sphincter impairment. ATM is the presenting manifestation in approximately 2% of MS cases and occurs in many MS patients during the course of the disease. Nevertheless, there are many other potential causes of ATM (Table 21.5), and 75% to 90% of cases not associated with MS follow a monophasic course. Patients presenting with ATM should undergo spinal cord imaging to exclude compressive etiologies, tumors, and AVMs. Brain imaging also is indicated to look for evidence of disseminated demyelination. CSF analysis is used to detect infectious etiologies, and blood studies can reveal evidence of systemic inflammation. In severe or rapidly progressive cases, empiric treatment includes administration of **high-dose glucocorticoids** and **intravenous acyclovir** while definitive diagnostic tests are pending. Plasma exchange is indicated in cases that are glucocorticoid-nonresponsive.

TABLE 21.5	Differential Diagnosis of Acute Transverse Myelitis
V	**Vascular:** spinal dural arteriovenous malformation, stroke
I	**Infectious:** viral: Herpetoviridae (varicella zoster virus, herpes simplex 1 and 2, Epstein-Barr virus, cytomegalovirus), group B arboviruses (West Nile and dengue), exanthemas (measles, mumps, rubella), rare causes (enteroviruses; hepatitis A, B, C; lymphocytic choriomeningitis virus) Mycobacterial and bacterial: *Mycobacterium tuberculosis* (tuberculosis), *Mycoplasma pneumoniae, Chlamydia pneumoniae, Borrelia burgdorferi* (Lyme disease), *Treponema pallidum* (syphilis), *Brucella melitensis* (brucellosis), *Bartonella henselae* (cat-scratch disease), bacterial meningitis, intraparenchymal abscess, and epidural abscess Parasitic: *Schistosoma haematobium, S. mansoni, S. japonicum, Toxocara* species
T	**Trauma:** cord compression secondary to trauma, herniated disk, or extradural mass lesion (metastatic disease to the spine, epidural abscess, Pott disease)
A	**Autoimmune:** Sjögren syndrome, systemic lupus erythematosus, mixed connective tissue disease, anticardiolipin autoantibodies, primary angiitis of the central nervous system, p-ANCA autoantibodies, Hashimoto encephalopathy (myelopathy), linear scleroderma, sarcoidosis, NMOSD
M	**Metabolic/toxic:** chemotherapy
I	**Idiopathic/hereditary:** multiple sclerosis, acute disseminated encephalomyelitis (postvaccination), neuromyelitis optica
N	**Neoplastic:** lymphoma, leukemia, and other infiltrating tumors; Paraneoplastic: Hodgkin lymphoma, other tumors
S	**Psychiatric:** conversion disorder

ANCA, Antineutrophil cytoplasmic antibody; *NMOSD,* neuromyelitis optica spectrum disorder.

NEUROMYELITIS OPTICA SPECTRUM DISORDER

Historically, the co-occurrence of ATM with optic neuritis, a normal brain MRI study at onset, and spinal cord lesions spanning three or more vertebral segments of the cord were the hallmarks of neuromyelitis optica (NMO), which is a rare demyelinating disease. This has now been broadened to NMOSD, which encompasses six core clinical characteristics, and serologic and imaging features appear in the diagnostic criteria revised in 2015. Acute attacks are treated with a combination of **glucocorticoids** and **plasma exchange.** There are no FDA-approved treatments that alter the course of the disease, although immunosuppressants such as azathioprine and mycophenolate mofetil are broadly used, as is the anti-CD20 monoclonal antibody **rituximab.** See Table 21.6 for core clinical characteristics. If AQP4-IgG Ab is positive, only one

TABLE 21.6	Neuromyelitis Optica Spectrum Disorder Diagnostic Criteria

Core Clinical Characteristics:
1. Optic neuritis
2. Acute myelitis
3. Area postrema syndrome (intractable vomiting or nausea/vomiting)
4. Acute brain stem syndrome
5. Narcolepsy or acute diencephalic syndrome with typical brain lesions
6. Cerebral syndrome with typical brain lesions

Adapted from Wingerchuk DM, et al. International consensus diagnostic criteria for neuromyelitis optica spectrum disorders. *Neurology.* 2015;85:177–189.

core clinical characteristic is needed. With a negative or unknown AQP4-IgG Ab, two characteristics must be positive, one of which is ON, acute myelitis, or area postrema syndrome (hiccups, nausea, and/or vomiting in conjunction with an area postrema demyelinating lesion), and those must be disseminated in space, and meet additional MRI requirements.

ACUTE MULTIPLE SCLEROSIS

Acute MS, or Marburg variant MS, is a rare fulminant demyelinating disease. Brain MRI shows large edematous contrast-enhancing lesions with mass effect, similar to a brain tumor, and many patients undergo brain biopsy. Historically, acute MS was a fatal disease, with death occurring within a year of onset, often secondary to extensive brain stem demyelination. Treatment recommendations, based on anecdotes, include **plasma exchange** in conjunction with high-dose **glucocorticoids** (e.g., 1 to 2 g/day of methylprednisolone for 10 days followed by a slow taper). High-efficacy immunotherapy is indicated thereafter, which may include cyclophosphamide, alemtuzumab, or mitoxantrone.

ACUTE DISSEMINATED ENCEPHALOMYELITIS

ADEM is a monophasic illness characterized by multifocal inflammation and demyelination and is most common in children. ADEM can be associated with recent rabies or smallpox vaccination (postvaccination encephalomyelitis) and recent infection (postinfectious encephalomyelitis). Common antecedent infections include childhood exanthemas such as measles and varicella (chickenpox), as well as *M. pneumoniae,* mononucleosis, rubella, mumps influenza, and parainfluenza. Acute hemorrhagic leukoencephalitis (Hurst disease) is a fulminant and devastating form of ADEM associated with microvascular hemorrhagic lesions. ADEM is distinguished from MS by a history of antecedent vaccination or infection, a rapid onset, and multifocal symptomatic involvement of the cerebrum, brain stem, cerebellum, and spinal cord. Alterations in consciousness and seizures are common in ADEM. Brain MRI in ADEM shows multiple areas of abnormal signal change that are acute and often enhance with gadolinium-DPTA. CSF findings are similar to MS. Treatment consists of **high-dose glucocorticoids.** When patients do not respond to glucocorticoids, **plasma exchange** (1.5 to 2 volumes) or intravenous immunoglobulin (**IVIG**) is used. In children, behavioral disorders, learning disorders, and epilepsy may be sequelae.

NEURO SARCOIDOSIS

Sarcoidosis is a systemic chronic inflammatory condition disease characterized histopathologically by multiple noncaseating granulomas affecting one or more organ systems. The condition is idiopathic but may reflect a granulomatous reaction to an as yet unidentified pathogen. It most commonly affects the lungs, mediastinal lymph nodes, and skin. Systemic features include fever, malaise, lassitude, erythema nodosum, polyarthralgia, mediastinal hilar lymphadenopathy, uveoparotid fever (Heerfordt syndrome: parotitis, uveitis, and facial palsy), keratoconjunctivitis sicca, hepatosplenomegaly, anemia, cardiac conduction defects, phalangeal bone cysts, and hypercalcemia.

Sarcoidosis affects the nervous system in 10% of patients, primarily the leptomeninges, producing a syndrome consistent with chronic meningitis. The clinical presentation relates to the site of involvement and may include headache, vertigo, impaired vision, isolated cranial nerve lesions (e.g., bilateral facial palsy), intracranial mass lesions, hemiparesis, ataxia, paresthesias, diabetes insipidus, or hypotestosteronism (from pituitary and hypothalamic dysfunction), seizures, encephalopathy, psychosis, dementia, hydrocephalus, polyradiculopathy, peripheral neuropathy, or myopathy. Rarely the spinal cord is involved. Sarcoidosis is five times more common in women. The median age of onset of sarcoidosis is 25 to 30 years; however, the range is broad.

Diagnosis

Laboratory investigations in sarcoidosis may reveal hypercalcemia, hyperuricemia, a raised serum globulin level, and increased serum ACE. The CSF ACE is positive in 55% of patients with neurosarcoidosis. The CSF may be abnormal, with raised pressure, a slight pleocytosis, markedly raised protein, and hypoglycorrhachia in 20% to 30% of patients. An elevated IgG index is found in 33%

of patients. MRI with gadolinium classically shows nodular lepto-meningeal enhancement and parenchymal lesions. The diagnosis is made clinically and confirmed by a biopsy of a suitable granuloma revealing a focal collection of epithelioid histiocytes surrounded by a rim of lymphocytes, endothelial cells, and giant cells (Langhans type) without organisms or caseation. Isolated neurosarcoidosis, seen in only 2% to 3% of patients with CNS involvement, is a dif-ficult diagnosis to make. Meningeal and brain biopsy is necessary to confirm the diagnosis.

Management

Corticosteroids (**prednisone 100 mg daily**) and azathioprine (**1–3 mg/kg/day**) are the first-line treatments for CNS sarcoidosis, immu-nosuppression with cyclophosphamide is a second-line treatment, and tumor necrosis tumor necrosis factor (TNF) inhibition with infliximab also has shown benefit in controlling neurosarcoidosis.

BEHÇET DISEASE

Behçet disease is an inflammatory disorder of unknown etiology characterized by a relapsing iritis and uveitis associated with oral (100%) and genital (75%) aphthous ulceration. Systemic features include recurrent fevers, keratoconjunctivitis, hypopyon, migrating superficial thrombophlebitis (25%) that may present as deep venous thrombosis, erythema nodosum (65%), furunculosis, intes-tinal ulceration, epididymitis, systemic and pulmonary arterial aneurysms, and arthralgia of large joints (60%).

Neurologic manifestations, including abrupt onset of recurrent meningoencephalitis and cranial nerve palsies, occur in 5% to 30% of patients with Behçet disease. Papilledema, venous sinus occlu-sion, hemiparesis, quadriparesis, pseudobulbar palsy, and involve-ment of the basal ganglia, cerebellum, or spinal cord can occur. It is more common and more severe in men, and the peak age of onset is in the 20s.

Diagnosis

The diagnosis is chiefly clinical and is based on the occurrence of a meningoencephalitis in combination with the characteristic cuta-neous and ocular lesions. It may mimic MS or strokes, with tran-sient or persistent multifocal involvement of the nervous system. There is no single confirmatory test, but an ESR over 50 mm/h is common. CSF studies show a mild pleocytosis with a moderate increase in protein. Brain imaging may show infarction (25%), hypodense/hypointense-enhancing lesions, and leptomeningeal enhancement. Pathologically, inflammatory changes are found in the iris, choroid, retina, optic nerve, and meninges and in the peri-vascular spaces (vasculitis) of the brain.

Management

Treatment may include analgesics, anticoagulants, colchicine, dapsone, levamisole, thalidomide, glucocorticoids, and immunosuppression (azathioprine, chlorambucil, cyclophosphamide). Posterior uveal tract and neurologic lesions, if untreated, may lead to blindness or death.

CENTRAL PONTINE MYELINOLYSIS

This condition is characterized by symmetric destruction of the pontine white matter. Rapid correction of hyponatremia is associated with the onset of CPM in most cases. CPM occurs more frequently in patients with a history of alcoholism, malnutrition, and multiorgan failure. The lesion destroys the myelin sheath, sparing neurons and axons. It presents as a rapidly progressing spastic quadriplegia with facial, glottal, and pharyngeal paralysis in a debilitated patient suffering from an acute illness. When the pons alone is involved, the patient may become mute and paralyzed or "locked-in". In more severe cases, demyelination also involves white matter tracts in the basal ganglia, which is a condition termed *extrapontine myelinolysis*. MRI is the imaging modality of choice. Recovery from even the most severe cases is possible but may take 4 to 12 months. The disease is rarely directly fatal, but the mortality rate can be high as a result of secondary complications.

CPM is best avoided in severely hyponatremic patients by slowly correcting the serum sodium no faster than 0.5 mEq/L per hour (12 mEq/L per day), to a maximum level of 130 mEq/L (Table 21.7).

TABLE 21.7	Formula for Correcting Hyponatremia[a]

$$\text{Change in serum Na}^+ = \frac{\text{infusate Na}^+ - \text{serum Na}^+}{\text{total body water} + 1}$$

Infusates	Dosage (mEq/L)
3% saline	513
0.9% saline	154
Ringer's lactate	130
0.45% saline	77

[a]Equation yields the effect of 1 L of infusate on serum Na^+ concentration in milliequivalents (mEq) per liter. The rate of the infusion should be adjusted to correct the serum Na^+ no faster than 8 to 12 mEq/L per day. The suggested target Na^+ concentration is 130 mmol/L. Total body water in liters is estimated as a fraction of body weight in kilograms; the fraction is 0.6 in men and 0.5 in women.

Adapted from Adrogue HJ, Madias NE. Hyponatremia. *N Engl J Med.* 2000;342: 1581–1589.

Infections of the Central Nervous System

There are a broad number of organisms that can cause damage to the central or peripheral nervous system, either directly or indirectly. These conditions are often life-threatening. Diagnosis can be challenging because patients often present with nonspecific clinical syndromes that can be caused by infectious and noninfectious causes. Prompt diagnosis and treatment are essential to prevent death or permanent neurologic disability. **The combination of fever, headache, and neurologic signs or symptoms must be treated as a central nervous system (CNS) infection until proven otherwise.** A management algorithm (Fig. 22.1) should be followed for suspected cases of bacterial meningitis. Empirical treatment for bacterial causes is outlined in Table 22.1. Based on presentation and risk factors, antiviral (e.g., acyclovir) and antifungal agents should be included in the empirical treatment. Definitive treatment will later be based on the results of cultures or other diagnostic tests.

APPROACH TO THE PATIENT WITH SUSPECTED CENTRAL NERVOUS SYSTEM INFECTION

Historical Features

1. **Age is a major feature that can aide a clinician regarding risk of specific pathogens (table).**
2. **Ascertain the acuity and tempo of symptoms.**
3. **Identify any predisposing risk factors:**
   - **Immunosuppression:** diabetes, alcoholism, malignancy, steroids or other immunomodulatory medications, transplanted organs, chemotherapy, HIV infection
   - **Head trauma, otologic or neurosurgical procedures**
   - **Unusual exposures:** foreign travel, wooded areas, sick contacts, animals, or insects, ingestion including raw meats, recreational activities
   - **Vaccine history**

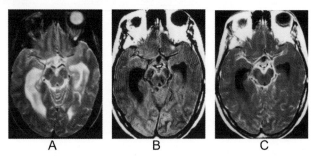

FIG. 22.1 Magnetic resonance imaging (MRI) findings of tuberculous meningitis. (A) T2-weighted and (B) precontrast T1-weighted images show hydrocephalus. (C) Postcontrast T1 image demonstrates thick enhancement of the basal meninges and exudates. (Reproduced with permission from Kapra P, et al. Infectious meningitis: Prospective evaluation with magnetization transfer MRI. *Br J Radiol.* 2004;77:387–394.)

Check for the following symptoms: fever, headache or neck pain, change in mental status, focal weakness, numbness, visual problems, back pain, urinary or bowel symptoms.

Examination Features

1. Check for evidence of infection elsewhere in the body: conjunctivitis, retinitis, uveitis, sinusitis, endocarditis, lymphadenopathy pneumonia, osteomyelitis, urinary tract infection, skin rash.
2. Always be sure to check for the following signs: vital signs, papilledema, meningismus, exanthem, sinus tenderness, otitis media, or spine tenderness.

Lumbar Puncture

Lumbar puncture (LP) is the most important test to confirm a CNS infection and identify the causative organism. The technique for performing LP is covered in Chapter 3. **If CNS infection is suspected, when deciding whether to perform an LP, the following clinical rule may be helpful (any two of these three require LP):**

1. Fever
2. Headache
3. Change in mental status

Because herniation is a serious but rare complication of LP, a computed tomography (**CT**) **scan** may be **required prior to LP.**

LP should not be performed before CT in patients with suspected bacterial meningitis when one or more of the following risk factors is present:

TABLE 22.1	Cerebrospinal Fluid Findings in Selected Infections of the Central Nervous System				
	Number of White Blood Cells (per mm^3)	Cell Type	Concentration of Protein (mg/dL)	Concentration of Glucose (mg/dL)	CSF Pressure (cm H$_2$O)
Normal	≤5	Lymphocytes and monocytes only	15–45	45–80	80–180
Bacterial meningitis	5–10,000	Polymorphonuclear leukocytes	Increased	Decreased	Increased
Viral meningitis	5–1000	Lymphocytes	Increased	Normal	Normal, occasionally increased
Tubercular meningitis	5–500	Lymphocytes	Increased	Decreased	Increased
Cryptococcal meningitis	5–100	Lymphocytes	Increased	Normal, occasionally decreased	Increased
Active neurosyphilis	5–500	Lymphocytes	Increased	Normal, occasionally decreased	Normal

- Altered mentation
- Focal neurologic signs
- Papilledema
- Seizure within the previous week
- A patient is immunocompromised

Relative contraindications to LP: Although there are no absolute contraindications to performing the procedure, caution should be used in patients with:

- Possible raised intracranial pressure (ICP)
- Thrombocytopenia or other bleeding diathesis (including ongoing anticoagulant therapy)
- Suspected spinal epidural abscess

ACUTE MENINGITIS

Acute Bacterial Meningitis

The classic triad of acute bacterial meningitis consists of fever, nuchal rigidity, and a change in mental status, although a number of patients do not have all three features. Most patients have high fevers, but a small percentage have hypothermia. Almost no patients have a normal temperature. Neurologic complications such as seizures, focal neurologic deficits (including cranial nerve palsies), and papilledema may be present early or occur later in the course. The presentation is usually dramatic but may be less obvious at the extremes of age (in infants and in the elderly), in whom change in mental status is often the only symptom.

Etiologies

Seeding of the leptomeninges usually occurs from hematogenous spread of the infecting organism (e.g., pneumococcal pneumonia complicated by meningitis); it also can result from a parameningeal infection (e.g., otitis media) or after trauma, cochlear implants, or neurosurgery (e.g., cerebrospinal fluid [CSF] leak). *Streptococcus pneumoniae* (50% of cases) and *Neisseria meningitidis* (25% of cases) are the most common causes of bacterial meningitis. Mortality is approximately 20%.

Laboratory Diagnosis

The diagnosis is established by abnormal CSF indices including polymorphonuclear pleocytosis, elevated protein level, and reduced glucose level (see Table 22.1). The organism is identified by CSF cultures. However, when CSF is sterile—for example, in cases in which antibiotics are given prior to LP—blood cultures often identify the causative organism. At least 50% of patients with bacterial meningitis have positive blood cultures. Interpreting CSF profiles in neurosurgical patients with recently placed ventricular drains can be difficult. A rising white blood cell (WBC) count and falling glucose level suggests an infection. Because of impaired CSF circulation in shunted patients, CSF should be sampled from the drain or shunt when possible. Radiographic findings of bacterial meningitis are often nonspecific and include evidence of enhancement of leptomeninges.

Treatment

The prognosis in bacterial meningitis depends on the interval between onset of disease and initiation of therapy. Selection of empirical antibiotics depends on age and risk factors, as shown in Table 22.1. Most adults with suspected community-acquired bacterial meningitis should be treated with **dexamethasone 6 mg intravenously (IV) every 6 hours for** 4 **days** (first dose given 15 minutes prior to antibiotics), and **ceftriaxone and vancomycin** until cultures provide for a definite diagnosis and antibiotic sensitivity. Treatment with dexamethasone blunts the acute inflammatory response and results in a 50% reduction in mortality; efficacy is greatest with pneumococcal meningitis. In neonates and older or immunosuppressed patients, **ampicillin** should be added as well to cover *Listeria monocytogenes* infection. Recently placed shunts or intracranial hardware should be removed.

Viral (Aseptic) Meningitis

Viral meningitis is typically a self-limited illness seen most frequently in children and young adults. The manifestations of viral meningitis are generally similar to bacterial meningitis but often less severe. Older children and adults may present with headache, fever, nausea, vomiting, stiff neck, and sensitivity to noise or light. In infants, the clinical presentation can be nonspecific, and may lead to irritability, vomiting, and diarrhea. They should be evaluated for nuchal rigidity and a bulging fontanelle.

Etiologies

A number of viruses produce aseptic meningitis including enteroviruses, herpes simplex virus (HSV), HIV, West Nile virus (WNV), varicella-zoster virus (VZV), mumps, and lymphocytic choriomeningitis (LCM) virus. Mollaret meningitis is a form of recurrent benign lymphocytic meningitis (RBLM), which is an uncommon illness characterized by greater than three episodes of fever and meningismus lasting 2 to 5 days, followed by spontaneous resolution.

Laboratory Diagnosis

The diagnosis is suggested by lymphocytic pleocytosis with a normal glucose level in the CSF (see Table 22.1) and negative CSF and blood bacterial cultures. In some cases of viral meningitis, the virus can be cultured or amplified (polymerase chain reaction [PCR]) from CSF, blood, nasal pharyngeal secretions, or fecal material. The presence of intrathecal production of virus-specific IgG antibodies acquired weeks after the onset of symptoms can establish a retrospective diagnosis (for WNV, immunoglobulin [Ig]M can be found as early as 1 week after onset of symptoms). The most common causes of viral meningitis include enteroviruses, arthropodborne viruses (especially WNV), HSV-2, LCM virus, and infection with HIV during the acute conversion period. Medications can cause aseptic meningitis simulating viral meningitis. The usual culprits include nonsteroidal antiinflammatory drugs (NSAIDs), metronidazole, carbamazepine, trimethoprim/sulfamethoxazole, and IV immunoglobulin (IVIG). Also in the differential are other infections including fungal and parasitic infections, as well as cancer of the leptomeninges. Treatment is supportive. Prognosis is excellent.

CHRONIC MENINGITIS

Chronic meningitis is defined as meningitis lasting for 4 weeks or more and is a complex entity with both infectious and noninfectious causes. A wide array of infectious agents can present as chronic meningitis, but a nearly identical syndrome can result from a number of inflammatory, malignant, or other noninfectious diseases. All patients with chronic meningitis should be questioned about travel or residence in geographic areas known to be endemic for possible causes of chronic meningitis including coccidioidomycosis, histoplasmosis, paracoccidioidomycosis, blastomycosis, schistosomiasis, trypanosomiasis, *Angiostrongylus cantonensis* infection, or cysticercosis. Analysis of CSF reveals abnormalities in patients with chronic meningitis, but these abnormalities are rarely diagnostic with some notable exceptions. The presence of eosinophilia can provide an important clue to the presence of a parasitic etiology or coccidioidomycosis. Antigen testing of the CSF for the presence of *Cryptococcus neoformans* and a Venereal Disease Research Laboratory (VDRL) test for syphilis should be performed on all patients with chronic meningitis. Here we discuss a few examples of causes of chronic meningitis.

Tuberculosis Meningitis

Tuberculosis (TB) meningitis, caused by the bacterium *Mycobacterium tuberculosis,* typically evolves over weeks to months, but the diagnosis is often overlooked until a fulminant syndrome develops. *Cranial nerve palsies, vasculitic small-vessel infarctions, and obstructive hydrocephalus* occur frequently and result from severe granulomatous inflammation of the basal meninges (see Fig. 22.1). TB can *cause focal abscess formation,* which can evolve into space-occupying mass lesions *(tuberculoma),* even without meningitis. Patients who are chronically exposed, immunosuppressed (AIDS or alcoholic patients), or at the extremes of age are particularly at risk. Morbidity and mortality are high unless treated early. *Hydrocephalus, seizures, and cognitive impairment* are frequent late complications.

Diagnosis

The CSF shows lymphocytic pleocytosis, elevated protein level, and moderately reduced glucose level (see Table 22.1). The diagnosis is established by observing *acid-fast* mycobacteria in the CSF; the yield exceeds 50% when multiple large-volume taps (10–25 mL) are examined. *M. tuberculosis* also can be *cultured* from the CSF, but the yield is low, and up to 6 weeks are needed for the organism to grow. *PCR* testing can establish the diagnosis by amplifying small amounts of tubercle bacillus DNA, but sensitivity is variable depending on the quantity of nucleic acid circulating in the CSF. Evidence of active pulmonary disease is found in only 30% of the cases; purified protein derivative (PPD) testing is too unreliable to be a useful diagnostic tool in working up TB meningitis. Common radiographic findings are basilar meningeal enhancement, cerebral infarcts in the basal ganglia, and evidence of hydrocephalus.

Treatment

Initial treatment consists of the four-drug regimen of **isoniazid** (also give **pyridoxine 50 mg per day**), **rifampin, pyrazinamide,** and **ethambutol**. There is evidence that higher doses of rifampicin in IV formulations and replacing ethambutol with a fluoroquinolone improve outcomes. Cotreatment with **dexamethasone 6 mg IV every 6 hours** also may be used in severe cases (with depressed level of consciousness, focal deficits, or multiple cranial nerve palsies) to inhibit the inflammatory response and limit damage. An infectious disease specialist should be consulted, given possible drug resistance and the high rate of unacceptable drug toxicity arising from these agents. After the intensive phase for 2 months, treatment with isoniazid and rifampicin should continue for 9 to 12 months. In patients with hydrocephalus, an external ventricular device may be needed.

Neurosyphilis

Syphilis is a chronic systemic infection caused by the spirochete *Treponema pallidum*. **Primary infection** is characterized by a chancre (firm, painless genital ulcer). A **secondary bacteremic stage** may occur 2 to 12 weeks later, resulting in generalized muco-cutaneous lesions (palmar and plantar rash) and lymphadenopathy. In up to 60% of cases, the CNS is seeded during the bacteremic stage; 10% of these patients will develop symptomatic early neurosyphilis (meningitis, meningovasculitis, cranial neuritis). Mild inflammatory CSF changes (elevation of cells and protein) can be detected at this stage.

After a latent period of 15 to 20 years, **tertiary syphilis** manifests as a slowly progressive, systemic inflammatory disease of the skin (gummas), heart (aortitis), eyes (chorioretinitis), or CNS. *Tertiary neurosyphilis* develops in 5% of patients with untreated primary syphilis. The classic manifestations include the following:

1. **General paresis**

   This condition results from chronic, diffuse encephalitis and manifests as dementia with prominent psychiatric features and bilateral upper motor neuron signs.
2. **Tabes dorsalis**

   Tabes dorsalis results from chronic spinal polyradiculitis with secondary dorsal root and column degeneration. Symptoms may include neuropathic shooting pains in the lower extremities, loss of posterior column sensation, and areflexia.
3. **Argyll Robertson pupils**

   These are small irregular pupils that react to accommodation but not to light and reflect chronic optic neuritis. Optic atrophy and blindness also may occur.

   In **HIV patients** the course of syphilis is often accelerated, and the early symptomatic forms of secondary syphilis (meningitis and meningovasculitis) predominate. Symptoms may occur during any stage of HIV infection.

Diagnosis

LP is required to rule out neurosyphilis in patients with a serum nontreponemal antibody (rapid plasma reagin [RPR] or VDRL) titer = 1:32, or in any patient with a positive serologic test and neurologic symptoms, no prior treatment, concurrent systemic tertiary syphilis, or HIV infection.

Standard CSF laboratory criteria to diagnose neurosyphilis do not exist. A positive CSF VDRL test is highly specific but only 50% sensitive. Many advocate routine testing of CSF fluorescent treponemal antibody absorption (FTA-ABS), which is highly sensitive but not specific. A negative CSF FTA-ABS and CSF VDRL virtually exclude the diagnosis of neurosyphilis. Some advocate treating if the CSF FTA-ABS is positive and there is either a CSF pleocytosis or elevated protein level.

In HIV patients laboratory diagnosis is more difficult because treponemal and nontreponemal tests are less reliable, and CSF indices can be difficult to interpret depending on the stage of HIV infection. Some advocate a positive CSF FTA-ABS along with a CSF pleocytosis as grounds for treating as neurosyphilis.

Treatment

Neurosyphilis, whether latent or active, is treated with penicillin G 3 to 4 million units IV every 4 hours for 10 to 14 days.

Lyme Disease

Lyme disease is caused by the spirochete *Borrelia burgdorferi*, which is inoculated into humans by the bite of an infected deer tick *(Ixodes dammini)*. A characteristic expanding erythematous "target" lesion, termed *erythema chronicum migrans*, develops at the site of the tick bite. Acute, chronic, and relapsing dermatologic, immunologic, rheumatologic, cardiac, and neurologic complications may occur. Both the peripheral and central nervous systems can be involved, either by direct effects of the infection or by immune-mediated processes, and are usually divided into early or late manifestations (Table 22.2).

Diagnosis

To diagnose CNS Lyme disease, there must be evidence of intrathecal production of IgG antibody (IgM during acute phase) to *Borrelia* using an enzyme-linked immunosorbent assay (ELISA) or Western blot. A PCR test for *Borrelia* DNA in CSF also is available

TABLE 22.2	Neurologic Manifestations of Lyme Disease

Early (less than 6 months after infection)
Mild meningitis or meningoencephalitis
Cranial neuropathy (particularly unilateral or bilateral facial nerve and optic nerve)
Myelitis
Radiculoneuritis
Mononeuritis multiplex
Acute polyneuropathy (resembles Guillain-Barré syndrome)

Chronic (months to years after infection)
Lyme encephalopathy (immune-mediated)
Recurrent or chronic meningoencephalitis
Chronic myelitis
Chronic axonal polyneuropathy

but is less sensitive than antibody testing. A lymphocytic pleocytosis with mildly elevated protein is found is meningitic forms or Lyme disease.

Treatment

Patients with CNS Lyme disease should receive ceftriaxone 2 g IV per day or penicillin G 4 million units IV every 4 hours for 2 to 4 weeks. Isolated facial palsy with normal CSF can be treated with doxycycline 100 mg by mouth (PO) two times a day or amoxicillin 50 mg PO three times a day for 7 to 21 days.

Fungal Meningitis

Fungal infection of the CNS is usually opportunistic, occurring in hosts with impaired cellular immunity (HIV/AIDS, organ transplant, malignancy, immunosuppressive therapy, diabetes, or alcoholism). *C. neoformans* accounts for most cases in the United States; other causes include *Coccidioides immitis* (southwestern United States), *Candida albicans, Histoplasma capsulatum,* and *Blastomyces* species. *Aspergillus* and *Mucor* species are unique in their tendency to invade local tissues and cause vasculitic infarction.

Diagnosis

The most consistent CSF abnormality is an elevated protein level. A lymphocytic pleocytosis and low glucose level are variably present. Eosinophils in the CSF may represent coccidioidal meningitis, although other parasitic etiologies should be considered. Detection of complement-fixing IgG antibodies or immunodiffusion tests for IgM and IgG in the CSF for coccidioidomycosis is nearly as specific as culture. 1,3-β-D-glucan in the CSF might be a useful adjunct test in patients with chronic *Candida* meningitis, as well as other etiologies of fungal meningitis. Diagnosis is based on demonstrating the organism by wet smear or culture. *Cryptococcus* infection is most rapidly diagnosed using the India ink stain or by detecting capsular antigen in the CSF. Sometimes, brain and/or meningeal biopsy is needed.

Treatment

All forms of fungal meningitis are treated with **fluconazole 400 to 800 mg PO daily** for mild cases or **amphotericin B 0.5 to 1.5 mg/ kg per day IV** for severe cases. Treatment should continue for 2 to 4 weeks. Non-HIV cryptococcal meningitis is treated with the combination of **amphotericin B** and **flucytosine (5-FC) 37.5 mg/kg PO every 6 hours** with dose adjustment to maintain a peak (70–80 mg/L) and trough (30–40 mg/L) levels. In the most severe cases, amphotericin B (0.1–0.3 mg daily) can be given intrathecally via a reservoir. Elevated ICP may respond to acetazolamide, but severe cases mandate frequent therapeutic LPs and, if refractory, lumbar or ventricular shunting.

BRAIN ABSCESS AND PARAMENINGEAL INFECTIONS

Bacterial Abscess

Brain abscess is a focal infectious collection within the brain paren-chyma and can arise as a complication of many types of infections; it is frequently seen in patients after trauma or surgery. Brain abscess most commonly presents with subacute progression of headache (in 75% of patients), altered mental status (in 50% of patients), focal neurologic signs (in 50% of patients), and fever (in 50% of patients). The infection usually begins as a focus of cerebritis, which develops into a localized collection of pus with a surrounding fibrovascular capsule. Most abscesses are formed by contiguous spread from a parameningeal infection (otitis media, osteomyelitis, sinusitis) or by hematogenous spread in patients with endocarditis, bronchiectasis, congenital cyanotic heart dis-ease, or pulmonary arteriovenous malformations. The most common organisms encountered are streptococci, *Staphylococcus aureus,* Enterobacteriaceae, and anaerobes such as *Bacteroides fragilis.* Polymicrobial infections are common.

Diagnosis

The diagnosis is suggested by a ring-enhancing lesion (Fig. 22.2) in the brain on CT or magnetic resonance imaging (MRI). The CSF may be normal or may show a mild pleocytosis; a pathogen is iso-lated from CSF cultures in less than 10% of cases. Blood cultures, echocardiography, chest X-ray, HIV testing, and a dedicated skull CT scan (to rule out sinusitis, otitis, or tooth abscess) should be performed. LP is contraindicated in a patient with focal symptoms or signs because there is a risk of herniation in these cases. The location of brain abscess reflects the site of the primary infection that spreads to the cerebral cortex. Cultures of pus obtained from a surgical drainage procedure are often the only way to establish the diagnosis, but even these cultures are negative in 20% of cases.

Treatment

For broad-spectrum empiric coverage of suspected bacterial abscess, treat with (1) **penicillin G 4 million units IV every 4 hours** or **ceftriaxone 2 g IV every 12 hours** *and* (2) **metronidazole 15 mg/kg IV every 12 hours.** For postsurgical or posttraumatic cases or if *S. aureus* is a consideration (positive blood culture), **van-comycin** should be added until sensitivities are known. When the

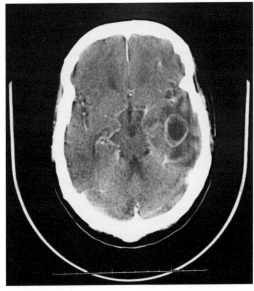

FIG. 22.2 Ring-enhancing lesion on computed tomography (CT) scan, characteristic of bacterial abscess.

pathogen underlying the abscess is in doubt, one must consider broadening coverage to include TB (see the previous section Tuberculosis Meningitis), fungus (amphotericin B), and toxoplasmosis (see the section on Neurologic Complications of AIDS). Aggressive organisms can cause the abscess to quickly expand, leading to rapid neurologic deterioration and herniation. Therefore neurosurgical consult is mandatory for possible emergent drainage and decompression. Patients with depressed level of consciousness also should be treated with **dexamethasone 4 to 10 mg IV every 6 hours** for 4 to 6 days to reduce edema.

Subdural Empyema

Subdural empyema is a closed-space infection between the dura and arachnoid, usually over the hemispheric convexity. In adults, spread of infection from a contiguous source (e.g., sinusitis or otitis) is the cause in most cases, whereas in children, subdural empyema often occurs as a complication of meningitis. The organisms most often cultured are similar to those for brain abscess, and empirical antibiotic coverage is the same. Surgical drainage at the earliest opportunity is essential for successful treatment.

Cranial and Spinal Epidural Abscess

Epidural CNS infection almost always results from infection from a contiguous source and is often seen in combination with osteomyelitis. The CSF often shows mild signs of inflammation (elevated WBC and protein levels) but is sterile.

Cranial epidural abscess usually presents with localized pain and tenderness and can lead to cranial nerve deficits. For example, infection of the petrous temporal bone (Gradenigo syndrome) often results in cranial nerve (CN) 5 and CN 6 deficits. Common infecting organisms are the same as for brain abscess, and empirical antibiotic treatment is the same.

Spinal epidural abscess is most common in the thoracic region and often occurs in diabetics and IV drug users. Symptoms may include intense local pain and tenderness, local root irritation with referred pain, and cord compression, which is a neurologic emergency. *S. aureus* and streptococci account for 75% of the infections, and gram-negative organisms account for 20%; unusual causes include *M. tuberculosis* (Pott disease) and fungi. MRI of the spine is the diagnostic technique of choice. Treatment with high-dose steroids **(dexamethasone 60–100 mg IV push [IVP], followed by 10–20 mg IV every 6 hours)** and **surgical drainage** should be performed immediately to prevent cord compression. **Vancomycin** and **ceftriaxone** usually provide adequate empirical antibiotic coverage for bacterial infection (Table 22.3).

Cysticercosis

Cysticercosis is the most common parasitic CNS infection worldwide and typically presents with seizures. It is one of the most common treatable causes of epilepsy worldwide. Ova shed by the intestinal tapeworm *Taenia solium* in human feces can contaminate food ingested by the host or others, which leads to hematogenous dissemination of encysted larvae throughout the body, including the CNS. Most cases occur in Latin America (e.g., Mexico) and Southeast Asia. Neurocysticercosis can occur intraparenchymally or extraparenchymally. Extraparenchymal neurocysticercosis is caused by intraventricular cysts, subarachnoid cysts, spinal cysts, and ocular cysts.

Diagnosis

CT and MRI scans are usually highly characteristic. *Uninflamed cysts* appear as small (less than 1 cm) fluid-filled cysts. *Active, inflamed cysts* occur when the larvae are dying and are identified by the presence of contrast enhancement. *Inactive cysts* result once the inflammatory reaction to a dying larval cyst has resolved; they appear as small, punctuate, calcified lesions. In the *racemic form,* cystic membranes fill the ventricles and the subarachnoid space,

TABLE 22.3	**Empirical Antibiotic Therapy for Bacterial Meningitis**	
Risk Group	**Pathogen**	**Empiric Therapy**
Neonates (<1 month)	Group B streptococci, *Escherichia coli, Listeria monocytogenes, Klebsiella*	Cefotaxime or gentamycin + ampicillin
Infants to young adults (1 month to 50 years)	*Streptococcus pneumoniae, Neisseria. meningitides*	Ceftriaxone or cefotaxime + vancomycin
Adults >50 years old	*S. pneumoniae, Listeria monocytogenes*, gram-negative bacilli	Ceftriaxone + vancomycin + ampicillin
Postneurosurgical, head	*S. pneumoniae, Pseudomonas aeruginosa, Staphylococcus aureus*	Cefepime or ceftazidime or meropenem + vancomycin
Trauma/skull fracture, cochlear implant	*S. epidermidis*, Enterobacteriaceae	
Shunt-related ventriculitis or meningitis	*S. aureus, S. epidermidis, Propionibacterium acnes*, Enterobacteriaceae	Cefepime or ceftazidime or meropenem + vancomycin

Adult dosages: Ampicillin 2.0 g intravenously (IV) every 4 hours, cefepime 2 g IV every 8 hours, cefotaxime 2 g IV every 6 hours, ceftazidime 2 g IV every 8 hours, ceftriaxone 2 g IV every 12 hours, meropenem 2 g IV every 8 hours, vancomycin 1 g IV every 8 hours, and dexamethasone 0.15 mg/kg IV every 6 hours.

resulting in hydrocephalus. Identification of a scolex in a cystic lesion is the only pathognomonic finding; they are rounded or elongated bright nodules within the cyst cavity. Plain radiography or CT can evaluate extraneural cysticercosis, which often is present in the muscle or subcutaneous tissue. Detection of *serum antibody titers* to *Cysticercus* can confirm the diagnosis, but sensitivity is less than 100% in patients with inactive disease or with a single enhancing lesion. Patients and family members should undergo stool examinations for ova and parasites because treatment can prevent reinfection. Other cystic lesions in the brain may be causes by echinococcosis, coenurosis, cystic glioma, and glioblastoma.

Treatment

Patients with inactive (calcified) neurocysticercosis or with few viable or degenerating cysts and minimal symptoms (e.g., seizures controlled with anticonvulsants and a nonfocal examination) do not require antimicrobial treatment. In the latter case, follow-up neuroimaging 6 to 10 weeks later usually shows progression of the enhancing lesion to a small, calcified nodule. For those with many cysts, giant cyst(s), or intraventricular/subarachnoid cysts, give **praziquantel 25 mg/kg PO three times daily** or **albendazole 7.5 mg/kg PO twice daily, for 14 days.** For patients undergoing treatment with a large lesion burden, give **dexamethasone 4 to 6 mg PO every 6 hours for 5 days** to attenuate the inflammatory reaction and an antiseizure medication (e.g., **phenytoin 300 PO daily**) to minimize symptoms related to the inflammatory response caused by dying cysts. Surgical resection is often more effective than ventriculoperitoneal shunting for treating intraventricular cysticercosis resulting in hydrocephalus.

VIRAL ENCEPHALITIS

Herpes Simplex Encephalitis

HSV-1 encephalitis is the most common cause of sporadic viral encephalitis and is fatal in up to 70% of untreated patients. Patients present with fever, altered mental status, headache, and seizures. The disease results from reactivation of dormant HSV-1 within the trigeminal ganglion, with viral spread via sensory pathways into the brain, rather than the more common picture of retrograde viral expression leading to perioral herpetic lesions.

Diagnosis

The CSF may show mild lymphocytic pleocytosis, increased red blood cells, and increased protein, but it may be normal, particularly early in the disease. A positive CSF HSV PCR confirms the diagnosis, but false-negative results occur, particularly if CSF is acquired after acyclovir use and within 1 week of symptom onset. The presence of intrathecal HSV antibody (IgM or IgG) from CSF acquired at least 1 week after onset of symptoms assists in making a retrospective diagnosis. CSF cultures usually do not yield the virus. Focal necrotizing lesions of the inferior frontal and medial temporal lobes are highly characteristic and are best seen with contrast MRI. An electroencephalogram (EEG) often shows periodic lateralized epileptiform discharges, consistent with structural temporal lobe lesions. Definitive diagnosis is made by brain biopsy, which demonstrates eosinophilic intracellular (Cowdry type I) inclusions but is rarely necessary when the clinical, radiologic, and EEG findings are highly characteristic.

Treatment

All patients with suspected viral encephalitis should be treated empirically with **acyclovir 10 mg/kg IV every 8 hours for 14 to 21 days.** *Because efficacy depends on early treatment, acyclovir should be started as soon as possible and should never be withheld pending the results of diagnostic studies. A lack of response to treatment should raise one's suspicion for acyclovir resistance, and further testing is often required.* Anticonvulsants (e.g., **phenytoin**) should be given to all critically ill patients and discontinued after 2 weeks if no seizures occur. Continuous EEG monitoring to rule out nonconvulsive seizure activity is recommended in patients with abnormal mental status.

West Nile Virus Infection

WNV, an arthropod-borne virus transmitted by the bite of the *Culex* mosquito, is the most common cause of epidemic encephalitis in the United States. Disease activity is now concentrated in the western United States, with outbreaks occurring predominately in the summer and fall months when mosquito activity is highest. Transmission has been reported via blood transfusion, organ transplantation, and breast-feeding; of those infected, only 20% become symptomatic and less than 1% develop neurologic complications (neuroinvasive WNV). The majority of neuroinvasive cases manifest as *meningoencephalitis* (60% to 75%), characterized by altered mental status, focal neurologic deficits, and tremor, or *meningitis* (25% to 30%), characterized by headache, neck pain, and occasionally cranial nerve palsy's (facial nerve particularly). Less commonly *myelitis and polyradiculitis* occur, characterized by the acute onset of asymmetric limb weakness, the absence of sensory less, and lower motor neuron signs.

Diagnosis

Neuroinvasive WNV is a diagnosis based on clinical suspicion (risk of exposure and suggestive signs and symptoms) and the presence of WNV IgM in the blood or CSF. A negative WNV IgM antibody test should be repeated in 7 days to allow for seroconversion after an acute infection. Serum WNV IgM antibody, which does not cross the blood–brain barrier, also should be present, and a fourfold change in acute to convalescent titers indicates a recent infection. Both serum and CSF IgM antibody can persist for months; therefore a single positive test does not necessarily imply recent infection. False–positives also can occur when antibodies to St. Louis encephalitis virus and Japanese encephalitis virus are present. CSF typically shows a mild pleocytosis, elevated protein level, and normal glucose level. West Nile poliomyelitis should be considered in cases of rapidly ascending paralysis with an inflammatory CSF profile. Isolation (culture) or amplification (PCR) techniques have a low sensitivity.

Treatment

Treatment remains supportive, but clinical trials with IVIG and interferon (IFN)-α are in progress.

Other Causes of Encephalitis

Causes of viral encephalitis other than HSV-1 and WNV are listed next. PCR testing on CSF is available for most viruses, but the sensitivity of most assays, when used in a clinical setting, is unknown. Virus-specific antibody testing on CSF is the most reliable method of making a diagnosis, albeit retrospectively.

1. **Enteroviruses**

   This group includes **coxsackievirus, echovirus,** and **poliovirus**. Outbreaks of meningitis and, to a lesser extent, encephalitis occur during the fall/winter months. The course is usually mild. CSF viral cultures and PCR are sensitive.

2. **Arboviruses (arthropod-borne viruses)**

   These viruses are transmitted to humans via a variety of vectors including mosquitoes and ticks and are restricted by geography and season:

   - **Eastern equine virus** (Gulf and Atlantic coast) causes a severe encephalitis with high morbidity and mortality.
   - **Western equine virus** (western United States) causes a mild meningoencephalitis.
   - **St. Louis encephalitis virus** (entire United States) causes a severe encephalitis with occasional epidemics.
   - **California encephalitis virus** (eastern and central United States) may simulate HSV-1 encephalitis.
   - **Colorado tick fever virus** (Rocky Mountains) is transmitted from the bite from a *Dermacentor andersoni* tick.
   - **Powassan virus** (Northeast United States) is transmitted from *Ixodes cookei,* or woodchuck tick.
   - **Japanese encephalitis virus** (Asia), transmitted by the *Culex* mosquito, is the most common cause of encephalitis worldwide and is not endemic to the United States. The mortality rate is approximately 30%.

3. **Herpes family viruses**

   - **HSV-2** is a common cause of encephalitis in neonates and meningitis in children and adults.
   - **Epstein-Barr virus (EBV)** is typically associated with polyradiculitis or cerebellitis.
   - **VZV** can cause encephalitis in association with a systemic primary infection (chickenpox), or a focal granulomatous

vasculitis of the brain or spinal cord after a zoster eruption in the corresponding vascular territory.

- **Cytomegalovirus (CMV)**-related neurologic complications are seen only in those with impaired cellular immunity (see the section on Neurologic Complications of AIDS).
- **Human herpes virus 6 (HHV-6)** can cause severe encephalitis in patients on immunosuppressive treatment.

4. **Measles virus**

Along with causing acute encephalitis 1 to 14 days after a viral exanthem (rubeola), the measles virus can cause (1) a relentlessly progressive subacute encephalitis in immunosuppressed patients, (2) postinfectious immune-mediated demyelinating encephalomyelitis, and (3) *subacute sclerosing panencephalitis (SSPE),* which is a "slow" viral infection characterized by progressive dementia, ataxia, myoclonus, periodic sharp waves on EEG, elevated titers of antimeasles virus antibodies in the CSF, and pathologic intracellular viral inclusion bodies.

5. **Rabies virus**

Rabies is spread by the bite of an infected (rabid) animal. After a variable incubation period (1–3 months), rabies encephalomyelitis invariably leads to delirium, seizures, paralysis, and death. After inoculation, the virus travels to the CNS via retrograde axonal transport. Negri bodies and dark intracellular viral inclusions are the characteristic pathologic lesion.

VIRAL MYELITIS

Acute Viral Myelitis

Acute myelitis, a relatively rare disease, may occur in isolation or concomitant with meningitis or encephalitis. Herpes family viruses (e.g., HSV-2, EBV, CMV, VZV), enteroviruses, and WNV are the most common causes. Acute viral myelitis presents with acute onset of weakness, sensory loss, and autonomic (particularly bladder) dysfunction. WNV and poliovirus are exceptional in that they infect motor neurons, causing asymmetric flaccid weakness (poliomyelitis). A polio-like illness of unknown etiology has been reported in the United States, commonly affecting young children. Many of the acute flaccid myelitis cases were temporally associated with outbreaks of respiratory illness attributed to enterovirus D68. Clinically discriminating viral from autoimmune, toxic, and vascular causes of acute myelitis can be difficult, but as a general rule, viral myelitis is more likely to affect only one spinal cord level.

Diagnosis

CSF typically reveals a mild lymphocytic pleocytosis with an elevated protein level. Many of the viruses can be amplified by virus-specific PCR assays, although the sensitivity of the assays in clinical practice is unproven. The presence of virus-specific antibody in CSF acquired weeks after the onset confirms the diagnosis. MRI typically shows focal area of increased T2-weighted signal that enhances with contrast.

Treatment

Antiviral treatment needs to be tailored to the specific causative virus, when known. EBV, VZV, or HSV type 1 or 2 is treated with **acyclovir 10 mg/kg IV every 8 hours,** and CMV is treated with **ganciclovir 5 mg/kg IV every 12 hours** and/or **foscarnet 90 to 120 mg/kg/day.** Corticosteroids are not indicated for viral myelitis but should be given when immune-mediated causes are a diagnostic consideration. Particular attention must be paid to bladder and bowel dysfunction.

Chronic Viral Myelopathy

Human T-cell lymphotropic virus type 1 or 2 (HTLV-1/2) and HIV, and less commonly HSV-2 and VZV, are recognized causes of chronic viral myelopathy. HTLV infection, which causes a myelopathy formerly known as tropical spastic paraparesis, is endemic in the Caribbean basin, Brazil, Japan, and parts of Africa. Symptoms include subacute to insidious onset of spastic paresis, sensory loss, and autonomic (erectile, urinary, and bowel) dysfunction.

Diagnosis

CSF may show mild nonspecific abnormalities including a lymphocytic pleocytosis and elevated protein level. HSV-2 and VZV infection can be confirmed by virus-specific PCR or IgG antibody in the CSF. HTLV-1/2 is confirmed by the presence of IgG antibody in the CSF. HIV myelopathy is a clinical diagnosis. Neuroimaging may be normal or show atrophy of the cord.

Treatment

Acyclovir 10 mg/kg IV every 8 hours should be given for HSV or VZV myelopathy. HIV myelopathy may respond to virologic control with highly active antiretroviral therapy (HAART). Antiviral therapy has not been shown to be effective in HTLV-associated myelopathy; otherwise, treatment is supportive, and particular attention must be paid to bladder and bowel dysfunction.

NEUROLOGIC COMPLICATIONS OF AIDS

Both the peripheral and central nervous systems are vulnerable to HIV-related complications. HIV is a neurotropic virus that directly invades the brain shortly after infection. The risk for *opportunistic infection* is greatest in those with CD4⁺ T helper lymphocyte counts less than 200/mm³, whereas *immune-mediated conditions* and *medication-related toxicities* can occur at any time. *Patients with AIDS are at risk for multiple, simultaneous opportunistic infections.*

Opportunistic Infections

1. **CNS toxoplasmosis**

   Toxoplasmosis, the most common cause of a space-occupying mass lesion in HIV patients, usually presents with fever, subacute encephalopathy, focal neurologic deficits, and seizures. A presumed diagnosis is based on brain imaging showing one or more ring-enhancing mass lesions that respond to antitoxoplasmosis treatment within 2 weeks. The clinical and radiographic response is typically quite dramatic. Ocular and spinal cord abscesses may occur; meningoencephalitis from a ruptured abscess is rare. The presence of serum toxoplasma IgG antibody at presentation raises the probability of the diagnosis. CSF analysis does not assist in making the diagnosis but may help exclude others.

   Patients with suspected toxoplasmosis should be treated empirically with **sulfadiazine 25 mg/kg PO every 6 hours and pyrimethamine 200 mg PO on day 1, followed by 75 to 100 mg per day for 6 to 8 weeks. Folinic acid 10 to 20 mg PO every day** also should be given to minimize hematologic toxicity. Clindamycin 600 mg IV or PO four times a day can be used instead of sulfadiazine in patients who are allergic to sulfa drugs. **Dexamethasone 6 mg IV every 6 hours** should be restricted to patients with large-mass lesions with impending herniation because its use may obscure the diagnosis. Repeat imaging, preferably MRI, with contrast should be performed 10 to 14 days after initiation of treatment. Nonresponders require a biopsy for definitive diagnosis and differentiation from malignant (e.g., CNS lymphoma) or other infectious (e.g., TB, bacterial) lesions.

2. **Cryptococcus meningitis**

   This diagnosis should be considered in any AIDS patient with a headache. Patients also may present with signs of increased ICP including nausea, vomiting, and confusion. Because this is a systemic infection, the presence of serum cryptococcal antigen is a sensitive (95%) but not specific screening test for meningitis. The diagnosis can be easily made or excluded with CSF analysis for cryptococcal antigen or fungal culture. CSF WBC count may be normal or minimally elevated. All HIV patients should undergo brain imaging before LP to rule out a space-occupying mass lesion. Treatment depends on the severity of infection. ***Mild cases*** (normal neurologic examination, CSF cryptococcal antigen <1:1024) can be treated with **fluconazole 400 mg PO each day for 8 to 10 weeks.** *More severe cases* require **amphotericin B 0.7 to 1.0 mg/kg per day IV for 2 weeks or until the CSF is sterile** followed by **fluconazole 400 mg PO every day** to complete a treatment course of at least 10 weeks. **5-FC, 25 mg/kg PO every 6 hours for 2 weeks,** may be added, but this requires drug-level monitoring (peak 70–80 mg/L, trough 30–40 mg/L) and is associated with bone marrow toxicity. Steroids have not been found to reduce morbidity and mortality in cryptococcal meningitis, and there are data to delay initiation of antiretroviral therapy. One complication of cryptococcal meningitis is elevated ICP, defined as a CSF opening pressure >250 mm H_2O, and prior literature suggested that there is higher mortality among cryptococcal patients with raised ICP. Therapeutic LPs after the diagnostic LP are recommended for those with baseline CSF opening pressure >250 mm H_2O or symptoms of raised pressure

3. **Progressive multifocal leukoencephalopathy (PML)**

PML is a demyelinating disorder caused by the JC virus and presents with subacute onset of focal neurologic deficits and dementia; the peripheral nervous system is spared. MRI typically shows striking white matter hyperintensities on T2-weighted images, with sparing of the cortical gray matter. Enhancement is typically seen in the context of immune reconstitution syndrome. CSF profile is often normal. PCR for JC virus in CSF is not a sensitive test but can help confirm the diagnosis. The most important treatment is HAART to reconstitute the immune system. There is no specific treatment that has been shown to reverse the effects of PML.

4. **CMV infection**

CMV can affect both the central and peripheral nervous systems. CMV retinitis, which presents with slowly progressive, painless visual loss, is the most common neurologic complication. Other complications are rare and usually occur in very advanced AIDS (CD4 < 50). *Ventriculoencephalitis* presents with rapidly progressive cognitive and behavioral changes; *myelitis* with acute onset of weakness, urinary dysfunction, and a sensory level; *polyradiculitis* with acute onset of back pain, asymmetric flaccid paresis of legs, paresthesia (often in a "saddle" distribution), and urinary dysfunction; and *mononeuritis multiplex* with asymmetric motor and sensory deficits conforming to a peripheral nerve distribution. CNS infection is accompanied by CSF pleocytosis (often numbering in the 1000s and with polymorphonuclear predominance), elevated protein level, and low glucose level. CMV PCR is highly sensitive for both systemic (blood) and CNS (CSF) infection. MRI typically shows inflammation and enhancement of affected areas, including a distinctive pattern of ependymal enhancement. CMV infections involving the CNS can rapidly progress; suspected cases require immediate treatment with **ganciclovir 5 mg/kg IV every 12 hours,** although efficacy is variable. **Foscarnet 60 mg/kg IV every 8 hours for 14 days** can be used as a second-line agent.

5. **Primary CNS lymphoma (PCNSL)**

    PCNSL lymphoma is caused by EBV and presents with subacute focal neurologic and cognitive deficits. Brain imaging shows one or more enhancing mass lesions, simulating toxoplasmosis abscesses. If not contraindicated, LP can help establish the diagnosis with the presence of amplifiable EBV by PCR. Thallium single-photon emission computed tomography (SPECT) showing increased local uptake ("hot" spot) or positron emission tomography (PET) imaging revealing a hypermetabolic lesion also can help discriminate PCNSL from an abscess such as toxoplasmosis. In most patients, however, the diagnosis is established by biopsy after failure to respond to empirical treatment for toxoplasmosis. Because malignancies and abscesses alike may respond favorably to steroids, **dexamethasone should be withheld** unless absolutely necessary until a definite diagnosis is ascertained. Whole-brain radiation, methotrexate, and HAART are the mainstays of treatment. Prognosis is variable from months to years, often depending on the patient's response to HAART.

6. **Herpes zoster (shingles)**

    Herpes zoster radiculitis/ganglionitis, caused by the reactivation of VZV, is a common HIV-related complication. Multiple dermatomes are often involved. In contrast to other infections, zoster may occur when the CD4 count is well above 200. VZV also causes a CNS vasculopathy, presenting with strokelike syndromes or myelopathy and often heralded by a zoster eruption. Uncomplicated zoster can be treated with **acyclovir (800 mg PO five times daily)** or **valacyclovir (1000 mg PO three times daily)** along with analgesics. If CNS vasculopathy is suspected or multiple dermatomes are affected, then further workup with LP and MRI is warranted, and **IV treatment (acyclovir 10–12.5 mg/kg every 8 hours)** should be given.

7. **Syphilis**

The course of syphilis is often accelerated in HIV-infected patients, and the early symptomatic forms of secondary syphilis (meningitis and meningovasculitis) predominate. Symptoms may occur during any stage of HIV infection. There is a higher rate of both false-positive and false-negative treponemal and nontreponemal tests in HIV patients. Treatment may require a more prolonged course of **penicillin G** (>10 days) than in immunocompetent patients.

8. **HIV (aseptic) meningitis**

HIV frequently causes a self-limited meningitis and rarely meningoencephalitis during primary viremia. CSF may show a mild pleocytosis, and HIV is readily amplifiable with PCR. Only symptomatic treatment is necessary.

Nonopportunistic Nervous System Complications of AIDS

1. **Distal sensory polyneuropathy (DSP)**

DSP is the most common HIV-related neurologic complication and is caused by immune-mediated pathways or antiretroviral toxicity (ddI, ddC, and d4T). Symmetric, painful paresthesias, sensory loss, allodynia in a stocking-and-glove distribution, and loss of ankle jerks are the clinical features. Antiretroviral toxicity tends to have a more abrupt onset, occurring shortly after initiation or dose escalation. Treatment of the neuropathic pain is symptomatic (see Chapter 18); the mainstay of treatment is improved virologic control with HAART. ARV-mediated DSP usually improves with cessation of the offending agent.

2. **HIV-associated cognitive disorder**

HIV invades the CNS and infects nonneuronal cells shortly after primary viremia. Years later, in the setting of immune failure (CD4 < 200) and dysregulation, chronic encephalitis ensues, manifesting with insidious onset of cognitive impairment (executive function), motor slowing, and behavioral changes (depression, apathy) resembling a subcortical dementia. The presence of neurocognitive deficits in certain HIV-infected individuals without alternative explanation other than HIV infection has long been recognized.

The diagnosis is clinical. There are three categories of HIV-associated neurocognitive disorder (HAND):

- **Asymptomatic neurocognitive impairment** (ANI) is determined by neurocognitive testing and is not apparent clinically.

- **Mild neurocognitive disorder** (MND) is a diagnosis of exclusion; it may be made clinically if neurocognitive testing is not available, and it involves mild functional impairment.
- **HIV-associated dementia** (HAD) involves moderate-to-severe functional impairment.

    Patients with HAD who are not on antiretroviral therapy often have elevated CSF protein and elevated HIV levels in the CSF. MRI typically shows central atrophy and leukopathy, and the CSF may show a mild pleocytosis. Virologic control with HAART can slow the dementing process (see Chapter 28).

3. **HIV-associated myelopathy**

    This uncommon disorder occurs in the advanced stages of HIV (CD4 < 200). It is characterized by an insidious onset of spastic paraparesis; sensory ataxia (posterior column dysfunction); and bowel, bladder, and erectile dysfunction. The syndrome resembles that seen with B_{12} deficiency. Infections (e.g., HTLV-1 CMV, HSV, TB, toxoplasma, bacterial abscess) and malignancies should be considered in the differential diagnosis. MRI of the spine may show atrophy and abnormal signal in the posterior columns but is usually normal. Somatosensory-evoked potentials are typically prolonged. Virologic control with HAART and symptomatic management is the only treatment available.

4. **HIV-associated myopathy**

    Despite its myriad causes (infectious agents, immune-mediated processes, or azidothymidine [AZT] toxicity), HIV-related myopathy is rare. Subacute onset of proximal muscle weakness, creatine kinase (CK) elevation, and myalgias characterize most cases. Diagnosis but not etiology can be confirmed by electromyography (EMG). Treatment depends on the cause.

5. **HIV-associated neuromuscular weakness syndrome**

    A severe sensorimotor neuropathy can develop in the setting of nucleoside reverse transcriptase use, particularly d4T. The syndrome is characterized by rapidly progressive weakness, simulating a Guillain-Barré syndrome, and constitutional symptoms (fever, general malaise, nausea, headache). Serum lactate levels are almost always elevated. CSF may show nonspecific abnormalities but is indicated to rule out other infectious causes (e.g., CMV). Electrophysiology studies typically show both axonal and demyelinating pathology, and muscle biopsy may show a myopathy suggestive of mitochondrial disease. Treatment consists of withdrawal of all nucleoside antiretrovirals and supportive care.

6. **Acute demyelinating polyneuropathy (AIDP)**

This complication is clinically indistinguishable from Guillain-Barré syndrome (see Chapter 16) and occurs shortly after HIV seroconversion. CSF is characterized by a lymphocytic pleocytosis, in contrast to the acellular CSF seen with seronegatives with AIPD, and an elevated protein level. CMV polyradiculitis should be ruled out with PCR. Treatment consists of **IV immunoglobulin (0.4 mg/kg every day for 5 days)** or **plasmapheresis** and supportive care in a monitored setting.

Neurooncology

Tumors of the central nervous system (CNS) are a significant cause of morbidity and mortality. In the United States, it is estimated that 22,000 new cases and 13,000 deaths caused by primary malignant CNS malignancies occur annually. Additionally, 28,000 new cases of meningiomas, which are more than 90% benign tumors, are diagnosed each year. Metastatic CNS tumors significantly outnumber primary tumors; an estimated 170,000 cases of brain metastases are diagnosed in the United States yearly. Fig. 23.1 lists the most common primary CNS neoplasms in adults by location.

SYMPTOMATIC MANAGEMENT IN NEUROONCOLOGY

Corticosteroids

The primary indication of corticosteroids in CNS tumors is to control brain and spinal cord vasogenic edema. Corticosteroids have significant side effects such as insomnia, hyperglycemia, myopathy, psychiatric effects, and opportunistic infections, and some studies suggest that they may decrease overall survival in glioma patients. Patients with asymptomatic CNS tumors and those with symptoms unrelated to vasogenic edema do not benefit from or require corticosteroids. In suspected cases of primary CNS lymphoma (PCNSL), corticosteroids should be avoided whenever possible because they decrease the diagnostic yield of biopsies. Dexamethasone is the standard corticosteroid in CNS tumors because of its virtual lack of mineralocorticoid effect and lower serum protein binding, which leads to higher CNS levels. There are no specific dexamethasone dosing guidelines; patients should receive the smallest amount needed to control the neurologic symptoms caused by vasogenic edema. **A standard starting dose for brain vasogenic edema is dexamethasone 4 mg twice daily**. Patients should not be reflexively started on proton pump inhibitors when started on corticosteroids, and this should be reserved for patients with a history of gastritis or gastric or duodenal ulcers. If corticosteroids

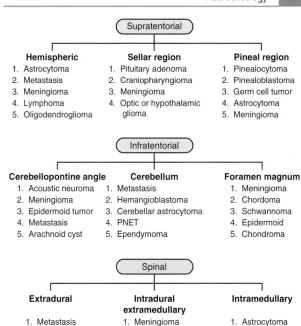

FIG. 23.1 Radiographic differential diagnosis of solitary CNS neoplasms in the adult patient, by location. PNET, primitive neuroectodermal tumor.

are used in a high dose ($\geq$20 mg of prednisone or approximately 3.2 mg of dexamethasone daily) chronically ($\geq$ 4 weeks), prophylaxis for *Pneumocystis jiroveci* must be started.

Antiepileptic Drugs

Although seizures are frequent in both primary and metastatic brain tumors, prophylactic antiepileptic drugs are not indicated in patients with CNS tumors who have never had a seizure. Primary seizure prophylaxis is only recommended in the immediate postoperative period after a brain tumor resection. Prophylactic antiepileptic drugs in patients undergoing brain tumor resection can reduce the risk of seizures by 40% to 50% in the first postoperative week, but they do not prevent seizure incidence afterward and should be quickly tapered off. On the other hand, antiepileptic drugs should be started in any patient who has experienced a seizure at tumor presentation or during the CNS tumor disease course, including after a single seizure episode. In general, nonenzyme-inducing antiepileptic drugs are preferred to avoid interactions with chemotherapies or targeted therapies.

Anticoagulants

Patients with CNS malignancies have an increased incidence of venous thromboembolic events. CNS tumor without acute hemorrhage is not a contraindication for prophylactic doses of unfractionated or low-molecular-weight heparin during hospitalization. Up to 30% of patients with high-grade gliomas develop symptomatic deep venous thrombosis or pulmonary embolism. CNS malignancy is not an absolute contraindication for full-dose anticoagulation when active or acute intracranial hemorrhage has been excluded. In fact, chronic anticoagulation is preferred over inferior vena cava (IVC) filters, which have frequent complications such as recurrent embolic events, IVC or filter thrombosis, severe postphlebitic syndrome, and chronic leg swelling.

GLIOMAS

The histopathologic criteria for the diagnosis of gliomas are based on the World Health Organization (WHO) classification. Grade I gliomas (pilocytic astrocytoma) are rare in adults and the only potentially curable glioma with a gross total resection. Grade II (low-grade) and grade III (anaplastic) gliomas can be subdivided into astrocytomas and oligodendrogliomas based on the morphology and molecular features; oligodendrogliomas must have both isocitrate dehydrogenase (IDH) mutation and 1p/19q chromosome codeletion. Glioblastomas (grade IV gliomas) are the most common and most aggressive primary brain tumors in adults; they are characterized by the presence of microvascular proliferation, necrosis, or both on pathology.

Epidemiology

Gliomas are the most common primary brain tumor in adults, with approximately 18,000 people diagnosed in the United States each year. Their incidence is slightly higher in men than women, and in Caucasians compared with African Americans. Glioblastomas account for more than 50% of cases of gliomas; incidence increases with age and peaks in the seventh decade of life. Anaplastic glioma peak of incidence is in the fifth decade of life, whereas low-grade gliomas are more common in patients between ages 30 and 40.

Diagnosis

Low-grade gliomas are nonenhancing infiltrative tumors with minimal or no vasogenic edema (Fig. 23.2). Oligodendrogliomas can have calcification or hemosiderin deposits from prior bleeding.

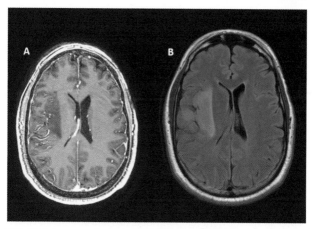

FIG. 23.2 Low-grade glioma. (A) Post-gadolinium T1-weighted image showing a hypointense mass within the right frontal lobe without significant enhancement. (B) Fluid attenuation inversion recovery (FLAIR) image showing a hyperintense mass within the right frontal lobe with mass effect.

Anaplastic gliomas have variable degrees of vasogenic edema, and about 50% show some signs of contrast enhancement on magnetic resonance imaging (MRI) scans. Glioblastomas have irregular borders, almost always enhance, and often have central necrosis and vasogenic edema (Fig. 23.3). Biopsy (or, whenever feasible, surgical resection) is required for histologic diagnosis because imaging features have limited predictive value. Histologically, low-grade gliomas show mild nuclear atypia and increased cellularity, whereas anaplastic gliomas are characterized by the presence of mitoses, and glioblastomas have microvascular proliferation and tumor necrosis.

Treatment

Newly Diagnosed Gliomas

SURGERY

Maximal safe resection is recommended for all glioma grades and subtypes whenever the tumor is surgically accessible and there are no absolute medical contraindications to surgery. A complete macroscopic resection, however, is almost never curative because grade II–IV gliomas infiltrate the normal brain. Nevertheless, surgical resection provides tissue for accurate diagnosis and molecular studies, can improve neurologic symptoms, decreases dependence on corticosteroids, and improves quality of life. Moreover, retrospective and prospective nonrandomized studies

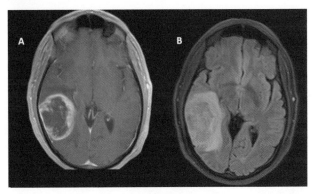

FIG. 23.3 Glioblastoma. (A) Post-gadolinium T1-weighted image showing an enhancing mass with irregular border and necrotic center within the right temporal lobe. (B) Fluid attenuation inversion recovery (FLAIR) image showing a hyperintense mass within the right temporal lobe with mass effect and vasogenic edema.

suggested that more extensive tumor resection is associated with longer survival in both low-grade and high-grade (grade III and IV) gliomas.

Because of tumor location, not all gliomas are amenable to resection, but, if feasible, a biopsy should be performed to provide histologic diagnosis. Neurosurgical advances such as neuronavigation, intraoperative brain mapping techniques, awake craniotomies, and intraoperative MRI allow neurosurgeons in specialized centers to resect CNS tumors previously considered unresectable successfully. Certain tumors located in the brain stem may have a high risk of biopsy complications, and the diagnosis and treatment decision may be based on neuroimaging and clinical features only.

RADIOTHERAPY

Radiotherapy increases median survival in patients with glioblastomas from approximately 4 months with supportive care only to about 12 months. **The most used protocol for anaplastic gliomas and glioblastomas delivers 200-cGy fractions of focal radiation over a 6-week period to a total dose of 6000 cGy.** For low-grade gliomas, lower total doses (a total of 4500 to 5400 cGy fractionated over 5–6 weeks) are more commonly used. The best timing for radiotherapy in low-grade gliomas, however, remains controversial. For patients with low-grade gliomas who had an optimal resection, tumors <6 cm, no neurologic symptoms other than seizures, and age <40 years, the recommendation is close surveillance with brain MRI scans, because upfront radiation or chemotherapy likely does not improve survival.

CHEMOTHERAPY

The most commonly used chemotherapy in gliomas is the alkylating agent **temozolomide**. Temozolomide is considered standard of care in the initial treatment of both anaplastic astrocytomas and glioblastomas. For low-grade gliomas and oligodendrogliomas, the role of temozolomide is less established. For newly diagnosed glioblastoma and anaplastic astrocytoma, radiotherapy and temozolomide (**75 mg/m² daily during radiotherapy followed by 6–12 cycles at 150–200 mg/m² on days 1–5 of 28-day cycles**) are recommended.

The tumor DNA damage caused by temozolomide and other alkylating agents can be reversed by a DNA repair enzyme encoded by the *O*-6-methylguanine-DNA methyltransferase (*MGMT*) gene. Glioblastomas with methylation of the *MGMT* promoter, and consequently less transcription of *MGMT* gene and lower levels of this DNA repair enzyme, have better outcomes on temozolomide than those with the unmethylated *MGMT* promoter. For glioblastomas with unmethylated *MGMT* promoter, withholding temozolomide is acceptable because of the low likelihood of benefiting from alkylating chemotherapy.

Oligodendrogliomas are more sensitive to chemotherapy compared with other gliomas. The best timing for chemotherapy for oligodendrogliomas, however, is not defined. It is unclear if chemotherapy can safely replace radiotherapy as the initial treatment of newly diagnosed anaplastic oligodendrogliomas. An old chemotherapy regimen called **procarbazine**, **CCNU** (also called lomustine), and **vincristine (PCV)** in addition to radiotherapy improves outcomes in oligodendrogliomas compared with radiotherapy alone; nevertheless, PCV has significant toxicity, and its use has been declining over the years.

Wafers containing the alkylating agent **carmustine (Gliadel)** implanted in the surgical cavity at the time of tumor resection are approved by the Food and Drug Administration (FDA) for recurrent or newly diagnosed high-grade (grade III or IV) gliomas but are rarely used. Gliadel's clinical benefit is quite limited, and it has unique side effects (surgical infection, cerebrospinal fluid [CSF] leak); moreover, Gliadel has not been directly compared with systemic chemotherapy in a clinical trial.

TUMOR-TREATING FIELDS

Tumor-treating fields (TTFields) are a noninvasive therapeutic modality that delivers low-intensity alternating electric fields through arrays over the scalp. TTFields have antimitotic activity, and they have been approved for treatment of glioblastoma; TTFields usually start about 4 weeks after the completion of radiation and temozolomide. The recommendation is to use TTFields for about 18 hours daily in conjunction with adjuvant temozolomide. TTFields can be used up to 2 years, and they improve overall survival in this population.

Recurrent Gliomas

There is no accepted standard of care for recurrent gliomas. A subset of patients may benefit from another surgical resection at the time of recurrence. Patients with low-grade gliomas who did not undergo radiotherapy at the time of diagnosis should receive radiation at the time of recurrence or progression. Reirradiation for recurrent high-grade gliomas may be an option for patients with a long interval from the initial radiotherapy and smaller tumors. **Bevacizumab**, a monoclonal antibody with antiangiogenic activity by blocking vascular endothelial growth factor (VEGF), is approved by the FDA for recurrent glioblastoma. Bevacizumab, however, does not improve survival in recurrent or newly diagnosed glioblastomas. Despite having no long-term benefit for glioma patients, bevacizumab is still used because it has potent antivasogenic edema control and can help symptom control. The approved regimen for glioblastomas is **10 mg/kg intravenously (IV) every 2 weeks**.

Other chemotherapy options for recurrent gliomas include nitrosoureas (lomustine and carmustine) and carboplatin. TTFields are also approved for recurrent glioblastomas. Enrollment in a clinical trial including immunotherapies, oncolytic viruses, and new treatment modalities should be encouraged because standard options have insufficient efficacy.

Prognosis

Tumor grade is a significant prognostic factor, because the median survival of patients with glioblastoma (grade IV glioma) is only 15 to 18 months, whereas the survival rate of patients with anaplastic gliomas varies between 2 and 5 years. The survival of patients with low-grade gliomas ranges from 3 to 10 years. Oligodendroglial tumors have a better prognosis than their astrocytic counterparts of the same grade. Nevertheless, patients with identical tumor histology and grade can have markedly different clinical courses and survival, likely reflecting the significant molecular heterogeneity of these tumors. Clinical factors associated with better outcomes, other than histology and tumor grade, include younger age at diagnosis, better performance status, and more extensive resection.

PRIMARY CENTRAL NERVOUS SYSTEM LYMPHOMA

PCNSL is an extranodal non-Hodgkin lymphoma involving the brain, eyes, meninges, or spinal cord in the absence of systemic lymphoma. Histologically, the vast majority of cases are diffuse large B-cell lymphomas.

Epidemiology

PCNSL is relatively uncommon, with approximately 1300 new cases diagnosed in the United States each year. Immunosuppression caused by HIV or iatrogenic causes (i.e., medications to prevent solid organ transplant rejection) markedly increases the risk of PCNSL. The incidence of PCNSL in HIV patients has declined significantly since the introduction of highly active antiretroviral therapy. PCNSL associated with immunosuppression is an Epstein-Barr virus (EBV)–mediated malignancy. EBV has tropism for B lymphocytes; immortalizes B lymphocytes; and, under immunosuppressive conditions, its infection may result in transformation to B-cell lymphoma.

Diagnosis

In immunocompetent patients with PCNSL, the brain MRI usually shows a diffusely enhancing tumor in the deep white matter or basal ganglia with surrounding vasogenic edema. The most typical characteristics of PCNSL on MRI scans are diffuse enhancement on T1 post gadolinium with absence of necrosis, hypointense tumor on T2-weighted imaging, and tumor restriction on diffusion-weighted imaging (Fig. 23.4). In immunosuppressed patients, tumors may

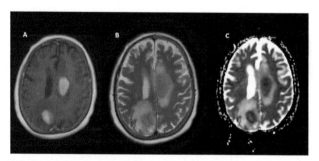

FIG. 23.4 Primary central nervous system lymphoma. (A) Postgadolinium T1-weighted image showing diffusely enhancing masses without necrosis. (B) T2-weighted image showing a hypointense mass with surrounding vasogenic edema. (C) Apparent diffusion coefficient image showing hypointensity of the lesions, which is a sign of water diffusion restriction.

have central necrosis. The diagnostic procedure of choice is a stereotactic brain biopsy. In rare circumstances, diagnosis can be made through vitreal biopsy or CSF cytology, but these tests have low diagnostic yield and should only be considered if there is no brain parenchymal lesion amenable to biopsy. In immunosuppressed patients, EBV polymerase chain reaction (PCR) in the CSF in conjunction with increased uptake on positron emission tomography (PET) or singe-photon emission computed tomography (SPECT) may suggest lymphoma, but diagnostic confirmation with a brain biopsy is preferable.

An ophthalmologic exam with slit-lamp to exclude ocular lymphoma should be performed in all patients. Patients with spinal symptoms should undergo a total spine MRI scan with gadolinium. Patients with presumed PCNSL must undergo HIV serology and a body computed tomography (CT) or PET to exclude systemic involvement. Testicular ultrasound in older men and bone marrow biopsy may be useful in selected cases.

Treatment

PCNSL should be treated with systemic high-dose **methotrexate-based chemotherapy**. The best dose of methotrexate and combination chemotherapy regimen is still not established. Multidrug regimens improve outcomes compared with high-dose methotrexate alone, and some of the commonly used drugs are rituximab, temozolomide, cytarabine, procarbazine, vincristine, and thiotepa. Radiation has short-lasting efficacy and can cause radiation neurotoxicity, which is characterized by progressive dementia, gait apraxia, incontinence, and death. Because of these reasons, radiation is becoming less frequently used in PCNSL.

Prognosis

The most important prognostic factors in PCNSL are age and performance status. Patients <50 years had a median survival of about 8 years, whereas patients ≥50 years old and good performance status had a median survival of 3 years, and those ≥50 years old and poor performance status survived only 1 year.

MENINGIOMAS

Meningiomas are the most common benign primary intracranial tumors; they are extraaxial tumors arising from meningothelial cells. Meningiomas are classified into grade I (benign, >90% of cases), grade II (atypical, approximately 5% of cases), and grade III (anaplastic or malignant, about 3% of cases) according to morphologic characteristics and number of mitoses. Although most meningiomas are benign lesions, these tumors can cause significant morbidity and occasional mortality secondary to their specific anatomic location within the CNS.

Epidemiology

The annual incidence of meningiomas is about 28,000 new cases per year in the United States, corresponding to approximately one-third of all primary CNS tumors. Meningiomas are twice as common in women than they are in men; it is uncommon in children, and its incidence rises steadily with advancing age.

Etiology

There is no clear etiology for most meningiomas. Ionizing radiation and genetic syndromes such as neurofibromatosis 1 and 2 are definite risk factors but correspond to only a small percentage of meningioma cases.

Diagnosis

Meningiomas are extraaxial masses that typically enhance diffusely after contrast and often have a dural tail constituting the thickening and enhancement of the dural perimeter of the mass. Also, on T2-weighted images, a CSF cleft separating the tumor from the brain parenchyma can be visualized (Fig. 23.5). Necrosis, vasogenic edema, and brain invasion can suggest a more aggressive

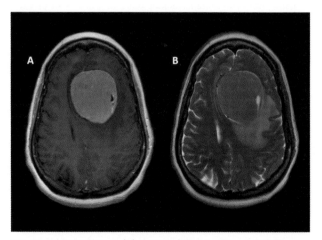

FIG. 23.5 Meningioma. (A) Post-gadolinium T1-weighted image showing an extraaxial diffusely enhancing mass. (B) T2-weighted image showing an extraaxial mass with surrounding vasogenic edema. Note the thin rim of cerebrospinal fluid (CSF) around the mass, confirming that the lesion is extraaxial (CSF cleft).

meningioma. Atypical meningiomas (grade II) are characterized by the presence of 4 or more mitoses per 10 high-power fields, whereas malignant meningiomas have more than 20 mitoses per 10 high-power fields.

Treatment

The best therapeutic approach for meningiomas requires individualization according to the patient's age, the presence of symptoms, comorbidities, tumor location, and grade.

Active Surveillance

Many meningiomas are incidentally found on neuroimaging studies for other reasons or symptoms unrelated to the tumor. Meningiomas can remain unchanged or grow so slowly that in some cases, especially in the elderly, they may never become symptomatic. An accepted approach to the management of small, asymptomatic meningiomas is to follow with MRI scans every 3 to 6 months; if the patient remains asymptomatic and there is no tumor growth, then conservative management with surveillance neuroimaging is recommended. This strategy is especially appropriate for elderly patients and those with high surgical morbidity risk.

Surgery

Patients with symptomatic meningiomas or those with progressively enlarging tumors should be considered for surgical resection. Complete surgical resection of the meningioma and its dural attachments is the best treatment option if it can be safely accomplished. For grade I meningiomas, complete resection alone is curative. In contrast, grade II and III meningiomas have higher recurrence rates of 20% to 40%. Meningiomas in the cerebral convexities, anterior falx, and tentorium and some posterior fossa tumors may be completely resected. In contrast, meningiomas adjacent to the cavernous sinus and some at the skull base are not amenable to complete resection.

Radiotherapy

Radiotherapy is an accepted treatment for partially resected or unresectable symptomatic meningiomas, recurrent meningiomas, and atypical or malignant meningiomas. Disease stabilization or prevention of recurrence are the goals of radiotherapy because tumor shrinkage is uncommon after radiation. Grade II meningiomas with a complete resection can be followed with surveillance MRI scans, whereas grade III meningiomas often are treated with postoperative radiation. Fractionated radiotherapy is the standard treatment for optic nerve sheath meningiomas, because surgery causes blindness and observation leads to progressive visual loss.

Stereotactic radiosurgery has gained acceptance as an effective treatment for selected patients with small meningiomas and those with small residual tumor postoperatively (<3 cm in diameter). Stereotactic radiosurgery is especially useful in patients who have high surgical risk because of medical comorbidities or tumor location but have small but symptomatic, progressive or recurrent meningiomas.

Medical Therapy

Chemotherapy or targeted therapies have no established role in the initial management of meningiomas. Patients with multiple recurrences who are no longer candidates for further surgery or radiation may try to enroll in a clinical trial, as medical treatment options are limited.

Prognosis

Patients with grade I meningiomas who undergo complete resection are often cured and have a normal life expectancy. In contrast, patients with grade II meningiomas have a 5- and 10-year survival rate of 78% and 33%, respectively, whereas patients with grade III meningiomas have 5- and 10-year survival rates of, respectively, 48% and 23%.

BRAIN METASTASES

Brain metastases are the most common CNS malignancy and usually appear late in the course of systemic cancer. The incidence of brain metastasis may be increasing because better systemic treatments for metastatic cancer prolong survival but leave the CNS vulnerable because of the poor drug penetration through the blood–brain barrier. Systemic cancer can also affect the nervous system through the remote effects of cancer, which are also known as paraneoplastic syndromes (Table 23.1).

Epidemiology

The incidence of brain metastasis varies significantly according to the primary cancer. Primary malignancies most commonly associated with brain metastases are lung cancer, breast cancer, melanoma, colon cancer, and renal cell carcinoma. The incidence of brain metastasis is also dependent on the histologic subtype. For example, small-cell lung cancer is more likely to metastasize to the brain than non–small-cell lung cancer, and HER-2–expressing

TABLE 23.1   Paraneoplastic Syndromes

Clinical Syndrome	Associated Tumor(s)	Autoantibodies
Multifocal encephalomyelitis/ Sensory neuronopathy	Small cell lung carcinoma	Anti-Hu (ANNA-1), anti-CV2 (CRMP-5), anti-amphiphysin, ANNA-3
	Various carcinomas	Anti-Ma, anti-Hu, anti-CV2
Cerebellar degeneration	Breast, ovarian, others	Anti-Yo, anti-Ma, anti-Ri (ANNA-2)
	Lung, others	Anti-Hu, anti-CV2, PCA-2, ANNA-3, anti-Ri, anti-VGCC, anti-Zic4
	Hodgkin's lymphoma	Anti-Tr, anti-mGluR1
Limbic encephalitis	Small cell lung carcinoma	Anti-Hu, anti-CV2, PCA-2, ANNA-3, anti-amphiphysin, anti-VGKC, anti-Zic4
	Testicular, breast	Anti-Ma2
	Thymoma	Anti-VGKC, anti-CV2
Opsoclonus-myoclonus	Breast, ovarian	Anti-Ri, anti-Yo
	Small cell lung carcinoma	Anti-Hu, anti-amphiphysin
	Neuroblastoma	Anti-Hu
	Testicular, others	Anti-Ma2
Extrapyramidal syndrome	Small cell lung carcinoma	Anti-CV2, anti-Hu
Brain stem encephalitis	Lung carcinoma	Anti-Hu, anti-Ri, anti-Ma
	Breast	Anti-Ri
	Testicular, others	Anti-Ma2
Stiff person syndrome	Breast, small cell lung	Anti-amphiphysin
	Breast	Anti-GAD
Optic neuritis	Small cell lung	Anti-CV2
Retinal degeneration	Small cell lung, others	Anti-recoverin
	Melanoma	Anti-bipolar cell
Neuromyotonia	Thymoma	Anti-VGKC
Sensorimotor polyneuropathy	Small cell lung carcinoma, others	Anti-Hu, anti-CV2, ANNA-3
Autonomic insufficiency	Small cell lung carcinoma	Anti-Hu
Lambert-Eaton myasthenic syndrome	Small cell lung carcinoma	Anti-VGCC

Only the most frequent associations are listed. For each of the clinical syndromes a number of other tumor types may be associated. A varying proportion of patients with each of the syndromes is "antibody negative," or has one or more autoantibody specificities that do not fit the well-characterized patterns listed.

GAD, glutamic acid decarboxylase; mGlu, glutamate receptor; VGCC, voltage-gated calcium channel; VGKC, voltage-gated potassium channel. (Reproduced with permission from Dropcho EJ: Curr Op Neurol 2005;18:331–336).

breast cancer also has a higher incidence of brain metastasis compared with HER-2–negative breast cancer.

Diagnosis

Brain metastases usually appear as ring-enhancing lesions in the gray–white matter junction with prominent surrounding vasogenic edema (Fig. 23.6). Intratumoral hemorrhage can be present, especially in brain metastasis caused by melanoma, renal cell carcinoma, and choriocarcinoma. Patients with known active and widely metastatic systemic cancer and typical lesions on brain MRI are usually diagnosed through imaging alone.

Treatment

The treatment of brain metastases depends on the number of lesions ($\leq$4 versus multiple lesions), CNS location, patient's performance status, extent of systemic cancer, and presumed radiosensitivity of underlying histology. **Whole-brain radiotherapy (WBRT)** was the main treatment modality for decades, but a subset of patients with $\leq$4 brain metastases, good performance status, and controlled systemic cancer can benefit from more aggressive treatment with surgical resection or stereotactic radiosurgery.

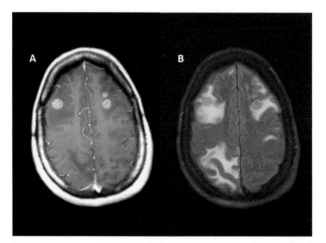

FIG. 23.6 Brain metastases. (A) Post-gadolinium T1-weighted image showing multiple enhancing masses in the gray–white matter junction. (B) Fluid attenuation inversion recovery (FLAIR) image showing prominent vasogenic edema, which is out of proportion to the size of the enhancing lesions.

WBRT is still considered the standard of care for patients with multiple (>4) brain metastases. Patients with disseminated systemic cancer without reasonable systemic treatment options or poor performance status should undergo WBRT or be offered palliative care only. WBRT can be associated with cognitive decline, which is a significant long-term side effect that impairs function and quality of life.

Patients with limited systemic cancer or those with effective systemic treatment options, good performance status, and ≤4 brain metastases should be considered for more aggressive focal therapy treatment with either surgical resection or stereotactic radiosurgery, or a combination of both. Stereotactic radiosurgery delivers a high-dose radiation fraction to a very precise target, but it should be limited to tumors ≤3 cm in diameter secondary to an increased chance of symptomatic cerebral edema and radiation necrosis.

Histology-specific or molecular-specific medical treatment is the best recommendation after surgery or radiation if the patient has a good performance status and is a candidate for systemic antitumor treatment. In general, the best medical option (chemotherapy, targeted therapy, and immunotherapy, among others) should be chosen independently of concerns about drug blood–brain barrier penetration. Brain metastases have significant breakdown of the blood–brain barrier, and even antibodies with large molecular weight can have efficacy in the appropriate setting (for example, immune checkpoint blockers in melanoma brain metastases).

Prognosis

The prognostic factors for patients with brain metastases associated with shorter survival are poor performance status, higher number of brain metastases, uncontrolled systemic cancer, absence of effective systemic antitumor therapies, and older age.

LEPTOMENINGEAL METASTASES

Leptomeningeal metastases occur in up to 5% of patients with cancer, usually at advanced and end stages of cancer. The most common malignancies that metastasize to the leptomeninges are breast cancer, lung cancer, melanoma, and lymphoma.

Diagnosis

Lumbar puncture with CSF cytology is considered the gold standard for diagnosis but has a sensitivity of only 54% after a single spinal tap and 85% after three spinal tap procedures. Gadolinium-enhanced MRI of the entire neuroaxis (brain and cervical, thoracic, and lumbosacral spine) can be diagnostic of leptomeningeal metastases without the need for a lumbar puncture in the appropriate clinical context. MRI can show tumor nodules on spinal and cranial nerves or enhancement of the leptomeninges.

Treatment

Because of its extremely poor prognosis, patients with poor performance status are usually offered supportive care only. Radiotherapy to the more symptomatic areas such as **WBRT** for increased intracranial pressure or lumbosacral radiotherapy for patients with cauda equina syndrome can provide palliation. A subset of patients with good performance status, no CSF flow obstruction, and normal intracranial pressure can benefit from **intrathecal or intraventricular chemotherapy, usually with methotrexate or cytarabine;** the benefit of intra-CSF chemotherapy is better established for hematologic malignancies and has an unclear role in solid tumors.

Prognosis

Patients with leptomeningeal metastases and poor performance status have a survival of only 4 to 6 weeks. A recent series of patients treated more aggressively achieved a median survival of just 2 months. The prognosis seems to be slightly better in patients with hematologic malignancies (lymphoma, leukemia) and possibly breast cancer.

METASTATIC EPIDURAL SPINAL CORD COMPRESSION

Metastatic epidural spinal cord compression occurs when cancer spreads to the spine and epidural space and then compresses the spinal cord or cauda equina. Up to 5% of patients with cancer develop epidural spinal cord compression; tumors most associated with this complication are prostate, lung, and breast cancers followed by non-Hodgkin lymphoma, renal cell carcinoma, and multiple myeloma.

Diagnosis

The most common and earliest symptom of epidural spinal cord compression is back or neck pain. Patients with known cancer and back or neck pain should undergo an MRI scan of the entire spine (cervical, thoracic, and lumbosacral) to rule out metastatic epidural spinal cord compression. Weakness, sensory changes, and bowel or bladder incontinence are common and often irreversible, so early diagnosis is critical to preserving neurologic function.

Treatment

High-dose corticosteroids should be promptly started in patients with metastatic epidural spinal cord compression. A randomized trial of high-dose **dexamethasone (IV bolus of 96 mg followed by 96 mg orally for 3 days and taper over 10 days) and radiotherapy** compared with radiotherapy without dexamethasone in patients with solid tumors showed improvement in ambulatory status from 33% to 59%.

External beam radiotherapy has been considered the mainstay treatment modality for metastatic spinal cord compression for several decades. Radiation provides pain relief, maintains stable neurologic function, or improves neurologic function if the onset of neurologic deficit is recent (<48 hours). The standard radiotherapy field includes two vertebral levels above and below the site of spinal metastasis, and the radiation is usually delivered in 10 fractions of 3 Gy over 2 weeks. Abbreviated radiation regimens of single or two fractions of 8 Gy may be similarly effective and more appropriate for patients with short life expectancies.

Surgery with direct circumferential decompression of the spinal cord may benefit a very select group of patients with metastatic epidural spinal cord compression. Patients with radiosensitive tumors such as lymphoma, leukemia, multiple myeloma, and germ-cell tumors usually do not benefit from surgery because radiotherapy is highly effective in these cases. Selected patients with symptomatic metastatic epidural spinal cord compression caused by radioresistant cancers restricted to a single spine level and good performance status may benefit from surgery. Also, patients with unstable spine or large bone fragments in the spinal canal caused by metastatic spinal disease need to be considered for decompressive surgery and spine fixation.

Prognosis

Prognostic factors include performance status, tumor type, the status of systemic cancer, and ambulatory status at presentation. The median survival is only approximately 4 months, even for patients treated with surgery and radiotherapy.

PITUITARY ADENOMA

Epidemiology

Pituitary adenomas account for approximately 15% of all brain tumors and occur most frequently in young adults (twenties and thirties). They arise from the adenohypophysis within the sella turcica, where they frequently remain. When large they can extend into the suprasellar region through an incompetent diaphragma sella.

Pathology

These histologically benign tumors tend to be slow growing and compress rather than invade surrounding neural tissue. Anatomically, pituitary adenomas can be divided into microadenomas (<10 mm in diameter), macroadenomas (>10 mm in diameter but surrounded by dura), and invasive adenomas (infiltrating dura, bone, or brain). Histologically, cells may appear chromophobic (most common), acidophilic, or basophilic (least common). However, the light microscopic appearance correlates poorly with secretory activity. The majority of pituitary adenomas are nonsecretory or prolactinomas.

Presentation

Pituitary adenomas may present via one of three mechanisms:

Pituitary hormone hypersecretion: Functional or secretory pituitary adenomas may present as (1) Cushing's disease, from ACTH secretion, (2) amenorrhea/galactorrhea, from prolactin secretion, or (3) acromegalic gigantism, from growth hormone secretion. Production of sex hormones (LH, FSH) or TSH by a pituitary adenoma is extremely uncommon. Secreting tumors are most frequently diagnosed when quite small (<1 cm), as severe endocrinologic disturbances bring them to medical attention early.

Mass effect: Nonsecreting tumors rarely cause symptoms until they have attained a large size. They can then cause panhypopituitarism by compressing the normal pituitary, visual disturbances (bitemporal hemianopia) by compressing the optic apparatus, and headache.

Pituitary apoplexy: This syndrome results from acute infarction or hemorrhage into a large, highly vascular tumor and can be life-threatening. Patients present suddenly with headache, visual loss, ophthalmoparesis, and mental status changes. Emergency decompression may be required. This mode of presentation is particularly common during pregnancy.

Diagnosis

MRI is more sensitive than CT for detecting microadenomas and is the imaging study of choice. Gadolinium normally causes enhancement of the pituitary gland, and tumor enhancement can be variable. Nonetheless, secretory adenomas are sometimes too small to be seen, even on MRI. In these cases the diagnosis is made on careful endocrinologic evaluation, which should include the following: T3, T4, TSH, GH, prolactin, LH, FSH, fasting glucose, serum cortisol, and estradiol (women) or testosterone (men) levels. Formal ophthalmologic testing should be performed in all cases of macroadenoma.

Treatment

With the exception of prolactinomas, surgery is generally indicated if signs of mass effect on the optic chiasm or cranial nerves are present. *Trans-sphenoidal surgery* has the lowest morbidity and mortality rates and results in visual improvement in approximately 75% of cases. Complication rates including cranial nerve and chiasmal injury may be further reduced with the use of intraoperative high-field MRI. Adrenal insufficiency or diabetes insipidus may occur postoperatively but is usually temporary. It is often impossible to completely remove a tumor with suprasellar extension, and in these cases the tumor usually recurs. Focused *radiation* (40 to 60 Gy over 4 to 6 weeks) reduces the postoperative recurrence rate and is indicated if the tumor could not be completely removed.

Medical therapy with a dopamine agonist is the treatment of choice for prolactinomas. **Bromocriptine 2.5 to 5 mg three times a day,** a synthetic dopamine agonist that inhibits pituitary secretion of prolactin, is the first line of treatment for prolactinomas regardless of size. The ultralong-acting D2-receptor agonist **cabergoline, given as 1.5 mg once a week,** appears to be as effective as bromocriptine and is better tolerated, but is not currently FDA-approved for this indication. In approximately 80% of cases, prolactinomas shrink dramatically with dopamine agonist therapy, with resolution of visual field and endocrine disturbances. If significant deficits persist, surgery may then be performed with the added benefit of bromocriptine pretreatment.

Prognosis

The overall recurrence rate following surgical resection of pituitary adenoma is approximately 12%, with most tumors recurring after 4 years. In patients treated surgically for Cushing's disease, a positive dexamethasone suppression test during the first week after surgery (AM serum cortisol <3 µg/dl following 1 mg of dexamethasone PO given the night before) predicts a >90% chance of remaining disease-free after 5 years.

ACOUSTIC NEUROMA

This tumor arises from the Schwann cells of the vestibular division of the eighth cranial nerve; hence, a more appropriate name is "vestibular schwannoma." This benign tumor arises within the internal acoustic canal and follows the path of least resistance, growing into the cerebellopontine angle.

Epidemiology

These tumors account for 8% of all brain tumors and occur mainly in middle-aged adults. Approximately 5% to 10% of patients have neurofibromatosis type 2 and may harbor bilateral acoustic neuromas, cranial or spinal meningiomas, schwannomas, and gliomas.

Presentation

The most common presenting symptom is unilateral tinnitus or hearing loss. As the tumor grows it compresses the adjacent cranial nerves, including the trigeminal (facial numbness, reduced corneal reflex), facial, and vestibular (vertigo) nerves. Ataxia from compression of the pons and cerebellum is a late sign.

Diagnosis

Gadolinium-enhanced MRI can reveal even small intracanalicular tumors. Both *audiography* and *brain stem auditory-evoked potentials* are important for quantifying the extent of damage to the cochlear nerve.

Treatment

Surgical resection is curative in most cases, particularly when the tumor is small (<2 cm in diameter). The main difficulty of surgery is preservation of the cochlear and facial nerves, something that becomes progressively difficult with increasing tumor size. Conventionally administered radiation is not effective in the treatment of these tumors, but *stereotactic radiosurgery* (i.e., gamma knife) shows promise in treating patients with small tumors, in which medical comorbidity precludes surgery.

Cerebrovascular Disease

Cerebrovascular disease includes a wide spectrum of disorders, all sharing an acquired or inherited pathology of the cerebral vasculature. Stroke syndromes range in scope from a minor hemisensory loss in a single limb to hemiplegia, cognitive changes, and coma. The onset of deficits usually occurs in seconds to minutes. The **physical examination** can give an impression of the size and a fair estimate of the location of the infarct and can thus guide the urgency of subsequent management steps. **Brain imaging** is necessary in almost all evaluations of stroke. Magnetic resonance imaging (MRI) should identify all but the smallest lesions and is superior to computed tomography (CT) for brain stem and small, deep infarcts. CT is the equal of MRI in detecting acute hemorrhage and is superior for assessing bony abnormalities. Whereas CT may miss an infarct within the first several hours of onset, MR diffusion-weighted imaging (DWI) can show ischemia within minutes of onset. The brain can tolerate only a few hours of ischemia before becoming irreversibly infarcted. The window of opportunity for acute intervention therefore is narrow. This chapter focuses on the presentation of acute stroke, with attention to the pathophysiologic mechanisms that drive the management decisions discussed in Chapter 6.

Classification

Acute stroke comprises three broad categories: **ischemic stroke, intracerebral hemorrhage (ICH),** and **subarachnoid hemorrhage (SAH).** The clinical presentations may be similar, yet the pathophysiology and consequent management algorithms are distinct.

SUBARACHNOID HEMORRHAGE

Clinical Presentation

Sudden, severe ("thunderclap") headache is the classic presentation of SAH from a ruptured cerebral aneurysm. When asked, patients usually classify the headache as the worst they have ever had or rate it a 10 on a scale of 1 to 10. Stiff neck and photophobia are often present, requiring a consideration of acute bacterial meningitis in the differential diagnosis. Preceding minor headache may occur from a sentinel bleed as a preamble to a major hemorrhage. Trauma is a more common cause of hemorrhage in the subarachnoid space, but the clinical presentation is then usually obvious. The most common neurologic finding in SAH is altered mental status. If focal signs or symptoms appear, it is often because of the presence of a local, intracerebral clot or because of direct compression of the aneurysm on a cranial nerve (causing, for example, a CN 3 palsy).

Missing the diagnosis of SAH can be disastrous. Untreated SAH may be fatal in up to 50% of patients. A large percentage of the deaths may be an immediate consequence of the hemorrhage, but secondary vasospasm, rerupture of the aneurysm, and obstructive hydrocephalus can add significantly to the morbidity and mortality. The rate of rerupture is 4% within the first 24 hours and 1% to 2% per day for the first 2 weeks. Early diagnosis and surgical clipping or endovascular embolization of the aneurysm are therefore essential.

Diagnosis

1. **A CT or MRI should be obtained as soon as possible.**

    Both CT and MRI are good at detecting acute hemorrhage. CT hyperdensity in the sulci, major fissures, or around the brain stem is diagnostic. Particular attention should be paid to the basal cisterns. Subarachnoid blood pooling in the quadrigeminal plate cistern, for example, may appear only as a subtle hyperdensity in this space and may even appear isodense with brain if the blood is 5 to 7 days old. Fig. 24.1 shows an example of SAH on CT. Other causes of SAH that may be detectable on CT or MRI include vascular malformation, venous thrombosis, and tumor.

2. **A negative CT or MRI scan does not rule out the diagnosis of SAH.**

    If there is clinical suspicion, and if CT or MRI is negative, a lumbar puncture should be performed. Cerebrospinal fluid (CSF) will show greater than 1000 red blood cells (RBCs) per cubic millimeter that do not clear in later tubes. Pathognomonic for SAH is *xanthochromia*, which is a straw-colored appearance of the CSF supernatant after centrifugation. Lumbar puncture can also rule out a diagnosis of bacterial meningitis.

3. **Patients should be classified according to the SAH grading scale of Hunt and Hess** (Table 24.1).

    Grading SAH patients not only will help monitor the clinical course but also will allow more accurate determination of

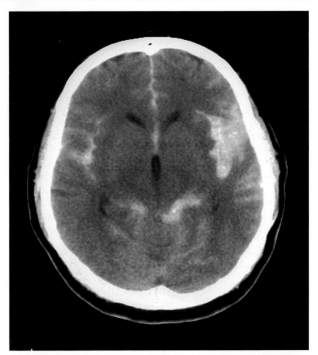

FIG. 24.1 Subarachnoid hemorrhage on computed tomography.

TABLE 24.1	Hunt and Hess Grading Scale for Aneurysmal Subarachnoid Hemorrhage		
		Hospital Mortality (%)[a]	
Grade	Clinical Findings	1968	2002
I	Asymptomatic or mild headache	11	7
II	Moderate to severe headache, or oculomotor palsy	26	2
III	Confused, drowsy, or mild focal signs	37	10
IV	Stupor (localizes to pain)	71	35
V	Coma (posturing or no motor response to pain)	100	65
Total		35	20

[a]Data from 275 patients reported by Hunt and Hess in 1968, and 404 patients treated at Columbia University Medical Center between 2000 and 2002.

Reproduced with permission from Mayer SA, Bernardini GL, Solomon RA, Brust JCM. Subarachnoid hemorrhage. In Rowland, LP, ed. *Merritt's Textbook of Neurology*. 11th ed. Baltimore, MD: Lippincott Williams & Wilkins, 2005:328–338.

prognosis and will guide management decisions. SAH of Hunt and Hess grades 1 and 2 has a good prognosis. Patients with grades 3 and 4 have a worse prognosis, and grade 5 patients are moribund. Aggressive, early intervention can yield good results even in poor-grade patients.

4. **Once a diagnosis of SAH is made, a four-vessel cerebral angiogram should be performed as soon as possible.**

   MR or CT angiography (MRA or CTA) is often used if emergency surgery is planned to evacuate a massive hematoma, but these tests have lower sensitivity than catheter angiography, particularly for small aneurysms. If an MR or CT angiogram is positive, this will help guide surgical treatment, but if catheter-based coiling is planned, or if the CTA or MRA is negative, a conventional angiogram will still be necessary. A second, unruptured aneurysm may also be present in up to 15% of cases. The most common sites for aneurysm formation are at vascular branching points around the circle of Willis (Fig. 24.2) (see Box 24.1 for management of unruptured aneurysms). Nonaneurysmal causes for SAH that may be detectable on angiogram include arteriovenous malformation (AVM), angiopathies such as vasculitis and fibromuscular dysplasia, vertebral artery dissection, and venous thrombosis.

5. **If both MRI and angiogram are negative, then the SAH may have arisen from a venous rupture around the midbrain (perimesencephalic SAH).**

   A coagulation profile and toxicology screen for cocaine should also be obtained if the diagnosis is still unclear. Cervical MRI may reveal a dural AVM, but this is rare. All patients with a negative initial angiogram require follow-up angiography within 2 weeks unless the patient is grade 1 or 2 and the initial CT shows a classic perimesencephalic pattern.

Management

For patients with aneurysm identified by angiography, management is two-pronged. First, early intervention by clipping or coiling the aneurysm (see the following) will improve short- and long-term morbidity and mortality. Because the rerupture rate is as high as 20% in the first 2 weeks, treating a ruptured aneurysm acutely will remove a substantial secondary risk. Many centers have adopted a policy of early antifibrinolytic therapy (Table 24.2) with ε-**aminocaproic acid** (United States) or **tranexamic acid** (Europe) to prevent early rebleeding prior to aneurysm repair, or until 72 hours after onset. The second major aspect of management is the prevention of delayed ischemic deficits from vasospasm, which affects 20% to 30% of patients. Fluid and blood pressure management are crucial both preoperatively and postoperatively to

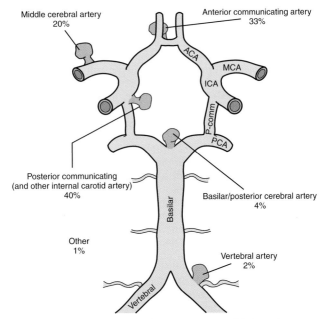

FIG. 24.2 Most common sites for aneurysms. *ACA*, Anterior communicating artery; *ICA*, internal carotid artery; *MCA*, middle cerebral artery; *PCA*, posterior cerebral artery; *P-comm*, posterior communicating artery.

BOX 24.1	Unruptured Intracranial Aneurysms

Intracranial aneurysms are uncommon in children but occur with a frequency of 2% in adults, suggesting that approximately 2 to 3 million Americans have an aneurysm. IUAs may be discovered incidentally or detected in patients who present with another symptomatic aneurysm (e.g., SAH cranial nerve compression, headache, seizure). Because surgical or endovascular aneurysm repair carries a 2% to 5% risk of stroke or death, the management of these aneurysms (which in most cases remain asymptomatic throughout life) is controversial. The annual risk of rupture of an IUA is approximately 0.7%, but this risk is higher in patients with large aneurysms (>10 mm), prior SAH, cigarette use, a family history of cerebral aneurysm, or a midline aneurysm (anterior communicating or basilar apex). Generally, treatment is strongly recommended for all patients with symptomatic IUAs or prior SAH and in young patients (<50) with large aneurysms. In light of their low risk of bleeding, incidental small IUAs (<10 mm) should be managed conservatively and followed with serial imaging, although treatment should be considered in younger patients with a larger (6- to 9-mm) midline aneurysm, a positive family history, or evidence of aneurysm growth. In addition, all patients should be counseled to avoid cigarette smoking.

IUA, Unruptured intracranial aneurysm; *SAH,* subarachnoid hemorrhage.

TABLE 24.2	Emergency Department and Intensive Care Unit Management Protocol for Acute Subarachnoid Hemorrhage
Blood pressure	• Control elevated BP during the preoperative phase (SBP < 60 mm Hg) with IV labetalol or nicardipine to prevent rebleeding
Antifibrinolytic therapy IV drip	• ε-aminocaproic acid (Amicar) 4 g IV on diagnosis, then 1 g/h until aneurysm repair, or a maximum of 72 h after onset
IV hydration	• Preoperative: normal (0.9%) saline at 80–100 mL/h • Postoperative: normal (0.9%) saline at 80–100 mL/h, and 250 mL 5% albumin every 2 h if the CVP is ≤5 mm Hg
Laboratory testing	• Periodically check complete blood count; transfuse for hematocrit ≤7 mg/dl in stable patients, or ≤10 mg/dl in patients with symptomatic vasospasm • Periodically check electrolytes to detect hyponatremia • Obtain serial ECGs and check admission cTI level to evaluate for cardiac injury; perform echocardiography in patients with abnormal ECG findings, or cTI elevation
Seizure prophylaxis	• Fosphenytoin IV load (15–20 mg/kg); discontinue on postoperative day 2 unless patient has seized or is unstable
Vasospasm prophylaxis	• Nimodipine 60 mg PO every 4 h for 21 days
Physiologic homeostasis Ventricular drainage Vasospasm diagnosis	• Cooling blankets to maintain temperature ≤ 7.5°C • Insulin drip to maintain glucose 120–180 mg/dL • Begin trials of clamping external ventricular drain and monitoring ICP on day 3 after placement • Transcranial Doppler sonography every 1 to 2 days until the eighth day after SAH • CT perfusion on days 4–8 after SAH if high risk
Therapy for symptomatic vasospasm	• Place patient in Trendelenburg (head down) position • Infuse 500 mL 5% albumin over 15 min • If the deficit persists, raise the SBP with norepinephrine until the deficit resolves, up to a maximum of 180–220 mm Hg • 250 mL 5% albumin solution every 2 h if the CVP is ≤8 mm Hg or if the inferior vena cava is collapsible on ultrasound • If refractory, place pulmonary artery catheter and add dobutamine to maintain cardiac index ≥ 4.0 L/min/m² • Emergency angiogram for possible cerebral angioplasty unless the patient responds well to the previous measures

BP, Blood pressure; *CT*, computed tomography; *cTI*, cardiac troponin; *CVP*, central venous pressure; *ECG*, electrocardiogram; *ICP*, intracranial pressure; *IV*, intravenous; *PADP*, pulmonary artery diastolic pressure; *PO*, by mouth; *SAH*, subarachnoid hemorrhage; *SBP*, systolic blood pressure.

Adapted with permission from Mayer SA, Bernardini GL, Solomon RA, Brust JCM. Subarachnoid hemorrhage. In Rowland LP, ed. *Merritt's Textbook of Neurology*. 11th ed. Baltimore, MD: Lippincott Williams & Wilkins, 2016:328–338.

maintain adequate cerebral blood flow in the presence of cerebral ischemia from vasospasm (see Table 24.2).

Surgery

Surgical clipping of the aneurysm is generally done as early as possible after the hemorrhage, but it cannot be done without substantial risk if cerebral vasospasm is present. Vasospasm is rare in the first 3 days, and it peaks around day 7. If, within the first 5 days after hemorrhage, an angiogram shows the aneurysm clearly and shows no vasospasm, surgery should be done within the following 24 hours. Transcranial Doppler ultrasonography (TCD) is an important means of monitoring vasospasm both preoperatively and postoperatively, checking for increases in flow velocity in the major vessels around the circle of Willis. Identification of impaired cerebral vasoreactivity with TCD by a blunted vasodilatory response to inhaled CO_2 may be an early marker of impending symptomatic vasospasm.

Endovascular Embolization

As an alternative to surgical clipping, packing the aneurysm with Guglielmi detachable coils (GDC) is an effective way to prevent rebleeding. In a large trial of predominantly good-grade patients with small anterior circulation aneurysms, coil embolization was found to be associated with better 1-year outcomes compared with clipping, presumably because it is associated with fewer complications. In this procedure, the tiny coils are delivered to the aneurysm by superselective angiography catheterization. Thrombosis of the aneurysm is induced by the presence of the coils.

Medical Management

Patients with SAH are best managed in an intensive care unit. Abnormalities of fluid and sodium homeostasis after SAH favor free-water retention and sodium loss. The emphasis on fluid management is therefore on maintaining normal or increased intravascular volume using isotonic fluids and on avoiding all potential sources of free water. A central venous or pulmonary artery catheter may be helpful in assessing volume status, particularly when there is symptomatic vasospasm (see Table 24.2). **Nimodipine 60 mg by mouth (PO) 60 mg q4h** should be given for 21 days after SAH.

Treatment of Vasospasm

Angiographic vasospasm affects 70% of patients with SAH, and 20% to 30% will experience delayed focal or global neurologic

TABLE 24.3	Modified Fisher Computed Tomography Rating Scale for the Prediction of Symptomatic Vasospasm			
Grade	Criteria	Percentage of Patients (%)	Delayed Cerebral Ischemia (%)	Frequency of Infarction (%)
0	No SAH or IVH	5	0	0
1	Minimal/thin SAH, no biventricular IVH	30	12	6
2	Minimal/thin SAH, *with* biventricular IVH	5	21	14
3	Thick SAH, no biventricular IVH	43	19	12
4	Thick SAH, *with* biventricular IVH	17	40	28
	All patients	100	20	12

Thick subarachnoid hemorrhage refers to subarachnoid clot > 5 mm in width completely fills at least one cistern or fissure. Delayed cerebral ischemia is defined as symptomatic deterioration, cerebral infarction, or both resulting from vasospasm.

IVH, Intraventricular hemorrhage; *SAH,* subarachnoid hemorrhage.

Data are based on a prospectively studied cohort of 276 patients at Columbia University Medical Center. From Claassen J, et al. Effect of cisternal and ventricular blood on risk of delayed cerebral ischemia after subarachnoid hemorrhage: the Fisher scale revisited. *Stroke.* 2001;32:2012–2020. With permission.

deficits related to cerebral ischemia resulting from this process. The risk of developing symptomatic vasospasm can be predicted by the modified Fisher CT rating Scale (Table 24.3), with the highest risk occurring in patients with both thick cisternal clot and significant intraventricular hemorrhage. In addition to hypertensive hypervolemic therapy (see Table 24.2), which results in some degree of clinical improvement in approximately 70% of patients, angioplasty of intracranial vessels that are narrowed by vasospasm has become an important treatment modality in centers with appropriate interventional neuroradiologic expertise. Angioplasty is increasingly being performed as a first-line intervention for acute symptomatic vasospasm, rather than as salvage therapy for medically refractory cases; the best outcomes occur when angioplasty is performed within 2 hours of the onset of a new significant neurologic deficit.

ISCHEMIC STROKE

Clinical Presentation and Diagnosis

Both ischemic stroke and ICH typically present with focal signs. The syndrome produced by infarction depends on the location of the lesion. Pain of any kind is uncommon with ischemic stroke, although headache may occur with larger stroke or hematoma. One of the most difficult aspects of managing acute stroke patients is that focal symptoms, particularly minor ones, are often attributed by the patient to some nonneurologic cause and ignored. Visual changes may be interpreted as a need for new glasses. Sensory loss or weakness in an extremity may be brushed off as the result of lifting a heavy package or bumping into the door the day before. Transient symptoms (i.e., transient ischemic attack [TIA]) may portend stroke but may be identified as important only retrospectively (Box 24.2). Delay in treatment beyond

| BOX 24.2 | Transient Ischemic Attacks |

TIAs are defined as transient symptoms of vascular etiology that do not result in infarction. Although the standard clinical definition includes symptoms lasting up to 24 hours, most TIAs last from minutes to a few hours. Deficits lasting longer than 1 to 2 hours may show a lesion on MRI, even if the symptoms resolve completely by 24 hours. **The clinical importance of TIA is highlighted by the high incidence of subsequent strokes.** Up to 50% of patients with TIA proceed to have an infarction within 5 years, if they are untreated, with up to 18% occurring in the first 90 days. *Age greater than 60 years, diabetes mellitus, symptoms lasting longer than 10 minutes,* and the *symptoms of weakness or speech impairment* all raise the likelihood of subsequent stroke. The most important etiology of TIA is high-grade carotid stenosis, producing hemodynamic failure or microemboli in the territory of the affected artery. TMB (amaurosis fugax) or a hemispheric syndrome such as unilateral weakness or sensory changes is a common presentation. Although TIAs also may arise from cardiac embolism or, rarely, from lacunar disease, the most important initial management step is to evaluate the internal carotid arteries, either with duplex Doppler ultrasonography or MRA. If stenosis greater than 70% is found, then the patient should be considered for early carotid endarterectomy or stenting. The rate of subsequent stroke is up to 1% per day in the first 2 weeks. If no large-vessel stenosis is identified, the algorithm for investigating etiology of ischemic stroke should be followed. If no carotid stenosis or cardioembolic source is identified, **ASA 81 mg or 325 mg per day** is the first line of treatment.

MRA, Magnetic resonance angiography; *MRI,* magnetic resonance imaging; *TIA,* transient ischemic attack; *TMB,* Transient monocular blindness.

the first several hours can result in a missed opportunity for acute intervention with a thrombolytic or mechanical thrombectomy. Despite an overlap in clinical syndromes among the various pathophysiologic etiologies, one should try to identify the stroke subtype. The management algorithm for secondary prevention depends on the stroke mechanism. Four major categories of stroke mechanism are discussed.

Cardioembolic Stroke

Fifteen percent to 30% of strokes are embolic from a cardiac cause such as atrial fibrillation or valvular disease. The classic clinical presentation of cardioembolic stroke is of sudden deficit, maximal at onset. Syndromes more likely to be embolic include hemianopia without hemiparesis, pure Wernicke aphasia, and top-of-the-basilar syndrome (ocular dysmotility, altered mental status, visual impairment). Hemiparesis and forced gaze deviation suggest a large hemispheric (eyes look away from the side of weakness) or critical brain stem (eyes look toward the side of weakness) lesion, particularly if these signs are accompanied by decreased level of consciousness. Behavioral abnormalities such as aphasia or hemineglect without a gaze preference or altered level of consciousness suggest smaller hemispheric lesions. CT and MRI scans that show a single cortical branch territory infarct are also consistent with an embolic cause because atheroma rarely extend into the surface vessels. Main stem branch occlusions also are often embolic as a clot traveling from one artery to another, but flow failure from local atherostenosis is also a possibility in such a setting. A potentially misleading scenario is one in which the initial CT scan shows a deep-lying lucency involving the internal capsule and basal ganglia approximately 2 to 3 cm in size, apparently sparing cortex, which can be misidentified as a large lacune. Often such instances are of embolic origin, involving several lenticulostriate branches of the middle cerebral artery after occlusion of the middle cerebral stem. Rapid collateralization from anterior or posterior cerebral branches or recanalization of the occlusion with distal migration of the embolus reperfuses the cortex, sparing it from infarction. A right-to-left intracardiac shunt, usually a patent foramen ovale, can be inferred when TCD ultrasonography shows microbubbles in the intracranial vessels after injection of 10 mL of agitated saline in the antecubital vein. Contrast transesophageal echocardiography can usually locate the defect in the intraseptal atrial wall. If atrial fibrillation is suspected but is not apparent on routine electrocardiogram (ECG), longer-term cardiac monitoring with a Mobile Cardiac Outpatient Telemetry (MCOT) device or a subcutaneous insertable loop recorder may pick up occult atrial fibrillation.

Large-Vessel Stenosis

In 15% of cases, severe large-vessel atherosclerosis is present and appears to be responsible for the stroke, particularly when there is severe extracranial internal carotid artery stenosis or occlusion and a "distal field" lesion is imaged on CT or MRI as an infarct high over the convexity, spreading caudally from the border zone between anterior and middle arterial territories. The most common clinical profile of this type of infarct is fractional weakness (the shoulder weaker than the hand, hip weaker than ankle). Male gender, hypertension, and diabetes mellitus appear significantly more frequently in this group than in patients with cardioembolic stroke. Intracranial atherosclerosis is more prevalent in non-Caucasian populations, whereas extracranial disease is more prevalent in Caucasians. Duplex Doppler ultrasonography readily delineates the severity of the internal carotid stenosis and shows high-velocity, turbulent flow. TCD ultrasonography often shows dampened pulsatility in the ipsilateral middle cerebral artery. Cerebral vasoreactivity as measured by a blunted TCD response to inhaled CO_2 is often impaired. Focal stenoses in the intracranial artery (ICA) or other major intracranial vessels also may be documented by TCD ultrasonography or MRA. Noninvasive imaging with MRA or CTA can now approach the resolution of the more invasive traditional cut-film angiography.

Artery-to-Artery Embolus

In another 15% of all stroke patients, significant large-vessel atherosclerosis is detected when, radiographically, the infarct appears embolic. In such a setting, embolic fragments may have arisen from atherosclerotic lesions in the ICA. Distinguishing interarterial embolism from a possible cardioembolic etiology may be difficult. The former usually produces a smaller cortical infarct, however, and the latter is more often associated with a decreased level of consciousness and an abnormal initial CT scan.

Lacunar Stroke (Small-Vessel Disease)

Small, deep lesions in the subcortical white matter, the thalamus, the basal ganglia, or the pons accompanied by an appropriate clinical syndrome suggest lacunar disease, accounting for 15% to 20% of all strokes. Arteriolar wall lipohyalinosis with fibrinoid necrosis or microatheroma are the most common pathologic findings, although microemboli may rarely produce small infarcts. Although more than 70 syndromes have been reported with small, deep infarcts, the classic lacunar syndromes are *clumsy hand dysarthria, pure motor hemiparesis, ataxic hemiparesis, sensorimotor syndrome,* and *pure hemisensory loss.* All are typically characterized by an absence of cortical signs or symptoms such as aphasia or hemineglect. CT scanning is positive in only 50% of acute lacunar stroke patients, with MRI almost always identifying the lesion in the hyperacute period with DW. Asymptomatic lacunes (silent strokes) occur in up to 20% of patients over age 65. Hypertension is the risk factor most associated with lacunar infarction.

Other Etiologies

Despite efforts to arrive at a diagnosis, the cause of infarction in up to 40% of cases remains undetermined after the standard workup is completed. This may result from an inability to perform appropriate laboratory studies because of the patient's advanced age or comorbidity or because of unwillingness on the part of the physician or patient. It may also result from inadequate timing of tests, such as an angiogram performed after an embolus has cleared or CT done before the infarction appears. In many cases, however, appropriate testing done at the proper time produces normal or ambiguous findings. Some of these cases may be explained by *hypercoagulable states* from protein C or protein S deficiency, abnormal fibrinogen levels, genetic mutations such as factor V Leiden or factor II prothrombin (G20210A), or by lupus anticoagulant or anticardiolipin antibodies. Other patients may have had emboli from *aortic arch atherosclerosis* that is >4 mm in thickness or ulcerated. Pain in the neck, side of face, teeth, jaw, or retroorbital area may indicate *vertebral or carotid artery dissection,* even without a history of neck trauma. Migraine, meningitis, arteritis, or inherited metabolic abnormality may explain rare cases. For the purposes of management, cases that cannot be categorized under one of the first four etiologies should be called "cryptogenic stroke." Additional diagnostic studies may be needed to secure a final diagnosis. Because of its grave prognosis, vasculitis of the central nervous system should not be missed (Box 24.3).

Management

1. All patients with suspected stroke should undergo a CT or MRI head scan.

2. All patients with stroke symptoms of less than 3 hours' duration should be considered for acute treatment with intravenous (IV) recombinant tissue plasminogen activator (rt-PA). If CT scan shows no hemorrhage, mass effect, delineated hypodensity, or edema, and if the patient meets inclusion and exclusion criteria guidelines, **IV rt-PA 0.9 mg/kg** should be given according to protocol (Box 24.4). An extended window of up to 4.5 hours is now acceptable to administer rt-PA.

BOX 24.3	Cerebral Vasculitis

Vasculitis is a rare cause of ischemic stroke. Infrequently appearing in the set-ting of a systemic collagen vascular disease such as polyarteritis nodosa, tem-poral arteritis, or Takayasu syndrome (aortic arch disease, pulseless disease), stroke may occasionally result from autoimmune disease restricted to the cen-tral nervous system. **Granulomatous angiitis of the brain** is a rare condition that produces multiple small infarctions or hemorrhages in the cortex and deep structures. The clinical presentation is usually one of fluctuating or stepwise progression of mental obtundation, with or without focal signs. CSF protein is elevated above 100 mg/dL, and a pleocytosis of up to 500 mononuclear cells per cubic millimeter is common. The typical arteriographic appearance is of multiple segmental areas of arterial narrowing followed by dilatations, often giving a "beaded" look. Clinical and radiographic data can be compelling in any given patient, but it is recommended that a brain and leptomeningeal biopsy specimen be obtained before embarking on the necessarily aggressive immu-nosuppressive treatment regimen. The diagnosis is secured if there are multi-nucleated giant cells infiltrating arterial walls. Because of the multifocal nature of the disease, however, biopsy results may be negative in up to 50% of cases. Progression of encephalopathy or new focal signs in combination with new areas of arterial narrowing on angiography may be sufficient to begin treat-ment if the biopsy yields negative results initially. The usual treatment regimen includes high-dose steroids and pulse doses of a steroid-sparing immunosup-pressive agent, such as cyclophosphamide, for more than a year. The prognosis is poor overall, but occasionally there is functional restoration approximating previous levels.

CSF, Cerebrospinal fluid.

3. If the patient's stroke symptoms are of less than 6 hours' dura-tion the National Institutes of Health (NIH) Stroke Scale is 8 or above; and if there is a large-vessel occlusion present on CT or MR angiography, catheter-based, intraarterial thrombectomy may be performed, provided that interven-tional radiologic expertise and experience are available. Newer CT and MRI algorithms can identify an area of hypoperfusion significantly larger than the area of infarction. A significant "diffusion-perfusion mismatch" may indicate that there is a larger area of ischemic but not yet infarcted territory of brain that is potentially salvageable if the large vessel that supplies the territory is recanalized. Even longer time windows may be allowable for revascularization procedures with imaging-guided algorithms. Hemorrhage after revascularization or after treatment with tPA alone remains the main risk of acute stroke treatment(see Fig. 24.3).

BOX 24.4	American Heart Association Guidelines for Use of Intravenous Recombinant Tissue Plasminogen

Inclusion Criteria
1. Symptoms are consistent with acute ischemic stroke
2. Timing of onset is clear; start rt-PA within 4.5 hours of symptom onset
3. CT is negative or shows only early signs of ischemic stroke (blurring of gray–white junction, minor hypodensity); if sulcal effacement, mass effect, or edema is present, rt-PA should not be given; CT should be read by an experienced neurologist, neurosurgeon, or neuroradiologist
4. Appropriate facilities must be available to handle bleeding complications should they occur (e.g., neurologic intensive care unit or stroke unit)
5. If treatment interval is 3-4.5 hours, age should be <80, NIHSS score ≤25, and there should be no concomitant history of diabetes and prior stroke.

Exclusion Criteria
1. Current use of oral anticoagulants, PT > 15 s or INR > 1.7
2. Use of IV heparin or IM low-molecular-weight heparin within 24 h or prolonged partial thromboplastin time
3. Platelet count < 100,000/mm^3
4. Large stroke or serious head injury within the past 3 months
5. Prior ICH
6. Major surgery within the past 14 days (relative contraindication)
7. Pretreatment SBP > 185 mm Hg or DBP > 110 mm Hg (must be treated before administration)
8. Blood glucose < 50 mg/dL or >400 mg/dL (relative contraindication)
9. Gastrointestinal or urinary bleeding within the preceding 21 days (warning only)
10. Recent myocardial infarction
11. Seizure at onset of stroke (relative contraindication)
12. Pregnancy (relative contraindication)

Administration of rt-PA
1. IV rt-PA (0.9 mg/kg, maximum 90 mg) with 10% of the dose given as a bolus followed by an infusion lasting 60 min
2. No anticoagulants or antiplatelet agents to be given within the first 24 h after administration of rt-PA
3. Blood pressure elevation to be treated by IV labetalol 10–150 mg (for SBP = 180–230 mm Hg or DBP = 105–120 mm Hg) or IV nitroprusside 0.5–10 µg/kg/min (for SBP > 230 mm Hg or DBP > 120 mm Hg)
4. Repeat brain imaging is required at 24 h to rule out hemorrhage after IV tPA; repeat earlier if there is any clinical deterioration

---

CT, Computed tomography; *DSB*, diastolic blood pressure; *ICH*, intracerebral hemorrhage; *IM*, intramuscularly; *INR*, international normalized ratio; *IV*, intravenous; *PT*, prothrombin time; *rt-PA*, recombinant tissue plasminogen; *SBP*, systolic blood pressure.

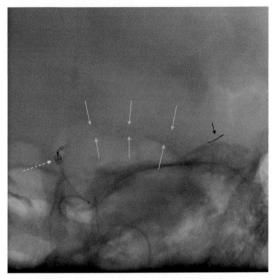

FIG. 24.3 Digital subtraction angiography image showing an endovascular stent-retriever expanded inside a left middle cerebral artery within a clot *(gray arrows)*. The microcatheter tip *(black arrow)* has been passed beyond the clot. The stent, clot, and microcatheter sheath *(dashed arrow)* will be pulled back through the artery to reopen it and restore flow.

4. If the clinical picture and CT or MRI appearances are consistent with a small-sized or moderate-sized ischemic stroke, and the suspected etiology is cardioembolic or large-vessel stenosis, IV **heparin may be administered** until the stroke subtype is confirmed, maintaining a partial thromboplastin time (PTT) of 1.5 to 2 times control. IV heparin has no proven efficacy in preventing early recurrent stroke or stroke progression but may be used as a bridge to long-term anticoagulation. Anticoagulation may be given if there is hemorrhagic infarction on brain imaging, *but only if the infarction is minor.* Resumption of anticoagulation in patients with atrial fibrillation generally requires 1 to 2 weeks for a hemorrhagic conversion within the infarct be to reabsorb.

5. ***Investigation of stroke etiology*** should focus first on cardioembolic sources and large-vessel atherothrombosis. Transthoracic echocardiography, carotid duplex Doppler ultrasonography, and TCD ultrasonography should be performed in nearly

all cases. MRA and transesophageal echocardiography may deliver a diagnosis when the previously mentioned studies are inconclusive.

6. Stroke patients with recent myocardial infarction, atrial fibrillation, valvular disease, or intracardiac thrombus should be given **oral anticoagulants such as warfarin, or a novel oral anticoagulant (e.g. Apixaban 5 mg twice daily [BI], rivaroxaban 20 mg once daily [QD], or edoxaban 60 mg once daily [QD])** for at least one year. The international normalized ratio (INR) of the prothrombin time (PT) should be targeted at 2.0 to 3.0 if warfarin is used. If there is atrial fibrillation, anticoagulation should be continued indefinitely, provided that reliable monitoring is available. Anticoagulation with **enoxaparin (Lovenox) 1 mg/kg subcutaneously (SC) BID** is an alternative to oral anticoagulation for those unable to swallow or in pregnant women to avoid teratogenicity of warfarin.

7. For patients found to have patent foramen ovale (PFO) without other potential etiology may benefit from catheter-based closure of the PFO by a qualified interventional cardiologist. Those with atrial fibrillation who have a contraindication to long-term anticoagulation may be considered for a catheter-delivered left atrial appendage occlusive device to reduce subsequent stroke risk. This treatment requires only short-term anticoagulation.

8. If the stroke is small, the heart is normal, and a duplex Doppler sonogram shows significant carotid stenosis (greater than 70%), a revascularization procedure should be considered. **IV heparin, ASA 325 mg PO QD, or clopidogrel 75 mg PO QD** should be continued until the exact degree of stenosis has been determined by MRA or CTA. Digital subtraction or cut-film angiography may be used in instances in which MRA or CTA is unavailable or noninvasive angiography results are equivocal. Prophylactic revascularization by *endarterectomy* (CEA) or *carotid artery stent angioplasty* (CAS) for patients with greater than 70% stenosis should be undertaken as soon as possible. CAS is indicated for cases of restenosis or radiation-induced stenosis in which surgery is riskier. Efficacy and procedural risk are otherwise similar for CEA and CAS. For stenting, interventionalists generally prefer patients to be on **clopidogrel 75 mg PO QD** for 3 days prior to the procedure, although a single loading dose of **clopidogrel 300 mg PO** may be used the day before the procedure. For patients with 50% to 69% stenosis, the benefit of surgery is lower compared with medical treatment but may still be considered. Doppler monitoring should be undertaken at intervals of 3 to 12 months to document those patients

whose stenosis increases to greater than 70%. Patients in whom asymptomatic carotid stenosis greater than 60% is identified should be considered for endarterectomy or stenting as well, provided the operation is done at a center at which the perioperative morbidity and mortality is less than 3%. The benefit from endarterectomy compared with medical therapy is a 6% versus an 11% chance of stroke in 5 years for the asymptomatic carotid stenosis group, and a 9% versus 26% chance of stroke in 2 years for the >70% symptomatic group.

9. If no cardioembolic source or operable carotid stenosis is identified, and if the patient is not considered at risk for hemorrhage, antiplatelet treatment with **aspirin 81 to 325 mg daily** should be given as chronic outpatient therapy. **Aspirin 25 mg/extended-release dipyridamole 200 mg twice a day** or **clopidogrel 75 mg PO once a day** also may be used, particularly if aspirin therapy has failed. Clopidogrel is often preferred when there is coronary artery disease or peripheral vascular disease. Some patients develop headache from ASA/extended-release dipyridamole.

INTRACEREBRAL HEMORRHAGE

Clinical Presentation

Primary ICH is defined as nontraumatic bleeding into the parenchyma of the brain. ICH accounts for approximately 15% of all strokes. Except for a higher frequency of headache and severe hypertension, the presentation of ICH may be identical to that for ischemic stroke occurring in the same location. Coma occurs with greater frequency, particularly when the hemorrhage is of larger volume or involves the brain stem. Patients with hematoma volumes less than 20 mL have an excellent prognosis, whereas those with volumes greater than 80 mL are usually fatal. Chronic hypertension is the most common cause of ICH and is presumed to result from rupture of the smallest penetrating arteries that have undergone degenerative changes such as lipohyalinosis, fibrinoid necrosis, and microaneurysm formation. Acute hypertension is present in 90% of the cases. Hypertension from sympathomimetics such as pseudoephedrine, amphetamines, or cocaine may also be seen. Hypertensive bleeds occur most commonly in the territory of small penetrating arteries, in the basal ganglia or thalamus (70%), in the brain stem (13%), or in the cerebellum (9%). In the 10% of cerebral hemorrhages that occur in the hemispheres, other causes must be suspected. The differential diagnosis of lobar ICH includes cerebral amyloid angiopathy (Box 24.5), primary or metastatic tumors

| BOX 24.5 | Cerebral Amyloid Angiopathy |

CAA results from the pathologic deposition of an amorphous eosinophilic amyloid material (that stains with Congo red) in small blood vessels of the cerebral neocortex and adjacent leptomeninges. CAA causes lobar hemorrhage in elderly adults with a mean age of 72. Recurrent hemorrhages are common. The amyloid protein precursor is a gene product from chromosome 21, stimulating interest about the role of amyloid in Down syndrome and Alzheimer's disease. The disease may occur in a familial trait or sporadically. More than 40% of patients with CAA have some degree of dementia. Hemorrhages are most common in the frontal and parietal lobes. MRI, particularly gradient echo sequences such as "susceptibility-weighted imaging," will often demonstrate microhemorrhages in a lobar distribution, along with superficial siderosis and small ischemic lesions. A diagnosis of "probable CAA" may be made in a patient older than 55 years with an appropriate clinical history and MRI findings of multiple hemorrhages of varying sizes and ages without other explanation. No definitive treatment is currently available.

CAA, Cerebral amyloid angiopathy; *MRI*, magnetic resonance imaging.

(melanoma, choriocarcinoma, bronchogenic carcinoma, or renal cell carcinoma), coagulopathies (disseminated intravascular coagulation, hemophilia, leukemia, thrombocytopenia, overdose of anticoagulant therapy), and vascular malformations.

Diagnosis

The cornerstone for diagnosis of ICH is neuroimaging. Both CT and MRI can detect fresh parenchymal blood in the hyperacute stage. Because the clinical presentation may be indistinguishable from ischemic stroke but the treatment strategies are quite different, any patient presenting with suspected ICH must undergo CT or MRI as soon as possible. In a patient under 60 years of age with a lobar hemorrhage of unclear etiology, an MRI with and without contrast material may disclose tumor or the abnormal vessels of a vascular malformation. For an AVM, cut-film angiography would then be necessary to make a definitive diagnosis and plan for treatment.

Distinguishing between ICH and ischemic infarction with hemorrhagic conversion may present a challenge. ICH on head CT tends to have a denser, homogeneous appearance, whereas the hemorrhagic infarction is usually spotted or mottled within a hypodense arterial territory. Hemorrhagic infarction most often occurs in the setting of embolic arterial occlusion and follows a branch artery territory. Intraventricular blood may be seen with ICH, particularly if the hemorrhage is in the thalamus or basal ganglia. Ventricular hemorrhage from embolic infarction does not occur. Significant mass effect may be present from the outset in ICH, whereas the mass effect from hemorrhagic infarction results from secondary edema formation, which peaks after 48 hours. The appearance of the hematoma on MRI follows a characteristic course from the acute to the subacute to the chronic stage (see Table 3.2). Coagulation studies (PT/PTT, platelet count) should be obtained at the time of diagnosis to rule out coagulopathy as a cause for the hemorrhage. Liver function tests should be obtained.

Management

1. **Correction of a coagulopathy** due to a vitamin K antagonist such as warfarin requires administration of **25–50 U/kg of prothrombin complex concentrate** and vitamin K 5–10 mg IV to terminate active bleeding. For those with hemorrhage associated with IV heparin or a low molecular weight heparin, these agents must be stopped and reversed with **protamine sulfate 1 mg per 100 U of heparin (maximum dose 50 mg)**. For the newer anticoagulants, specific reversal agents are available (see Chapter 6, page 98 for more details).

2. **Active control of blood pressure** to systolic levels of <140 mm Hg should be attempted and appear to be safe with oral or IV antihypertensives. Unlike in ischemic infarction in which reduction of blood pressure may result in decreased cerebral blood flow and consequent extension of infarction, reducing blood pressure in ICH may help prevent recurrent bleeding.

3. **Control of increased intracranial pressure** with pharmacologic measures and hyperventilation may allow the patient to pass through a critical phase until the hematoma begins to resolve, but these measures are limited in time scope (see Chapter 13).

4. **Placement of an intraventricular drain** may be necessary because intraventricular blood or direct compression of the cerebral aqueduct by a brain stem hematoma may cause obstructive hydrocephalus. If there is any clinical deterioration, a CT or MRI scan should be obtained to distinguish between hydrocephalus and worsening as a result of extension of the hemorrhage or edema.

5. **Surgical hematoma evacuation** and craniectomy remains controversial but may lower mortality. Minimally invasive approaches are being tested in clinical trials. Surgical hematoma evacuation should be strongly considered in patients with large ICH, and it is recommended in patients with cerebellar hematomas greater than 3 cm in diameter. For patients presenting in coma or for those with a severe and stable neurologic deficit, surgery is unlikely to help.

Movement Disorders

Movement disorders may be defined simply as *abnormal involuntary (i.e., uncontrollable) movements.* These movements are not the result of weakness or sensory deficits. Rather, they are generally the result of dysfunction of what may be defined anatomically as either the basal ganglia or cerebellum and functionally as the extrapyramidal motor system.

The diversity of movement disorders can be overwhelming, with movements including those that are commonly known (tremors, tics) and those that are less familiar to the beginner (dystonia, chorea, and hemiballismus). Despite this diversity, movement disorders may be conveniently categorized into two types:

1. *Hyperkinesias* are characterized by an excess of movement.
2. *Hypokinesias* are characterized by a paucity of movement.
   Several basic principles should be kept in mind when first approaching a patient with a movement disorder. These are outlined in the following.

BASIC PRINCIPLES

1. Take time to **observe** the patient. Some movements may be quite elaborate. Look at the pattern and quality of the movements.
2. **Describe** what you see. Do not label anything yet. For example, note that "the eyes seem to be intermittently squeezing closed" or that "there are jerking movements of the left arm every 5 seconds."
3. **Classify** the movement as a hyperkinesia or a hypokinesia, as defined earlier.
4. **Give the movement a name** (e.g., tremor, chorea). The list of different types of abnormal movements (see Step 4 in the following paragraphs) provides a glossary of terms. Read each term and its definition and try to decide which of these terms best describes what you have seen. Sometimes you may see more than one type of movement.

5. **Diagnose a specific disease** after naming the movement. For example, both tremor and bradykinesia are features of Parkinson disease.

6. Finally, think about the appropriate **treatment.** Table 25.1 lists the medications and dosages for treatment of movement disorders.

The most common error is for students to skip straight to diagnosis and treatment. It is important first to **observe, describe, classify, and name.**

The remainder of this chapter will follow the preceding six-step outline.

STEP 1: OBSERVE

Inform the patient that you are going to watch his or her movements and then *just observe the patient.* Some patients may be self-conscious and may try to inhibit their movements, particularly if these are embarrassing. If this is the case, ask the patient to allow the body to behave naturally and not stop any movements. You may need to ask the patient to perform certain maneuvers that will bring out the movement (e.g., writing may bring out a tremor, walking may bring out a dystonic foot movement). Some movements may be elaborate, and the period of observation may be lengthy before you get a sense of a pattern or before you can fully describe what you see.

STEP 2: DESCRIBE

Try to describe the movements. This is not easy. In fact, neurologists sometimes find it easier to use gestures, rather than words, when describing a movement.

Some descriptions may be straightforward. For example, you might describe Mr. H.'s movements in the following way: "The right side of Mr. H.'s face twitches every 5 seconds." Other descriptions may be elaborate. For example, you might describe Mrs. R.'s movements as follows: "Mrs. R.'s neck seems to be twisted and tilted to the left side and forward and the neck seems to have a slightly shaky quality, particularly in certain positions."

Avoid describing Mr. H. as having hemifacial spasm and Mrs. R. as having torticollis. These statements are not descriptions; they are diagnoses.

STEP 3: CLASSIFY

It is important to classify the movement as a hyperkinesia or a hypokinesia. This is the easiest step. One caveat is that some patients may simultaneously exhibit both types of movements. For example, a patient with Parkinson disease may have a tremor (hyperkinesia) and bradykinesia (hypokinesia).

TABLE 25.1 **Movement Disorder Medications and Dosages**

Medication	Dose	Condition Treated
Alprazolam (Xanax)	0.125–to 3 mg per day (two to three times a day)	Essential tremor
Amantadine (Symmetrel)	100–300 mg per day (two to three times a day)	Parkinson disease, chorea
Apomorphine (Apokyn)	Injection 2–6 mg/day as needed	Parkinson disease
Atenolol (Tenormin)	50–150 mg/day, once per day	Essential tremor
Aripiprazole (Abilify)	2–30 mg per day, once per day	Chorea
Baclofen (Lioresal)	10–to–120 mg per day (three times a day)	Dystonia
	30–60 mg per day (three times a day)	Tourette syndrome
Clonazepam (Klonopin)	0.5–6 mg/day (two times per day) for essential tremor, 1–4 mg per day (two to four times a day)	Tourette syndrome
Clonidine (Catapres)	0.2–0.3 mg per day, divided	Tourette syndrome
Diazepam (Valium)	2–10 mg per day, divided (two to three times a day)	Dystonia
Entacapone (Comtan)	200–1600 mg per day divided	Parkinson disease
Gabapentin (Neurontin)	1200 mg per day (three times a day)	Essential tremor
Guanfacine (Tenex)	600–1200 mg once per day	Restless leg syndrome
	1–6 mg per day, once per day	Chorea
Haloperidol (Haldol)	1–10 mg per day (two to three times a day)	Tics, chorea

TABLE 25.1   Movement Disorder Medications and Dosages—cont'd

Medication	Dose	Condition Treated
Levodopa/carbidopa (Sinemet)	300–2000 mg per day, divided	Parkinson disease
Metyrosine (Demser)	250–1000 mg per day (three to four times a day)	Chorea
Nadolol (Corgard)	120–240 mg/day, once per day	Essential tremor
Olanzapine (Zyprexa)	5–20 mg per day (once a day)	Chorea, Tourette syndrome
Oxycodone (Oxycontin)	10–40 mg qhs	Restless leg syndrome
Penicillamine (Cuprimine)	125–1500 mg per day	Wilson disease
Pimozide (Orap)	1–6 mg per day, divided	Tourette syndrome
Pramipexole (Mirapex)	1.5–4.5 mg per day (three times a day)	Parkinson disease *or*
	0.375–0.75 mg qhs	Restless leg syndrome
Primidone (Mysoline)	50–1000 mg per day (three to four times a day)	Essential tremor
Propranolol (Inderal)	40–320 mg per day (three to four times a day) or in a long-acting preparation (60–320 mg/day)	Essential tremor
Quetiapine (Seroquel)	25–100 mg per day, divided, two to three times a day	Chorea
Rasagaline (Azilect)	0.5–1 mg/day given once daily	Parkinson disease
Reserpine	0.5–8 mg per day (three to four times a day)	Tourette syndrome, chorea
Risperidone (Risperdal)	0.5–6 mg per day (two times a day)	Chorea, Tourette syndrome

Ropinirole (Requip)	3–24.0 mg per day (three times a day)	Parkinson disease *or*
	0.25 to 4 mg qhs	Restless leg syndrome
Rotigotine patch (Neupro)	4–8 mg/24 hours (patch)	Parkinson disease
Selegiline (Eldepryl)	5–10 mg per day (two times a day)	Parkinson disease
Sotalol (Betapace)	80–160 mg/day, divided, twice a day	Essential tremor
Tetrabenazine (Xenazine)	12.5–100 mg per day, divided, two to three times a day	Chorea
Topiramate (Topamax)	200–400 mg per day (two to three times a day)	Essential tremor
Trientine (Syprine)	750–1250 mg per day (two to four times a day)	Wilson disease
Trihexyphenidyl (Artane)	1–10 mg per day (three to four times a day)	Parkinson disease *or* Dystonia
	1–10 mg per day (adults), 1–120 mg per day (children), divided, three to four times a day	
Zinc acetate (Galzin)	150 mg per day (three times a day)	Wilson disease
Ziprasidone (Geodon)	20–100 mg per day, divided, two times a day	Chorea

qhs, Each night at bedtime.

STEP 4: GIVE THE MOVEMENT A NAME

The following is a list of different types of abnormal movements. Movements in **bold** letters are the hypokinesias; all other movements are hyperkinesias. The essential element of each movement is *italicized*.

Name of Movement	Definition or Description
Akathisia	A subjective *feeling of inner motor restlessness* that is relieved by movement; the movements are stereotypic and complex and convey restlessness (e.g., crossing and uncrossing legs, rocking back and forth, squirming and attempting to arise from the chair, and pacing)
Asterixis	Sudden periods of *cessation of muscle contraction* best seen when the patient's arms are extended in front of their body, as if stopping traffic
Athetosis	Slow, continuous, *sinuous, writhing* movements, usually of the distal parts of the limbs
Ballismus	Wild *flinging, flailing* movements of a limb or limbs that represent large-amplitude proximal choreiform movements; ballismus is often unilateral (hemiballismus)
Bradykinesia	Movements that are either *slow* or of *diminished amplitude*
Chorea	*Semipurposeful flowing* movements in a continuous and random pattern
Dyskinesia	General term for any excessive movement; the term dyskinesia is often used more specifically as an abbreviation for "tardive dyskinesia" (often manifests as repetitive oral movements; often seen in patients taking certain psychiatric medications)
Dystonia	*Twisting* movements or movements/postures that are often *sustained* for variable periods of time
Freezing	Brief episodes (usually lasting several seconds) during which a motor act is temporarily blocked or halted; talking is a motor act that is commonly affected
Myoclonus	Sudden, brief, shocklike *jerks*
Myokymia	*Quivering* or rippling of muscle

Rigidity	Muscle tone that is increased on passive motion; distinct from spasticity, it is present equally in all directions of movement (i.e., both in flexors and in extensors)
Tachykinesia	Movements or speech characterized by *continuous acceleration* or loss of amplitude
Tics	*Repetitive, stereotypic movements or sounds* that are suppressible and that relieve a feeling of inner tension
Tremor	*Rhythmic, oscillatory movements* that may be present at rest or with action; an intention tremor occurs when the patient's limb approaches a target during purposeful movements (e.g., finger-to-nose maneuver).

STEP 5: DIAGNOSE A SPECIFIC DISEASE

Parkinson Disease

Parkinson disease was first described by James Parkinson in 1817.

Types of Movements

The types of movements involved in this disease are tremor, rigidity, bradykinesia, freezing, and tachykinesia. The *tremor* of Parkinson disease is most commonly a *rest tremor.* This means that the tremor is present when the arms are resting in the patient's lap or at their side (while lying down, while standing with arms relaxed, or while walking). Many patients with Parkinson disease also have an *action tremor,* which is present when their arms are outstretched in front of their body *(postural tremor)* or when they are using their hands for purposeful movement *(kinetic tremor).* Sometimes it takes a moment for this tremor to appear, in which case it is called a *reemergent tremor.* The *rigidity* is often called *cogwheel* rigidity because it may have a ratchet-like quality. The *bradykinesia* is characterized by a decrease in the frequency of movements (diminished blink frequency, few facial expressions, or *masked facies*) and by slowness of movement, with loss of amplitude. *Postural reflexes,* lost later in the disease, may be tested by performing the *pull test.* Stand behind the patient and pull him or her backward. A normal response is for the patient to take one or two steps back without falling. Always stand behind the patient in the event that you need to catch him or her. *Freezing* is most commonly seen as *start hesitation* or *turning hesitation.* Walking in narrow, cramped quarters may bring on freezing. *Tachykinesia* may take the form of rapid accelerating speech *(tachyphemia)* or rapid accelerated walking *(festination).*

Diagnostic Tests

Parkinson disease is a clinical diagnosis. The cardinal features are tremor, rigidity, bradykinesia, and loss of postural reflexes. Lumbar puncture (LP), electroencephalogram (EEG), computed tomography (CT), and magnetic resonance imaging (MRI) are nonspecific. The DaTscan may reveal a reduction in dopaminergic neurons and may be a particularly useful diagnostic tool early in the disease when clinical features are difficult to discern.

Treatment

LEVODOPA

Levodopa-carbidopa (Sinemet) 300 to 2000 mg per day of levodopa, with administration of individual doses ranging from every 2 to 3 hours to two times a day. Controlled-release forms of levodopa-carbidopa may be given orally (Sinemet CR, Rytary) and nonorally (via dopamine intestinal infusion pump, DUOPA) as well.

DOPAMINE AGONISTS

Pramipexole (Mirapex) 1.5 to 4.5 mg per day, divided, three times a day
Ropinirole (Requip) 3 to 24 mg per day, divided, three times a day
Rotigotine patch (Neupro), 4 to 8 mg/24 hours (patch)
Apomorphine (Apokyn) injection 2 to 6 mg/day as needed

AMANTADINE

Amantadine (Symmetrel) 100 to 300 mg per day, divided, two to three times a day

ANTICHOLINERGICS

Trihexyphenidyl (Artane) 1 to 10 mg per day, divided, three times a day

COMT INHIBITORS

Entacapone (Comtan) 200 to 1600 mg per day, divided, as an adjunct to levodopa-carbidopa

MAO-B INHIBITORS

Selegiline (Eldepryl) 5 to 10 mg per day, divided, two times a day
Rasagaline (Azilect) 0.5 to 1 mg/day given once daily

Stimulation of the globus pallidus interna after implantation of *deep brain stimulation* electrodes improves bradykinesia, rigidity, rest tremor, impaired balance, and medication-induced dyskinesia and motor fluctuations in the limb contralateral to the electrode. Stimulation of the subthalamic nucleus is similarly beneficial, and selection of the optimal brain target is tailored to the patient's needs.

Stereotactic thalamotomy has been shown to decrease the severity of parkinsonian tremor and allow for reductions in dosages of levodopa. However, this procedure has largely been supplanted by electrical stimulation of the ventral intermediate nucleus of the thalamus after implantation of deep brain stimulation electrodes. The procedure is beneficial for the treatment of contralateral parkinsonian tremor or essential tremor.

Essential Tremor

One of the earliest reports of essential tremor was that of Charles Dana in 1887.

Types of Movements

The characteristic movement in this disease is tremor. The tremor or essential tremor is most commonly an *action tremor* of the arms. It is present when the patient holds his or her arms extended in front of the body (postural tremor) and with tasks such as writing, pouring water, and touching the finger to the nose (kinetic tremor). Kinetic tremor is generally of greater amplitude than postural tremor. Many patients with essential tremor have an *intention tremor* of the arms. The tremor also may involve the head, voice, and jaw in some patients; the head tremor generally resolves when the patient lies down. In cases of severe essential tremor, a tremor at rest may be present in the arms but not the legs. Patients also may have mildly ataxic gait, noted on tandem walking.

Diagnostic Tests

Essential tremor is diagnosed on the basis of the clinical features described previously. Other causes of similar tremor, including hyperthyroidism and certain medications (e.g., lithium or valproate), should be ruled out. The diagnosis may be confirmed by computerized tremor analysis with accelerometry.

Treatment

BETA BLOCKERS

Propranolol (Inderal) 0 to 320 mg per day, divided, three to four times a day or in a long-acting preparation (60–320 mg/day)
Atenolol (Tenormin) 50 to 150 mg/day, once per day
Sotalol (Betapace)80 to 160 mg/day, divided, twice a day
Nadolol (Corgard) 120 to 240 mg/day, once per day

MEDICATIONS THAT ENHANCE GABA-ERGIC TONE

Primidone (Mysoline) 50 to 1000 mg per day, divided, three to four times a day

Topiramate (Topamax) 50 to 300 mg per day, divided, two to three times per day

Gabapentin (Neurontin) 1200 mg per day, divided, three times a day

Alprazolam (Xanax) 0.125 to 3 mg per day, divided, two to three times per day

Clonazepam (Klonopin) 0.5 to 6 mg/day, divided, two times per day

Botulinum toxin (Botox) injected into selected muscles (hands, head and neck, vocal cords) several times per year

Electrical stimulation of the ventral intermediate nucleus of the thalamus after implantation of deep brain stimulation electrodes.

Huntington Disease

Huntington disease was first described by George Huntington in 1872.

Types of Movements

Chorea and dystonia are common features of the disease. The *chorea* of Huntington disease may involve the face, tongue, limbs, or trunk. It is often exacerbated by anxiety or stress and may be brought on by asking the patient to close the eyes, hold the arms extended in front of the body, and count backward or perform simple arithmetic. *Dystonia* and *tics* also may be present. The dystonia may take the form of fist clenching, shoulder elevation, or foot inversion during walking. Another feature of Huntington disease is *motor impersistence* (inhibitory pauses occurring during voluntary motion that account for the "milkmaid grips" seen when hand grasp is tested). In addition to involuntary movements, patients with Huntington disease often have psychiatric manifestations (depression, psychosis) and cognitive problems, changes in personality, and prominent disinhibition. Eye motion abnormalities (jerky smooth pursuits and slowed saccades) are an early feature of the disease, and agnosia (lack of awareness or frank denial of physical and mental changes) is a prominent feature as well.

Diagnostic Tests

Because the disease is transmitted in an autosomal dominant manner, a family history is an important feature of the diagnosis. One should rule out other causes of chorea including hyperthyroidism, use of anticonvulsants, and Sydenham chorea. The abnormal gene, on the short arm of chromosome 4, consists of an abnormally long CAG repeat fragment. CT or MRI scan may show atrophy of the caudate nuclei.

Management

In many cases, the movements are not bothersome to the patient, and the psychiatric manifestations are often the focus of treatment. However, treatment for the movements might consist of the following:

Tetrabenazine (Xenazine), 12.5 to 100 mg per day, divided, two to three times a day

Olanzapine (Zyprexa) 5 to 20 mg per day, once per day

Risperidone (Risperdal) 2 to 6 mg per day, divided, two times per day

Quetiapine (Seroquel) 25 to 100 mg per day, divided, two to three times a day

Haloperidol (Haldol) 1 to 10 mg per day, divided, two to three times a day

Amantadine (Symmetrel) 100 to 300 mg per day, divided, two to three times a day

Reserpine 0.5 to 8 mg per day, divided, three to four times a day

Metyrosine (Demser) 250 to 1000 mg per day, divided, three to four times a day

Idiopathic Torsion Dystonia (Dystonia Musculorum Deformans)

This illness is characterized by twisting dystonic movements and occasional tremor.

Types of Movements

The illness usually begins in childhood and has a progressive course. The *dystonia* often initially involves the foot and is most apparent with certain actions but not with others (e.g., intermittent spasmodic inversion of the foot while walking but not while running or walking backward). Eventually, involvement of other limbs and neck often occurs. Although the dystonia initially consists of twisting *movements* with action, sustained dystonic *postures* at rest become apparent eventually. Limbs with dystonia also may exhibit an irregular *dystonic tremor* that resembles the action tremor seen in patients with essential tremor.

Diagnostic Tests

The diagnosis is based on clinical history and examination. It should be distinguished from other secondary or symptomatic causes of dystonia (e.g., Wilson disease) and from adult-onset dystonia. The latter usually runs a more benign course and begins in adulthood with involvement of the neck, eyes, vocal cords, or hand, but it rarely involves the leg. A common gene for idiopathic torsion dystonia, the *DYT1* gene, is located on the long arm of chromosome 9 and is inherited in an autosomal dominant manner with a penetrance of 30%.

Management

Trihexyphenidyl (Artane) 1 to 10 mg per day (adults), 1 to 120 mg per day (children), divided, three to four times a day

Baclofen (Lioresal) 10 to 120 mg per day, divided, three times a day

Diazepam (Valium) 2 to 10 mg per day, divided, two to three times a day

Botulinum toxin (Botox) injected into selected muscles several times per year

Tourette Syndrome

Tourette syndrome was first definitively described by Gilles de la Tourette in 1885.

Types of Movements

This syndrome is characterized by multiple chronic motor and vocal tics that wax and wane over time. The tics may be *simple motor tics* (eye blinking, eyebrow raising), *complex motor tics* (head shaking, wrist shaking), *simple phonic tics* (throat clearing, grunting), or *complex phonic tics* (uttering words). *Coprolalia* (uttering obscenities) and *echolalia* (repeating sounds or words) are examples of the latter. As with most tics, these are voluntarily suppressible for brief periods and may vary in intensity over time. In addition to these motor features, patients with Tourette syndrome often have psychiatric manifestations including attention deficit hyperactivity disorder and obsessive compulsive disorder.

Diagnostic Tests

The diagnosis is clinical. This disorder usually begins in childhood with both motor and phonic tics. Coprolalia is not an essential feature of the diagnosis.

Management

Tetrabenazine (Xenazine) 12.5 to 300 mg per day, divided, three times a day

Clonazepam (Klonopin) 1 to 4 mg per day, divided, two to three times a day

Baclofen (Lioresal) 30 to 60 mg per day, divided, two to four three times a day

Risperidone (Risperdal) 0.5 to 6 mg per day, divided, two times a day

Ziprasidone (Geodon) 20 to 100 mg per day, divided, two times a day

Aripiprazole (Abilify), 2 to 30 mg per day, once per day
Olanzapine (Zyprexa) 5 to 20 mg per day, once per day
Pimozide (Orap) 1 to 6 mg per day, divided
Haloperidol (Haldol) 1 to 10 mg per day, divided, two to three
    times a day
Clonidine (Catapres) 0.2 to 0.3 mg per day, divided
Guanfacine (Tenex) 1 to 6 mg per day, once per day

Wilson Disease

Wilson disease was first described by Samuel Alexander Kinnier Wilson in 1912.

Types of Movements

The movements are protean. Tremor, rigidity, bradykinesia, dystonia, and chorea are all seen in this disease, and one or more of these movements may be present. A *parkinsonian form* of the illness may be characterized by rest tremor, rigidity, or bradykinesia. A *pseudosclerotic* form of the illness is associated with a *wing-beating tremor* (a large-amplitude, flapping, violent tremor that is present when the shoulders are abducted, elbows are flexed, and fingers are facing each other). *Dystonia* and *chorea* also may be present. Dysarthria occurs frequently and may progress to anarthria. Psychiatric manifestations (anxiety, depression, psychosis) are a common feature of the illness.

Diagnostic Tests

The diagnosis is based on clinical history and examination and is supported by the presence of Kayser-Fleischer rings (ring-shaped copper deposits in the cornea), low serum ceruloplasmin level, abnormalities in liver function tests, or hepatitis. Lesions in the basal ganglia may be seen on an MRI scan.

Management

Penicillamine (Cuprimine) 125 to 1500 mg per day, divided, two
    to four times a day
Trientine (Syprine) 750 to 1500 mg per day, divided, two to four
    times a day
Zinc acetate (Galzin) 150 mg per day, divided, three times
    a day

Restless Leg Syndrome

The syndrome is characterized by feelings of discomfort and restlessness in the legs and occasionally in the arms. These feelings, which occur primarily in the evening hours, are often relieved by movement (e.g., moving the legs in bed or getting out of bed to pace).

Types of Movements

The movements involved are fidgeting, kicking, or writhing movements of the legs and pacing the floor.

The discomfort is deep-seated and is often described as feelings of stretching, itching, crawling, or creeping in the bones, muscles, or tendons. These symptoms are most common when the patient first lies down in bed at night. The feelings may cause writhing movements in the legs, fidgeting, or kicking. Some patients need to pace the floor for temporary relief. Unlike akathisia, which also causes discomfort with a desire to move, restless leg syndrome initially occurs primarily at night.

Diagnostic Tests

Restless leg syndrome is a clinical syndrome that is diagnosed based on the clinical features described. Akathisia can resemble restless leg syndrome but is typically constant throughout the day, has a more generalized distribution (i.e., not just localized leg discomfort), and is confined to patients taking neuroleptic medications or patients with Parkinson disease.

Treatment

Gabapentin enacarbil (Horizant) 600 to 1200 mg, once per day
Pregabalin (Lyrica) 150 to 450 mg/day
Pramipexole (Mirapex) 0.375 to 0.75 mg each night at bedtime (qhs)
Ropinirole (Requip) 0.25 to 4 mg qhs
Rotigotine (Neupro) 1 to 3 mg per day, applied as a patch
Oxycodone (Oxycontin) 10 to 40 mg qhs

Miscellaneous Disorders

This section briefly discusses those movements from the list in **Step 4** that were not discussed under specific diseases.

Akathisia is most commonly seen as a side effect of certain psychiatric medications.

Asterixis, usually seen bilaterally in the arms, is most commonly a feature of toxic/metabolic states such as liver or renal failure. Patients are often encephalopathic.

Athetosis may appear in a variety of neurologic disorders ranging from cerebral palsy to paroxysmal kinesigenic choreoathetosis. Athetotic movements may merge with chorea (choreoathetosis).

Ballismus, most commonly unilateral (hemiballismus), is usually the result of a stroke in the contralateral subthalamic nucleus.

Myoclonus may occur anywhere in the body, including palatal myoclonus and ocular myoclonus. Myoclonus may be the result of anoxic ischemic injury (Lance-Adams syndrome), birth injuries, degenerative disorders (Ramsay Hunt syndrome), infections, tumors, strokes, or even medications (levodopa). Hiccups are a physiologic form of myoclonus.

Myokymia, most commonly seen in facial muscles, is often caused by pontine lesions, particularly plaques in multiple sclerosis or pontine gliomas.

Epilepsy and Seizure Disorders

Epilepsy, seizures, and related disorders are among the most commonly encountered problems in neurologic practice. Diagnosis and treatment of these disorders can be challenging for even the most experienced physicians, and for patients, these disorders can be the source of significant morbidity, emotional distress, and disability. This chapter will provide an overview to the diagnosis, differential diagnosis, and management of epilepsy and related disorders.

DEFINITIONS

A *seizure* is defined as transient neurologic signs or symptoms that are related to abnormal excessive synchronous activity of cortical neurons.

A *provoked (acute symptomatic) seizure* is defined as a seizure that occurs as a direct result of an acute brain insult, such as toxic, metabolic, traumatic, inflammatory, or infectious derangements. The provoking factor must occur in close temporal relationship to the seizure. For example, a seizure that occurred within a few hours of an acute ischemic stroke would be considered provoked, whereas a seizure that occurred 3 months later would be considered *unprovoked.* The exact length of time between the provoking factor and the seizure is the subject of some debate, and it depends on the specific factor, but it is generally in the range of hours to a few days.

Epilepsy is defined as a brain disorder characterized by at least two unprovoked seizures occurring at least 24 hours apart, or one unprovoked seizure combined with additional information (such as an abnormal electroencephalogram [EEG] or magnetic resonance imaging [MRI]) that would indicate a high likelihood (>60%) of seizure recurrence.

SEIZURE CLASSIFICATION

The classification system for seizures has undergone several changes over the years, and this can be a source of confusion among learners and nonneurologists. The most recent proposed international classification scheme divides seizures into focal seizures (those that start in one part of the brain), generalized seizures (those that arise from or rapidly involve both hemispheres), and seizures of unknown onset. Within each of these categories, there are a number of seizure types, which are outlined in Fig. 26.1. In clinical practice, the modern terminology is often used interchangeably with older terms, so in this chapter the older terms will be included in parentheses for the sake of clarity.

Generalized seizures

Generalized Tonic-Clonic ("Grand Mal") Seizures

This type of seizure can be seen in primary generalized epilepsy syndromes, but it also can occur as a result of diffuse propagation of focal-onset seizures ("secondary generalization"). There is a characteristic progression of features, usually starting with an ictal cry (generated by forced inspiration caused by contraction of the diaphragm combined with contraction of laryngeal muscles); followed by a tonic phase (contraction of muscles in the trunk and limbs); and followed by clonic jerking that generally starts as low-amplitude, high-frequency jerks and progressing to higher-amplitude, lower-frequency jerks. After offset, there is often diffuse decrease in muscle tone, as well as noisy, wet, slow ("stertorous") breathing. The typical duration of an event is 1 to 2 minutes. Patients are often sleepy or confused for 5 to 30 minutes afterward, sometimes even longer. Patients with rare generalized tonic-clonic seizures often report feeling unwell for hours to days afterward, with muscle soreness, headache, and fatigue. During the tonic phase, patients often develop lateral tongue bite because of tonic contraction of jaw muscles and can develop injuries such as posterior dislocation of the shoulder or compression fractures of thoracic vertebrae. In the absence of an experienced and observant witness, it can be difficult to distinguish this type of seizure from "mimics" such as psychogenic nonepileptic spells (PNESs) or syncope with convulsive features.

Absence ("Petit Mal") Seizures

These seizures have an abrupt onset; brief duration (typically 10 seconds, and almost always less than a minute); and are characterized by staring, behavioral arrest, amnesia, and sometimes eyelid fluttering or subtle oral automatisms. On EEG, they are associated with a run of 3-Hz generalized spike wave discharges. They

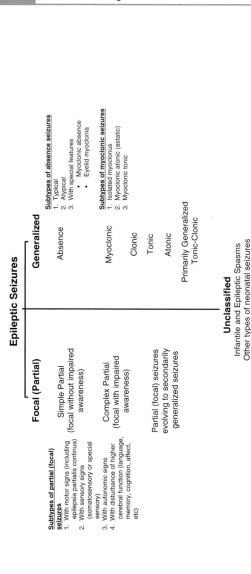

Epileptic Seizures

Focal (Partial)

Simple Partial
(focal without impaired awareness)

Complex Partial
(focal with impaired awareness)

Partial (focal) seizures evolving to secondarily generalized seizures

Subtypes of partial (focal) seizures
1. With motor signs (including epilepsia partialis continua)
2. With sensory signs (somatosensory or special sensory)
3. With autonomic signs
4. With disturbance of higher cerebral function (language, memory, cognition, affect, etc)

Generalized

Absence

Myoclonic

Clonic

Tonic

Atonic

Primarily Generalized Tonic-Clonic

Subtypes of absence seizures
1. Typical
2. Atypical
3. With special features
   • Myoclonic absence
   • Eyelid myoclonia

Subtypes of myoclonic seizures
1. Isolated myoclonus
2. Myoclonic atonic (astatic)
3. Myoclonic tonic

Unclassified

Infantile and Epileptic Spasms
Other types of neonatal seizures
Status Epilepticus

FIG. 26.1 International League Against Epilepsy classification of epileptic seizures. (Adapted from Moeller JJ, Hirsch LJ. Diagnosis and classification of seizures and epilepsy. In Winn HR, ed. Youmans and Winn Neurological Surgery. 7th ed. Philadelphia, PA: Elsevier; 2017:388–395.)

are most often seen in neurologically normal children, in disorders such as childhood and juvenile absence epilepsy. Atypical absence seizures usually occur in patients with symptomatic generalized epilepsy (such as in Lennox-Gastaut syndrome), and are longer, with less clear onset and offset.

Myoclonic Seizures

These seizures are seen most often in juvenile myoclonic epilepsy (JME) and can occur either in isolation or preceding a primarily generalized tonic-clonic seizure. They are often brief, lasting only a split second, and are associated with rapid synchronous jerking of proximal muscles, usually without impairment of awareness. In JME, they often occur in the context of sleep deprivation or alcohol use. On EEG, myoclonus is often associated with generalized or bifrontal polyspike-wave discharges.

Tonic Seizures

This type of seizure is seen most often in symptomatic generalized epilepsy syndromes, such as Lennox-Gastaut syndrome. It is associated with sudden, intense, bilateral contraction of proximal (and sometimes distal) muscles, possibly with brief impairment of awareness. They generally last only a few seconds, and there is rapid recovery afterward. On EEG, there is diffuse background attenuation, sometimes with superimposed diffuse, low-voltage, high-frequency (beta) activity. This type of seizure is particularly disabling because it is often associated with a sudden fall if the patient is standing.

Atonic Seizures

These also are most commonly seen in symptomatic generalized epilepsy syndromes. The patient has a brief (usually only a few seconds) loss of tone, resulting in a sudden fall. Patients can often have both tonic and atonic seizures, sometimes with single events that have features of both seizure types. These events are sometimes called "drop attacks" because they result in a sudden loss of posture or tone, which is particularly concerning when the patient is standing or walking. On EEG, there is typically diffuse attenuation, or diffuse low-voltage fast activity.

Focal (Partial) Seizures

Focal Seizures Without ("Simple Partial Seizures") or With Impairment of Awareness ("Complex Partial Seizures")

The clinical features of focal seizures depend on the region of the brain that is involved. These seizures can have motor manifestations (such as jerking, tonic posturing, loss of tone, widespread hyper motor activity) and can have sensory (including special sensory, such as smell, taste, vision, etc.), autonomic, cognitive, or emotional features, alone or in combination. The unifying feature of this type of seizure is that there is no impairment in the patient's ability to respond appropriately and remember the incident afterward. This type of seizure typically lasts up to a few minutes in duration, but some patients will feel fatigued for minutes or even hours afterward.

The term **aura** refers symptoms that occur at the onset of some focal seizures, most commonly sensory symptoms such as smell or taste, cognitive symptoms like déjà vu, or autonomic symptoms like nausea or flushing.

Focal seizures can progress to impairment of awareness, with or without preceding symptoms. The features during impairment of awareness can range from behavioral arrest to automatisms and other motor manifestations.

TEMPORAL LOBE SEIZURES

Focal seizures arising from the temporal lobe are the most common type of seizure in adults. Some temporal lobe seizures are preceded by aura, which is usually characterized by a rising epigastric sensation and other symptoms including déjà vu, smells, fears, stereotyped thoughts or mental images, or an indescribable cephalic sensation. When they progress to impairment of awareness, there is staring and unresponsiveness, with oral (chewing, lip-smacking) and manual (picking, rubbing, patting) automatisms. There may be clues that can help lateralize the seizure onset. Often, there is dystonic posturing of the hand or arm contralateral to seizure onset. After the seizure is over, there can be nose wipe with the ipsilateral hand (because the contralateral hand is weak). If the seizures arise from the dominant hemisphere, which is the left hemisphere in most patients, there is often postictal aphasia for at least a minute afterward.

FRONTAL LOBE SEIZURES

Typically, frontal lobe seizures are shorter than other types of focal-onset seizures, usually 15 to 40 seconds in duration. They frequently occur in clusters, and during sleep. Seizures arising from or adjacent to the primary motor cortex are associated with motor manifestations such as unilateral clonic jerking (sometimes spreading from one body region to another in a "Jacksonian march"). Seizures arising from the supplementary motor area are associated with bilateral, often asymmetric tonic posturing of the limbs, often with retained awareness. Seizures arising from the prefrontal regions can have hypermotor manifestations such as restless movements, bicycling of the legs, screaming or grunting, and other bizarre behaviors. It can be difficult to distinguish this type of seizure from a PNES.

OCCIPITAL LOBE SEIZURES

Seizures arising from the occipital lobe are less common than those arising from either frontal or temporal lobes. The manifestations of these seizures depend on where in the occipital lobe they arise. Seizures arising from the primary visual cortex are associated with simple visual phenomena, such as simple shapes, often with a flashing or strobelike character. Seizures arising from associative visual cortices may be more complex, manifesting in fully formed visual hallucinations. Seizures that start in the occipital lobe can propagate to either the temporal lobe or the parietal lobe, and, in either case, will progress to develop manifestations of seizures in those regions.

PARIETAL LOBE SEIZURES

This is the least common type of focal-onset seizure. Typically, patients have a sensory aura, which can be either tingling or less commonly a painful phenomenon. As with occipital seizures, they can spread to the temporal or frontal lobe and develop corresponding symptoms.

Seizures of Unknown Onset

Infantile (Epileptic) Spasms

This is the seizure type most commonly associated with West syndrome. When this type of seizure occurs in infants, it is called infantile spasms. In some cases, a similar seizure type persists into adulthood, and is called "epileptic spasms." There is some variability in the manifestations of the seizures, but they are typically extremely brief (a few seconds) and characterized by sudden tonic contraction of proximal flexor or extensor muscles, which is most intense at onset, and then gradually becomes less intense over the next few seconds. These spasms usually occur in clusters of several or even dozens of spasms over a period of several minutes. These are more frequent during wakefulness and sleep. On EEG, there is often a high-voltage, frontal-maximal slow wave followed by several seconds of diffuse attenuation ("electrodecremental response").

EPILEPSY SYNDROMES

Epilepsy syndromes are identified by combining the seizure type with other features, including EEG findings, other neurologic manifestations, genetics, and neuroimaging. The following are some of the common electroclinical syndromes.

Idiopathic Generalized Epilepsy Syndromes

All of the idiopathic generalized epilepsy syndromes have the common features of normal development, a normal neurologic examination, generalized seizures, and generalized discharges on EEG. These syndromes almost always have an onset in childhood, adolescence, or young adulthood. It is very rare for a patient to have generalized epilepsy with onset in later adulthood.

Childhood Absence Epilepsy

Age at onset: 4 to 10 years (peak 6 years).

Clinical course: Normal development and normal neurologic examination. Frequent seizures (up to hundreds per day), with resolution by puberty in the vast majority of patients. Can be misdiagnosed as attention deficit disorder.

Seizure types: Absence; generalized tonic-clonic seizures are rare.

EEG findings: 3-Hz generalized spike-wave discharges.

Treatments: Ethosuximide is the treatment of first choice. Alternatives include lamotrigine or valproic acid.

Juvenile Absence Epilepsy

Age at onset: 10 to 17 years (peak 12 years).

Clinical course: Normal development and normal neurologic examination. Seizures can occur daily, but they are less frequent than in childhood absence epilepsy (CAE). Can persist into adulthood, with need for lifelong antiepileptic drug (AED) therapy.

Seizure types: Absence; generalized tonic-clonic seizures in ∼80% of patients.

EEG findings: 3-Hz generalized spike-wave discharges.

Treatment: Lamotrigine, levetiracetam, valproic acid, zonisamide, topiramate, clobazam.

Juvenile Myoclonic Epilepsy

Age at onset: 12 to 18 years (peak 15 years).

Clinical course: Normal development and normal neurologic examination. Seizures occur in the morning, typically within 30 to 60 minutes of awakening. Can be precipitated by alcohol, sleep deprivation, or photic stimulation. Myoclonic jerks are often misrecognized as morning clumsiness. Seizures are usually well controlled on medication, but lifelong AED therapy is required in the vast majority of patients.

Seizure types: Myoclonic, generalized tonic-clonic; some patients have absence.

EEG findings: 4- to 5-Hz generalized spike-wave and polyspike-wave discharges. Generalized epileptiform discharges during photic stimulation ("photoparoxysmal response").

Treatment: Valproic acid is the most effective treatment, but it cannot always be tolerated, and it is not an ideal choice in women of childbearing age. Alternatives include levetiracetam, lamotrigine, topiramate, zonisamide, and clobazam. Myoclonic jerks can be exacerbated by some of the sodium channel blocking agents such as carbamazepine, lamotrigine, oxcarbazepine, and phenytoin.

Epilepsy With Generalized Tonic-Clonic Seizures on Awakening

This is a disorder that is similar to JME but without the myoclonic jerks. Treatment is similar.

Symptomatic Generalized Epilepsy Syndromes

West Syndrome (Infantile Spasms)

Age at onset: Almost always in the first year of life. Rare after age 18 months.

Clinical course: This syndrome can occur because of a large number of brain disorders, including genetic disorders, chromosomal abnormalities, inborn errors of metabolism, congenital infections, and perinatal brain insults. In some cases, there is no identified etiology ("cryptogenic"). Infants with this syndrome can have dozens or even hundreds of infantile spasms daily. Developmental regression is common.

Seizure types: Infantile spasms.

EEG findings: Hypsarrhythmia (high-voltage, disorganized background with abundant multifocal spikes), electrodecremental response during the spasms.

Treatment: Adrenocorticotropic hormone (ACTH) is the treatment of choice in most cases. Vigabatrin is often first-line therapy for patients with tuberous sclerosis.

Lennox-Gastaut Syndrome

Age at onset: 1 to 8 years (peak 3 to 5 years).

Clinical course: Patients have developmental delay and frequent seizures of multiple types, including drop attacks, which can be related to atonic, tonic, or myoclonic seizures. There are multiple etiologic causes, and many patients were previously diagnosed with West syndrome.

Seizure types: Multiple seizure types, including drop attacks.

EEG findings: "Slow" generalized spike-wave discharges at less than 2.5 Hz, paroxysmal fast activity during sleep, multifocal epileptiform discharges, diffuse slowing.

Treatment: Patients often require treatment with multiple AEDs, and complete seizure control is uncommon.

Idiopathic Localization-Related Epilepsy Syndromes

Benign Childhood Epilepsy With Centrotemporal Spikes ("Benign Rolandic Epilepsy")

Age at onset: 2 to 13 years (peak 7 to 9 years).

Clinical course: Patients are typically developmentally normal, and many have rare seizures, usually at night. Most patients do not have seizures after puberty.

Seizure types: Focal-onset seizures, often with sensory disturbance in oropharynx and drooling, which can progress to clonic jerks of the face, or even of the entire hemibody. Secondarily generalized tonic-clonic seizures can occur.

EEG findings: Central-temporal spikes, often bilateral, more frequent in sleep.

Treatment: For patients with rare seizures, AEDs may not be necessary. For patients with more frequent or severe seizures, multiple AEDs can be effective.

Childhood Occipital Epilepsy With Occipital Paroxysms

Age at onset: 2 to 17 years. Early-onset variant ("Panayiotopoulos syndrome") peak onset is 3 to 5 years. Late-onset variant ("Gastaut variant") peak onset is 7 to 9 years.

Clinical course: Patients are usually developmentally normal, and many have rare seizures, particularly with the early-onset variant. Patients with late-onset variant may have more frequent seizures, and seizures may persist into adulthood.

Seizure types: Early-onset variant: Focal seizures with vomiting and eye deviation, with other variable features. Late-onset variant: Focal seizures with visual symptoms, including loss of vision or hallucinations.

EEG findings: Occipital spikes, more frequent during sleep.

Treatment: For patients with rare seizures, AEDs may not be necessary. For patients with more frequent or severe seizures, multiple AEDs can be effective.

Febrile seizures

Up to 5% of children in the developed world will have a febrile seizure, and the incidence in other parts of the world is even higher. Typical age of occurrence is between 6 months and 5 years. **Simple febrile seizures** are defined as seizures that occur in close temporal relationship to a fever, are shorter than 15 minutes in duration (usually 3–4 minutes), have no focal features, and do not recur in the same 24-hour period. ***Complex febrile seizures*** are longer, may have focal features, or recur within 24 hours. Simple febrile seizures do not need to be treated, as long as the patient has recovered, and there is a clear association between the fever and the seizure. Complex febrile seizures often warrant additional investigations. There is an overall increase in lifetime risk of epilepsy in children with febrile seizures, but this risk is much higher in children with complex febrile seizures.

THE FIRST SEIZURE

A general approach to the evaluation of a patient with first seizure is shown in Fig. 26.2 The two most important elements are to ensure that the event was in fact a seizure (and not a seizure "mimic") and to determine whether or not the seizure was provoked.

Seizure "Mimics"

Several types of events can superficially resemble epileptic seizures. The most common differential diagnosis for seizures includes PNESs and syncope. It can be difficult to distinguish between these events and seizures, and the most important distinguishing information is usually based on the history and physical examination. Table 26.1 outlines some of the important distinguishing factors between generalized tonic-clonic seizures, PNESs, and syncope.

Several pieces of information have been traditionally associated with seizures, but they can be seen in other syndromes. For example, urinary incontinence can occur with syncope or with PNES, and on its own it will not necessarily be helpful in confirming a diagnosis of epilepsy. Tongue biting can occur with seizure mimics as well, although lateral tongue bite may be more commonly associated with seizures. Certain types of injuries may be helpful in clarifying the diagnosis. These include injuries that occur during the tonic phase of a generalized tonic-clonic seizure, such as posterior dislocation of the shoulder, vertebral compression fracture, or petechiae on the face and upper chest.

Some laboratory investigations may be helpful in distinguishing generalized tonic-clonic seizures from syncope and PNES, including anion gap metabolic acidosis, elevated white blood cell count, elevated ammonia level, or elevated creatine kinase (CK) level. An increase in serum prolactin also can occur, but this blood test has to be drawn within 10 to 20 minutes after the seizure and compared

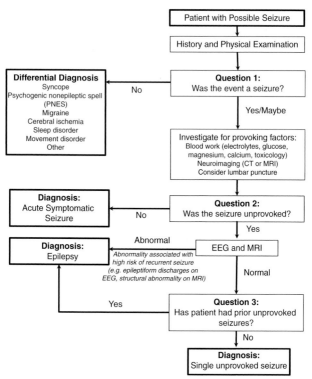

FIG. 26.2 An initial approach to the evaluation of a patient with suspected seizure. *CT*, Computed tomography; *EEG*, electroencephalogram; *MRI*, magnetic resonance imaging. (From: Moeller JJ, Hirsch LJ. Diagnosis and classification of seizures and epilepsy. In Winn HR, ed. *Youmans and Winn Neurological Surgery.* 7th ed. Philadelphia, PA: Elsevier; 2017:388–395.)

with a baseline level drawn later. Although these blood tests may be useful in narrowing the differential diagnosis, none of these tests on its own is sufficient to distinguish seizures from mimics.

Provoked Seizures

As mentioned previously, multiple factors can provoke a seizure. If there is an immediate provoking factor that can be identified by history or laboratory investigations, then the treatment is to avoid the provoking factor in the future. In these cases, additional investigations or treatments for epilepsy are generally not warranted.

TABLE 26.1	Clinical Features That May Help to Distinguish Generalized Tonic-Clonic Seizures From Two Common Seizure Mimics, Psychogenic Nonepileptic Spell, and Syncope		
	Before the Event	During the Event	After the Event
Generalized tonic-clonic seizure	Aura or other focal seizure Myoclonus	Prominent tonic phase "Ictal cry" Duration is typically 1–2 min	Noisy, wet ("stertorous") breathing Prolonged sleepiness or confusion Sore muscles, headache, lateral tongue bite
PNES	May have acute psychological stressor	Asynchronous, stopping and starting movements, with back arching, pelvic thrusting Eyes often closed Can have preserved awareness with bilateral movements Weeping	Shallow, rapid respirations Rapid recovery in some cases Emotional distress or weeping
Syncope	Lightheadedness, pallor, diaphoresis, tunnel vision, warmth Palpitations Provoked by position change, emotional distress, pain, etc.	Generally <15 s unless patient kept upright Myoclonus is common, but tonic posturing is much less common	Rapid recovery in most cases Can have urinary incontinence Prolonged confusion can sometimes result from head injury during fall

PNES, Psychogenic nonepileptic spell.

Adapted from Moeller JJ, Hirsch LJ. Diagnosis and classification of seizures and epilepsy. In Winn HR, ed. *Youmans and Winn Neurological Surgery*. 7th ed. Philadelphia, PA: Elsevier; 2017:388–395.

The following specific types of provoked seizures warrant individual consideration.

Traumatic Brain Injury

Some patients with mild traumatic brain injury will have an acute seizure immediately after the injury, and in many cases, this does not warrant treatment with an AED. Patients with more severe injury (skull fracture, penetrating wound, prolonged loss of consciousness or amnesia, intracranial hemorrhage) are at particularly high risk of seizures within the first 7 days after the injury. In these patients, prophylactic AED treatment for the first 7 days after injury reduces the likelihood of seizures during that time. However, this treatment does not prevent the subsequent development of epilepsy. If the patient remains seizure free for the first 7 days after head injury, then treatment should not be continued because it likely will not prevent subsequent seizures and may impair recovery.

Alcohol

Seizures secondary to alcohol withdrawal typically occur approximately 24 hours after the last drink. The treatment for alcohol withdrawal seizures is avoidance of alcohol. AEDs are not usually indicated because patients are not compliant, withdrawal of medications can lead to worsening seizures, and some AEDs are hepatotoxic. In some patients with chronic alcohol abuse, seizures can occur even after the patient has become abstinent. In these cases, AED therapy is indicated.

Stroke

Seizures can occur in 4% to 9% of patients with acute stroke, with higher rates in patients with hemorrhagic stroke than with ischemic stroke. Acute symptomatic seizures almost always occur within the first 48 hours of stroke, and they usually warrant early treatment with AEDs. Only a small minority of patients will develop subsequent epilepsy, so many patients can be weaned off AEDs at follow-up. Many patients with large strokes are at risk of subclinical or nonconvulsive seizures, and so if available, continuous video EEG monitoring should be considered in patients with large strokes and unexplained decreased level of consciousness.

Investigating the First Seizure

As outlined previously, a careful history can help distinguish seizures from mimics and can help determine whether there are any provoking factors. In addition, it is important to ask about other seizure types. In many cases, when a patient presents with a "first seizure," they are actually presenting with the first *recognized* seizure, but they may have had other seizure types that were not recognized as such in the past. These include symptoms suggestive of nocturnal seizures (such as awakening with disorientation, tongue bite, or muscle soreness), myoclonic seizures as in JME, staring spells or lapses in attention that might indicate unrecognized seizures with impairment of awareness, or symptoms suggestive of simple partial seizures. If other seizure types are identified by history, then there is a much stronger indication to treat with AEDs.

As mentioned previously, laboratory investigations and other tests can be helpful to differentiate seizures for mimics and to identify provoking factors for seizures. If there are symptoms of orthopedic injury, then X-rays of the thoracic spine or shoulder may be indicated. If the patient has focal neurologic symptoms after the seizure, then urgent neuroimaging (computed tomography [CT] or MRI) is indicated. Patients with signs or symptoms of central nervous system infection may need a lumbar puncture, which should be done only after imaging excludes any contraindication. Other diagnostic tests can be helpful in determining the likelihood of recurrent seizure, such as EEG and MRI, as discussed in the next section.

Risk of Recurrence

There are several features that can help determine the likelihood of recurrent seizure after a first unprovoked event. These include abnormalities on neurologic examination, the presence of epileptic abnormalities on EEG, abnormal MRI, and nocturnal convulsions. If there is more than one of these factors present on evaluation of a patient with first seizure, then the likelihood of a recurrent event over the next 2 years exceeds 70%, and in almost all cases, an AED should be started. If there are no risk factors, then the risk of recurrent seizure is approximately 20% to 30%, and in many situations, it is reasonable to defer starting an AED until there is a second event.

A normal EEG does not "rule out" the diagnosis of epilepsy. In patients with proven epilepsy, the likelihood of finding epileptiform discharges on a single routine EEG is in the range of 25% to 50%. The likelihood increases with multiple EEGs, recordings done immediately after the seizure, or prolonged EEGs. However, there are some patients with epilepsy who never have epileptiform discharges on EEG because of the location or extent of the epileptic focus. Therefore it is important to consider EEG findings in the appropriate clinical context.

Seizures and Safety

A discussion about safety should occur with every patient who has had a seizure. In patients with a single unprovoked seizure, the highest risk of subsequent seizures is in the first 6 months after the initial event, and patients should be particularly cautious during this period. Patients should be advised to use caution when performing any activities that would subject them to a particularly high risk of harm in the event of lost consciousness or awareness, such as climbing ladders, using firearms or power tools, working at heights or around heavy machinery, and driving. Providers should be aware of the laws pertaining to driving and epilepsy in their jurisdiction and should discuss these with the patient.

TREATMENT

Pharmacologic Treatment
General Principles

The choice of AED depends on a number of factors, including epilepsy syndrome and seizure type, side effect profile, comorbidities, drug interactions, and cost. In addition, there are several special considerations in women with epilepsy.

Choice of Antiepileptic Drug Depending on Epilepsy Syndrome and Seizure Type

The first step in determining an AED is to establish the likely epilepsy syndrome and seizure types. There is a more limited range of AEDs typically used to treat generalized seizure types, whereas a greater number of drugs are effective in preventing focal-onset seizures. Table 26.2 shows the AEDs that are effective for both generalized and focal seizure types ("broad spectrum") and those that are effective for focal-onset seizures ("narrow spectrum"). Ethosuximide is effective for absence seizures only. There is limited data regarding the comparative efficacy of AEDs, particularly many of the newer drugs. As such, the choice of AED may depend on other considerations, such as side effects and comorbidities, as outlined in the next section.

Side Effects and Comorbidities

All AEDs have the potential to cause side effects, especially at higher doses. Whenever possible, the lowest effective dose of the best-tolerated AED should be used. Each drug has particularly common side effects, and these should be considered in relation to the patient's comorbidities and preferences.

TABLE 26.2	Broad- and Narrow-Spectrum Antiepileptic Drugs

AEDs That Are Effective for Both Generalized and Focal-Onset Seizures ("Broad Spectrum")	AEDs That Are Effective for Focal-Onset Seizures, Including Secondarily Generalized Seizures ("Narrow Spectrum")
Brivaracetam	Carbamazepine
Clobazam	Eslicarbazepine
Felbamate	Gabapentin
Lamotrigine	Lacosamide
Levetiracetam	Oxcarbazepine
Perampanel	Phenobarbital
Rufinamide	Phenytoin
Topiramate	Pregabalin
Valproic acid	Vigabatrin
Zonisamide	

Refer to the On-Call Formulary starting on page 485 for dosages, side effects, and prescribing notes.

AED, Antiepileptic drug.

Skin rash and allergic reaction: AEDs that are most likely to cause an allergic skin reaction include lamotrigine, phenytoin, phenobarbital, oxcarbazepine, and carbamazepine. Patients who have had a skin rash with one of these medications are more likely to develop a rash with another medication. Therefore in patients with a history of skin rash or other allergic reaction caused by an AED, medications with low risk of rash, such as valproic acid, levetiracetam, pregabalin, or topiramate, should be considered.

Migraine: Several AEDs also are indicated for prevention of migraines, including topiramate and valproic acid. These medications may be considered as monotherapy or add-on therapy in patients with frequent migraines.

Psychiatric disease: Psychiatric comorbidities such as depression and anxiety are very common in patients with epilepsy. In patients with particularly prominent psychiatric disorders, medications with higher rates of psychiatric side effects (levetiracetam, vigabatrin, clobazam, perampanel, and possibly brivaracetam) should be used with caution. Patients with bipolar disorder may benefit from AEDs with mood-stabilizing effects, such as lamotrigine, valproic acid, carbamazepine, and oxcarbazepine.

Weight gain/obesity: Valproic acid and pregabalin have been associated with particularly high rates of weight gain, and they should be used with caution in patients with obesity. Zonisamide and topiramate can be associated with appetite suppression and weight loss, which may be a beneficial side effect in some patients.

Hepatic disease: Most AEDs undergo some hepatic metabolism. In patients with severe hepatic disease, medications with minimal or no hepatic metabolism, including gabapentin, levetiracetam, and pregabalin may be preferred. In the case of mild-to-moderate hepatic dysfunction, the doses of most other AEDs may require adjustments. Valproic acid should be avoided in patients with severe hepatic disease, and free levels of highly protein-bound AEDs, particularly phenytoin, should be monitored.

Renal disease: Several AEDs undergo significant renal clearance, including eslicarbazepine, felbamate, gabapentin, lacosamide, levetiracetam, oxcarbazepine, phenobarbital, pregabalin, primidone, topiramate, vigabatrin, and zonisamide. These AEDs will require dosage adjustments in the presence of renal failure. Several AEDs are removed with hemodialysis, requiring an additional dose after dialysis sessions. Careful monitoring of predialysis and postdialysis levels of these medications, if possible, is recommended.

AEDs in the elderly: The pharmacokinetics of AEDs can vary significantly in elderly patients. The clearance of most AEDs is reduced by 20% to 40% in elderly patients. Therefore in elderly patients it is recommended to start at the lowest possible effective dose and increase slowly as needed ("start low, go slow"). Adjustments should be made for decreased creatinine clearance or for other nonepilepsy medications with significant interactions.

Cognitive side effects: Several AEDs are associated with relatively high rates of cognitive side effects, particularly topiramate, zonisamide, phenytoin, and valproic acid. In patients with prominent underlying cognitive dysfunction, or in patients who are particularly sensitive to cognitive side effects, these medications should be used with caution.

Drug Interactions

Many AEDs have prominent drug interactions, including both inhibition and induction of hepatic enzymes. Patients should be aware if the medication they are taking has significant interactions, and the interaction profile should be reviewed with any new medication that is started. Table 26.3 shows the AEDs that are hepatic enzyme inducers and inhibitors.

Special Considerations in Women With Epilepsy

There are several important considerations for women with epilepsy, particularly those of childbearing potential. Contraception should be discussed with every woman of childbearing potential who is taking an AED. Medications that are inducers of hepatic

TABLE 26.3	Antiepileptic Drugs With P450 Enzyme-Inducing or Enzyme-Inhibiting Effects

Enzyme-Inducing AEDs	Enzyme-Inhibiting AEDs
May reduce effectiveness of warfarin, oral contraceptives, other AEDs, and many other medications.	Can increase levels of coumadin and other AEDs, resulting in toxicity.
Strong Enzyme Inducers Carbamazepine Phenobarbital Phenytoin Primidone	**Examples include:** Felbamate Valproic acid
Weaker Enzyme Inducers Eslicarbazepine Oxcarbazepine Perampanel (12 mg daily or higher) Topiramate (200 mg daily or higher)	

AED, Antiepileptic drug.

enzymes may reduce the effectiveness of combined oral contraceptive pills. Women taking these medications should be aware that they need an alternative method to ensure adequate contraception. Conversely, the oral contraceptive pill can profoundly decrease levels of lamotrigine. Therefore women who are on a steady dose of lamotrigine will likely require an adjustment in dose on starting or stopping an oral contraceptive pill.

A discussion about pregnancy and epilepsy is highly recommended for every woman with epilepsy of childbearing potential. It is best to have this discussion before pregnancy because unintended pregnancy in women with epilepsy is very common. All women with epilepsy of childbearing potential should take folic acid supplementation (1 mg daily at all times; 4–5 mg daily if planning pregnancy) to reduce potential teratogenic effects of AEDs. If at all possible, valproic acid should be avoided in women with epilepsy of childbearing potential because of high rates of teratogenicity and cognitive dysfunction. The teratogenic potential of other AEDs should be discussed with the woman, and the risks and benefits of continuing AEDs through pregnancy should be weighed. Medications such as lamotrigine and levetiracetam are associated with relatively low rates of major congenital malformations (~3%), and there are significant risks to both fetus and mother from recurrent seizures in pregnancy, particularly generalized tonic-clonic seizures. The levels of several medications should be monitored through pregnancy because they can decrease significantly. In particular, levels of lamotrigine can drop two- to 3-fold in pregnancy, requiring substantial increases in dose to ensure a therapeutic level. Levels of levetiracetam and oxcarbazepine also can drop during pregnancy, although not to the same degree as lamotrigine.

Dietary Therapy

The **ketogenic diet** is most often used for children with severe epilepsy syndromes. It is a high-fat, low-carbohydrate diet that results in production of ketone bodies and other metabolic changes that simulate starvation. The mechanism by which this diet improves seizures is unknown, but approximately two-thirds of patients have significant improvement in seizure frequency, and up to one-third have a profound reduction in seizures. This diet can be difficult to maintain, and it has many potential adverse effects. Other diets, including the *modified Atkins diet,* may be easier to implement and maintain, and it can result in substantial improvement in seizure frequency in some patients.

Surgical Treatment

Every patient with refractory epilepsy should be referred to a tertiary center for consideration of epilepsy surgery. A patient who has continued to have seizures in spite of treatment with two appropriate AEDs at therapeutic doses has only a 5% chance of becoming seizure free with a trial of a third medication. Therefore epilepsy surgery should be considered early in the course of refractory epilepsy.

Focal Resection

Patients may be considered candidates for resective surgery if (1) a focus of seizure onset can be identified and (2) that focus can be safely resected without resulting in neurologic disability. Many patients become seizure-free after resective surgery, with long-term seizure freedom rates of up to 70% to 80% in carefully selected patients with temporal lobe epilepsy. Rates of seizure freedom are lower in extratemporal epilepsy, but a meaningful improvement in seizure frequency can be achieved in most carefully selected patients. Patients with a lesion associated with epilepsy that can be identified on MRI (such as a low-grade tumor, vascular malformation, or malformation of cortical development) have higher rates of seizure freedom after epilepsy surgery than patients with no abnormality on MRI.

Other Neurosurgical Options

There are several options available to patients for whom a focal resection is not possible. In patients with a seizure focus that cannot be resected because of the risk of subsequent disability, *multiple subpial transections*, in which horizontal fibers are transected to prevent lateral spread of seizures, can spare the vertical descending fibers and thus preserve neurologic function. *Corpus callosotomy* can decrease drop attacks in patients with frequent injuries. *Hemispherectomy* is a treatment that can be used in severe unilateral epilepsy syndromes such as Rasmussen encephalitis and hemimegalencephaly. *Gamma knife stereotactic radiosurgery* can be effective for some types of vascular malformations and brain tumors. *Stereotactic laser ablation* is a promising minimally invasive technique that may be an option for the treatment of some types of focal lesions, but further research is necessary to elucidate the risks and benefits of this approach compared with traditional resective approaches.

Neurostimulation for Epilepsy

The *vagus nerve stimulator* is a device that provides periodic electrical stimulation of the vagus nerve through a pacemaker that is implanted in the upper chest. The stimulation parameters can be adjusted by the physician based on the patient's response and side effects. The mechanism of action of this device is unclear, although the vagus nerve has several afferent projections to areas of the brain that are important in seizure generation. Up to one-third of patients will have a significant reduction in seizures with this device, but it is rare for a patient to become seizure free. The effectiveness of this device may increase over time. There are minimal side effects, other than a change in voice, and cough during stimulation.

The *responsive neurostimulator (RNS) device* includes electrodes that are placed over seizure foci that can simultaneously record and stimulate to prevent propagation of seizures. This device may be particularly useful in patients with multiple epileptic foci (such as in bitemporal epilepsy) or in patients with an epileptic focus that cannot be resected because of concerns about subsequent neurologic dysfunction. Forty percent to 45% of patients will have a significant reduction in seizures with this device, but complete seizure freedom is uncommon. The RNS device has the initial advantage of providing long-term seizure recording, which can be useful in monitoring response to other treatments.

Pediatric Neurology

A developmental, social, and family history should be obtained for every pediatric patient seen as an emergency. The guardians' understanding of any preexisting diseases and of the cause of the current events also should be elicited. At first glance, determine the degree of neurologic compromise by estimating the level of alertness of the child and the need for rapid intervention. Then, direct the interview toward assessing the child's baseline neurologic performance and how the current event departs from it. Infants become more cooperative when they are spoken to in a pleasant voice, and children are less intimidated when the examiner appears to ignore them at first. When possible, children should be examined while resting on their caretaker's lap and should be engaged in conversation and play. Careful observation and holding of normal-appearing children may reveal unsuspected tone anomalies (Fig. 27.1) but should be reserved for the end of the examination. Both intellectual and motor milestones should be documented (Table 27.1). The basic anthropometric measures (weight, length and, most importantly, head circumference) also should be charted. Normative growth charts are available from the National Center for Health Statistics, Hyattsville, MD 20782 or at http://www.cdc.gov/growthcharts/.

BIRTH TRAUMA

Large (over 4500-g) infants, use of instrumentation during delivery, uncommon fetal presentations, augmented delivery, and first vaginal delivery are all associated with neurologic birth trauma. **Clavicular fracture,** the most common form of trauma, is diagnosed by palpation and, if needed, by radiographs. Spontaneous recovery is the rule.

Birth Injury of the Brachial Plexus

presents with flaccid paralysis as a result of injury to one or several brachial plexus roots. It occurs rarely and affects less than 1% of live

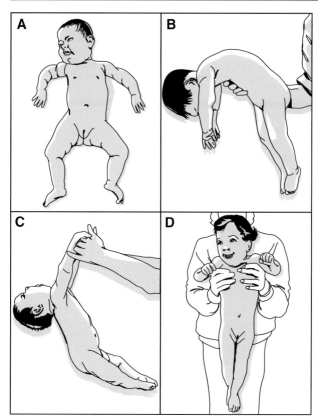

FIG. 27.1 Examination of tone. (A–C) Severe hypotonia in an infant with spinal muscular atrophy. (A) Hypotonic frog-legged posture with arms adducted, legs in external rotation, and knee flexion. All limbs make contact with the examination table. (B) Ventral suspension revealing limp arms and legs and poor neck extension. (C) Pulling maneuver demonstrating significant head lag and extended legs. (D) Hypertonicity after periventricular leukomalacia. The thumbs are in a "cortical" position, and the legs display "scissoring."

births, with an incidence of 0.04% to 0.4%. Obstetrical history, prolonged labor, or use of instrumentation are potential risk factors to explain the nature of brachial plexus injury. Shoulder dystocia and microsomia are the most common causes leading to brachial plexus injury.

TABLE 27.1	Normal Developmental Milestones

Age (Months)	Milestones
1 to 1½	Head control; identification of familiar persons
4	Smiling; attempts at lifting up the head briefly
6	Reaching for objects; rolling from prone to supine
8	Transfer between hands; sitting with support; combination of syllables
10	Standing held; fine grasp
12	Walking supported; two-word or three-word vocabulary
15	Walking unsupported
18	Command following
24	Phrases
36	Handedness develops

The clinical examination is essential to make the diagnosis of brachial plexus injury. Inspection of the newborn may reveal an asymmetry in spontaneous movements. During the examination mobilization of the affected extremity might be painful, particularly within the first week of life. However, asymmetry in the Moro reflex can elicit clinical signs of flaccid arm paralysis during the examination. Involvement of the upper roots, C5-C7, is seen in nearly 75% of the newborns presenting with brachial plexus injury. The affected limb presents with a characteristic position such as shoulder in adduction and internal rotation, elbow in extension, forearm in pronation, and wrist in extension. Paralysis of the hemidiaphragm can occur in the presence of phrenic nerve damage. Injury of the upper roots or proximal portion of the brachial plexus occurs in 50% to 80% of cases. Distal paralysis (Klumpke palsy) accounts for only 2% of the cases presenting with brachial plexus injury. In the presence of distal brachial plexus injury, flaccid paralysis involves the wrist and the hand, whereas the functions of elbow and shoulder are spared (Fig. 27.2).

Brachial plexus injury resulting secondary to birth trauma has a favorable outcome with the chance of complete recovery in 75% to 95% of the cases. The presence of total paralysis and Horner syndrome suggest poor prognosis.

Spinal Cord Injury

Spinal cord injury, sometimes caused by rotation of the head during forceps or forceful extraction, may be difficult to appreciate in infants with a low Apgar score. Long-term sequelae include hydromyelia and myelomalacia. C1-C2 subluxation, however, is more common and follows a benign course. Atlantoaxial rotatory subluxation may cause torticollis. When caudal dysraphism is

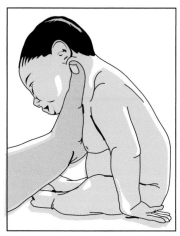

FIG. 27.2 Erb palsy in a newborn. The limb is adducted and internally rotated.

suspected, lumbosacral ultrasounds may be obtained until the sixth month of life. Magnetic resonance imaging (MRI) is the preferred diagnostic test for an accurate diagnosis.

Tentorial Subdural Hematoma

A tentorial subdural hematoma that resolves within the first weeks of life occurs predominantly in neonates who are extracted with a vacuum. **Subgaleal hemorrhage** is palpable as a soft collection that crosses skull sutures and may cause progressive anemia and consumption coagulopathy. **Cephalohematoma** is confined to the subperiosteum and therefore respects suture lines; it is firm to palpation and self-limited. Both should be differentiated from **caput succedaneum** caused by subcutaneous edema involving the presenting part during delivery.

HYPOTONIC NEWBORN

Extreme prematurity and **sepsis** are the leading causes of newborn hypotonia. When encephalopathy is caused by ischemia, and Down syndrome, Prader-Willi syndrome, and neurotransmitter disorders have been excluded, attention must be turned to the spinal cord, nerve, or muscle as the cause of hypotonia. **Infantile spinal muscular atrophy (SMA)** may occasionally present in the newborn period and is sometimes accompanied by arthrogryposis or respiratory failure. Lower motor neuron signs and tongue fasciculation are present. The first diagnostic step for SMA is the genotyping of the SMN gene for deletions. **Congenital myotonic dystrophy** can be associated with a diaphragmatic hernia and is usually maternally inherited in an autosomal dominant fashion; therefore mothers should be examined for myotonia. **Neonatal myasthenia gravis** is caused by placental antibody transfer from a mother afflicted by myasthenia gravis or inflammatory bowel disease. **Congenital myopathies** are characterized by their histologic appearance (with nemaline, central cores, or myotubules), whereas the **metabolic myopathies** mitochondrial DNA depletion syndrome, Pompe disease (with cardiomegaly, macroglossia, and anterior horn cell dysfunction), and cytochrome C oxidase deficiency exhibit specific metabolic abnormalities useful for diagnosis. **Congenital muscular dystrophies** may be associated with cerebral dysgenesis and signs of severe encephalopathy including seizures and hydrocephalus. The **congenital myasthenic syndromes** are caused by mutations in the neuromuscular junction apparatus, and some can manifest with diminished pupillary reactivity or recurrent apnea (the latter sometimes becoming prominent later in childhood), in addition to fatigability and weakness. Often, an "unexplained" elevation of serum aspartate transaminase (AST) and alanine transaminase (ALT) (originating from muscle instead of the liver) in a weak infant (or a child) is the first clue to a myopathy until creatine kinase (CK) is eventually measured.

CEREBROVASCULAR COMPLICATIONS OF PREMATURITY

Premature infants are susceptible to intraventricular hemorrhage, periventricular hemorrhagic infarction, and periventricular leukomalacia. Diagnosis by ultrasonography can be performed for as long as the anterior fontanelle remains open. **Intraventricular hemorrhage** is associated with extreme prematurity (or birth weight below 1500 g) and occurs within the first few days of life. It is divided into grades I (germinal matrix), II (intraventricular blood that does not distort the ventricular system), III (blood that causes ventricular enlargement), and IV (parenchymal infiltration). Higher-grade hemorrhages cause hydrocephalus, which is manifested as an abrupt increase in head circumference and a bulging fontanelle. Decreased tone or spontaneous movements, loss of pupillary reactivity, apnea, hypotension, and anemia may be associated features. Serial lumbar punctures relieve the hydrocephalus in some cases; the remaining hydrocephaluss may require ventriculoperitoneal or ventriculosubgaleal shunt. Long-term outcome correlates with the degree of parenchymal damage.

Periventricular Hemorrhagic Infarction

Periventricular hemorrhagic infarction, which must be distinguished from intraventricular hemorrhage type IV, is a venous infarct probably caused by compression of terminal veins located under the germinal matrix of the lateral ventricles. The infarct involves the dorsal and lateral aspect of the lateral ventricle and is usually asymmetric, evolving into a cavity that communicates with the ventricle. It is associated with a significant mortality rate and with spastic hemiparesis in survivors.

Periventricular Leukomalacia

Periventricular leukomalacia affects the white matter of the centrum semiovale. It is caused by perfusion failure at the border zone between the long penetrator vessels branching off the middle cerebral artery that enter the brain from its surface and the basal lenticulostriate arteries (short penetrators). It may cause spastic quadriparesis with predominant lower extremity involvement or paraplegia (see Fig. 27.1). The lesions tend to cavitate, causing a typical Swiss cheese ultrasound appearance of the white matter.

NEONATAL SEIZURES

The etiology, clinical, and electroencephalography (EEG) features of neonatal seizures are different from the seizures reported in the infants and older children. Neonatal seizures are considered "acute seizures" as a result of a specific etiology such as hypoxia, ischemia, and other metabolic derangements. Hypoxic ischemic encephalopathy remains the most common cause of neonatal seizures followed by ischemic stroke, intracerebral hemorrhage, infection, and metabolic abnormalities.

Newborns do not display generalized seizures, possibly because of immature myelination; however, focal cortical excitation in newborns affects the brain function diffusely. Causes of neonatal and early infantile seizures are listed in Table 27.2. In neonates, clinical diagnosis of seizures may not be straightforward, and EEG monitoring is required to assess baseline EEG findings and characterize the clinical events of interest. Approximately 50% of seizures in neonates present without clinical manifestations or with signs. Therefore recognition of nonconvulsive seizures by EEG is crucial to optimize the medical treatment.

Except in rare cases, neonatal convulsions are not a benign phenomenon. Newborns and infants younger than 3 months of age with unexplained new-onset seizures should be evaluated and treated for infection until blood, urine, and cerebrospinal fluid (CSF) cultures are negative for at least 2 days, even without fever. In the

TABLE 27.2	Causes of Neonatal and Early Infantile Seizures

Sepsis and meningitis
Intrauterine infection (TORCH)
Drug effect or withdrawal
Cerebral dysgenesis
Ischemic encephalopathy
Intraventricular hemorrhage of prematurity
Other intracranial hemorrhages
Biotinidase deficiency
Folinic-acid responsive seizures
Pyridoxine dependency
Glycine encephalopathy
Neonatal maple syrup urine disease
Hypoparathyroidism and hypocalcemia
Menkes disease
Cerebral venous thrombosis
Tuberous sclerosis
Fukuyama muscular dystrophy
Muscle-eye-brain disease
Infantile neuronal ceroid lipofucsinosis
Incontinentia pigmenti
Urea cycle defects
Familial benign neonatal seizures
Organic acidemia
Ketotic hyperglycinemia
Neonatal adrenoleukodystrophy and other leukodystrophies
Gaucher disease type 2
GM_1 gangliosidosis
Herpes simplex encephalitis
Sulfite oxidase deficiency
Glucose transporter type 1 deficiency
Pyruvate dehydrogenase deficiency
Pyruvate carboxylase deficiency

List is roughly in order of frequency. *TORCH*, Toxoplasmosis, other (syphilis, varicella-zoster, parvovirus B19), rubella, cytomegalovirus, and herpes infections.

absence of infection or of cerebral structural abnormality detectable by imaging, the single most important diagnostic procedure is the lumbar puncture. CSF protein levels can be as high as 150 mg/dL in normal newborns, but glucose should never fall below 40 mg/dL. Several polymorphonuclear cells also may be found in the CSF after delivery. A small volume of extra CSF may be stored in ice for specialized analyses for up to 16 hours. Continuous video EEG monitoring may reveal unsuspected ictal events and background rhythm abnormalities in neonates. Management also should include immediate evaluation of electrolytes with correction if needed.

Treatment

Currently, there is no consensus for the optimal treatment of neonatal seizures. **Phenobarbital** is given as a **20 mg/kg intravenously (IV)** load, followed by **5 mg/kg** daily orally or IV. Two repeat loading doses of **10 mg/kg** may be administered for refractory seizures. To avoid respiratory depression, care must be taken not to add a benzodiazepine while administering phenobarbital. **Fosphenytoin** at a loading dose of **20 mg/kg IV** may substitute or be added to phenobarbital. Levetiracetam is an alternative, although the efficacy of levetiracetam as a first-line treatment remains to be determined. In the case of refractory neonatal seizures, consider underlying metabolic encephalopathy, for which specific treatment may be warranted.

A number of metabolic disorders including mitochondrial disorders may be responsive to vitamin therapy. In pyridoxine-dependent epilepsy, pyridoxine administration is diagnostic for this epileptic encephalopathy Low EEG demonstrates the burst suppression pattern, which reverses with IV pyridoxine (50–100 mg). In suspicious cases, oral administration at 30 mg/kg/day divided into 2 to 3 doses may be given as a trial for 3 consecutive days. Diagnosis can be established by elevated alpha amino adipic acid and pipecolic acid, and by mutation in the ALDH7A1 by genetic test. Clinical management should include oral administration of pyridoxine with the daily dosage of 15 to 30 mg/kg/day divided into two or three doses.

Other vitamin-responsive epilepsies include pyridoxine-5 phosphate (PLP5)–dependent epilepsy treated with PLP 30 to 60 mg/kg/day divided into 4 to 6 daily doses, folinic acid–responsive seizures treated with folinic acid 3 to 5 mg/kg/day plus pyridoxine, and biotinidase deficiency, which responds to biotin supplement. Children diagnosed with biotinidase deficiency often present with infantile-onset seizures including infantile spasms.

INFANTILE SPASMS

West syndrome (infantile spasms) is age-specific epilepsy that affects predominantly infants between 4 and 6 months of age. Infantile spasms often present with autonomic changes such as cyanosis, pallor or sweating, vocalizations, nystagmus, eye deviation, or grimacing. The spasms are seizures characterized by an initial contraction followed by a more sustained tonic phase. They may be either abduction and extension of the extremities (extensor spasms), flexion and adduction of extremities (flexor spasms), or mixed. Other seizure types can accompany infantile spasms prior to the onset or follow the offset of infantile spasms such as focal seizures. There are a number of precipitating factors described to trigger infantile spasms, such as handling (diaper change, feeding), loud noise or tactile stimulus, excitement, anger, fever, and change in the environmental temperature. Differential diagnosis should include sleep myoclonus, myoclonic epilepsy of infancy presenting with myoclonic seizures, Sandifer syndrome (gastroesophageal reflux), spasticity, and excessive startle response (hyperplexia). EEG video recording will provide information to characterize the clinical seizures and to establish a definitive diagnosis of infantile spasms.

The underlying etiology may vary. Prenatal causes include chromosomal abnormalities, inborn errors of metabolism, and neurocutaneous syndromes (such as tuberous sclerosis, cortical malformations, and intrauterine infections). Perinatal causes include ischemic encephalopathy and birth trauma. Postnatal causes include central nervous system (CNS) trauma, infection, and intracranial hemorrhage. The smaller group is characterized by the lack of prior encephalopathy or of known cause, and it is associated with a better long-term outcome. Standard first-line treatments should include adrenocorticotropic hormone (ACTH) and/or vigabatrin, which will accomplish seizure control in approximately 60% to 70% of the patients.

FEBRILE SEIZURES

Febrile seizures are one of the most common seizure types reported in children between the age of 6 months and 5 years; they are often secondary to self-limitng viral infection caused by upper respiratory infections or gastrointestinal infections. Overall frequency was reported in 2% to 5% in the population. Simple febrile seizures are defined by duration less than 15 minutes without lateralizing features. Complex febrile seizures present with focal features such as eye deviation, arm or leg or face twitching, or unilateral stiffening. If a febrile seizure lasts longer than 30 minutes, it is classified as febrile status epilepticus, which requires immediate medical intervention. Approximately 90% of children have their first febrile seizure before the age of 3 years. Only 6% of febrile seizures occur before 6 months and 4% after 2 years of age. A majority of the children will have a history of normal growth and development. Approximately 25% to 40% have a family history of febrile seizures. Mutations in the subunit genes of neuronal voltage-gated sodium channels or GABA-A receptor subunit gene mutations have been reported, but with its benign course routine genetic testing is not recommended.

Risk of febrile seizure recurrence is about 30%, although more than three febrile seizures are seen in less than 5%. The younger the age at the time of the first febrile seizure, the higher the risk of febrile seizure recurrence: Febrile seizure recurrence is associated with younger age at the time of first febrile seizure. If a first febrile seizure is prolonged, then a subsequent febrile seizure can be prolonged as well.

Diagnosis

Regarding diagnostic workup, neuroimaging studies such as brain computed tomography (CT) or MRI is generally not indicated after a febrile convulsion unless focal clinical features are reported at the onset of the seizure. Similarly, EEG may be of limited use and may show transient EEG abnormalities after the seizure offset. Therefore routine EEG is not recommended for children presenting with febrile seizures.

Treatment

To eliminate febrile status epilepticus, diazepam rectal gel is recommended as an abortive treatment if a convulsion lasts longer than 5 minutes. However, because the risk for additional febrile seizures is higher when the first febrile seizure is prolonged, rectal diazepam can be administered earlier than 5 minutes. In case of prolonged or repeated seizures, caregivers should call 911. Long-term use of the anticonvulsant treatment is not recommended for febrile seizures or febrile status epilepticus. Administration of rectal diazepam does not pose any adverse reaction or respiratory depression other than drowsiness or sleepiness, which is expected to last 4 to 5 hours after the administration. Caregivers should be cautioned if the convulsion continues after rectal diazepam. Emergency medical services should be immediately contacted in that case.

A number of studies demonstrated that although antipyretics make the child more comfortable, the administration of antipyretics does not prevent recurrence of febrile seizures even at the onset of the febrile illness. Therefore antipyretic prophylaxis is not recommended to prevent febrile seizures. This condition may require a customized evidence-based plan of care to each child and family. Prolonged and daily antiepileptic drug treatment is not recommended to prevent febrile seizures.

Longitudinal studies demonstrated that the risk of developmental, behavioral, and academic disabilities in children with febrile seizures is no greater than in the general population.

DISORDERS THAT RESEMBLE SEIZURES

Syncope may be followed by automatisms and be pallid (thought to represent an exaggerated autonomic response) or cardiogenic (which may be caused by congenital heart disease or long QT syndrome). **Breath-holding spells** occur between 6 months and 2 years of age and are preceded by vigorous crying and followed by brief apnea and cyanosis. **Sandifer syndrome**, which is caused by gastric reflux, can mimic tonic seizures and be accompanied by autonomic dysfunction. **Hyperekplexia** results in loss of tone in response to a sudden stimulus with preserved consciousness. Excessive startle is a feature of some cerebral degenerations such as Tay-Sachs disease. **Benign myoclonus of infancy** occurs as an isolated phenomenon in a normal neurologic substrate and disappears by 12 months of age. Isolated **apnea** is rarely a seizure manifestation, but it can be prominent in nonketotic hyperglycinemia. **Paroxysmal dyskinesias** may be elicited by movement (kinesigenic) or occur at rest (nonkinesigenic). **Spasmus nutans** is a benign condition that usually occurs before 1 year of age and disappears within 2 years. It includes head nodding, torticollis, and nystagmus. When monocular nystagmus is the presenting sign, MRI must be performed to exclude optic nerve glioma. **Oculogyric crises** may last from seconds to hours and can be caused by a variety of agents that interfere with neurotransmitter function or by aromatic L-amino acid decarboxylase deficiency.

INFECTIONS OF THE CENTRAL NERVOUS SYSTEM

Children with CNS infections may present with acute meningitis syndrome; acute encephalitis syndrome; subacute or chronic meningitis syndrome; encephalopathy with systemic infections in which CNS is involved as part of the systemic infection such as malaria, endocarditis, typhoid fever; and postinfectious syndromes such as transverse myelitis or acute disseminated encephalomyelitis (ADEM).

Diagnostic Evaluation

The signs of meningitis may be absent in children who are younger than 3 years of age or neutropenic (absolute neutrophil count below $1000/mm^3$). In the newborn, the most common organisms causing meningitis are Group B *Streptococcus*, *Escherichia coli*, and *Listeria monocytogenes*. *Citrobacter koseri* is the cause for cerebral abscesses during the newborn period. During infancy and preschool age, the responsible microorganisms are *Haemophilus influenzae*, *Neisseria meningitidis*, and *S. pneumoniae* and in school age, *N. meningitidis* and *S. pneumoniae*.

Herpes simplex virus (HSV) is the most common cause of viral encephalitis. *Enteroviruses* are frequent in developing countries with higher incidence in summer and fall. *Japanese encephalitides* is a common encephalitis frequently reported in Asia, particularly in India, Nepal, Philippines, Vietnam, Thailand, Cambodia, and part of China. Early diagnosis and aggressive treatment are critical for CNS infections. High index of suspicion is required to establish early diagnosis and prompt treatment. Clinical history and physical examination are the important and essential first steps to approach diagnosis for CNS infections. The chronology of symptoms and signs will help to categorize the illness to one of the syndromes as described previously. The clinical history regarding trauma, surgery, travel, insect bites, contact, and sexual activity are important elements to determine the etiology. Prior history of viral illness, immune deficiency, presence of ventricular peritoneal shunts, history of respiratory tract infections or gastrointestinal infections, rash, and arthritis are the other important clinical symptoms that help identify the underlying etiology. Acute-onset headache, fever, vomiting, neck stiffness, seizure, and change in mental status are the common presenting symptoms. Neck stiffness, photophobia, bulging fontanel in infants, and positive Kernig sign or Brudzinski sign are the clinical features important for the diagnosis of acute meningitis syndrome. Specific clinical features such as petechiae, shock, and disseminated intravascular coagulation (DIC) are common in meningococcal meningitis. The presence of focal clinical features, alteration of mental status, and focal seizures should raise the concern for encephalitis. History of rash, enlargement of the lymph nodes, history of conjunctivitis or pharyngitis, and low-grade fever should raise the question for viral meningitis, whereas early alteration of mental status and rapid progression should raise the concern for encephalitis.

Diagnosis

After the clinical history and physical examination, spinal fluid examination remains the hallmark for the diagnosis of CNS infection. Lumbar puncture should be avoided in the presence of cardio-respiratory instability, increased intracranial pressure, prolonged seizures, focal neurologic findings on examination, the presence of thrombocytopenia or coagulation disorders, or local infection at the site of lumbar puncture. Lumbar puncture helps to identify the organism in a timely manner and to select appropriate antibiotics and to make the decision for how long to continue appropriate medical treatment. However, in the case of delay of the lumbar puncture, antimicrobial treatment should be administered in all cases of suspected CNS infection. Initial CSF examination should include cell count, measurement of protein and glucose, Gram stain, and culture. In the presence of acute bacterial meningitis, typical CSF findings include increased opening CSF pressure; a white blood cell count of more than 500 cells/μL (<100 cells/μL in early stages), with the majority being polymorphonuclear cells; and elevated protein and low glucose. A single polymorphonuclear cell in the spinal fluid will be consistent with meningitis in the right clinical setting. Most cases of viral meningitis present a clear CSF, normal or slightly elevated proteins, and normal glucose level with or without lymphocytic pleocytosis. The presence of red blood cells in CSF may raise the concern for HSV encephalitis. Gram stain of the CSF sample is a quick method to detect the organism accurately. Approximately 70% to 80% of untreated bacterial meningitis will demonstrate an abnormal positive smear. CSF culture is positive in the majority of untreated cases of meningitis. Polymerase chain reaction (PCR) in CSF is available for common microorganisms causing meningitis. PCR has replaced viral cultures for identification of viral agents including *HSV, JE virus, enterovirus, cytomegalovirus, Epstein-Barr virus, varicella-zoster virus, human herpes virus (HHV)-6, influenza, and adenovirus.* PCR identifies HSV in CSF with a sensitivity of 95% and a specificity of nearly 100%. Therefore PCR analysis for HSV remains the gold standard for the diagnosis of HSV encephalitis. It is important to remember that HSV PCR may be negative during the first 3 days of the illness and after 10 to 14 days of the illness. Spinal tap should be repeated in a few days if the initial assay is noncontributory to the diagnosis.

Neuroimaging has a limited role in the diagnosis of CNS infections. However, the presence of increased intracranial pressure, focal neurologic signs and rapid deterioration of neurologic status or mental status, and hydrocephalus requires immediate neuroimaging using CT scan. However, CT of the head should not be recommended routinely for patients before lumbar puncture. Brain MRI is superior to head CT to demonstrate meningeal enhancement, cerebral edema, and vascular complications in the cases of encephalitis.

EEG has a limited diagnostic value; however, it is a valuable diagnostic method to identify nonconvulsive seizures or status epilepticus in patients with sustained mental status changes. EEG should be performed in all patients presenting with focal neurologic findings and patients who have clinical features of encephalitis. The presence of periodic lateralized epileptiform discharges and focal temporal slowing should raise the concern for HSV encephalitis.

Treatment of Central Nervous System Infections

The diagnosis of CNS infection requires immediate attention for timely diagnosis and management. For empiric antibiotic coverage, see Table 22.2. All children diagnosed with CNS infections must be kept under close observation and monitoring. CNS infections may present with life-threatening complications such as raised intracranial pressure, DIC, shock, and status epilepticus. Therefore clinical features warrant the admission to the inpatient pediatric service or intensive care unit. In the presence of a Glasgow Coma Scale score of less than 8, early intubation and mechanical intubation should be considered. Shock could occur in the early stages or during the clinical course of CNS infection, which may be septic, neurogenic, or hypovolemic. Therefore hemodynamic status should be monitored closely, and fluid replacement should be considered if there is a sign of shock such as tachycardia, hypertension, or prolonged capillary refill time.

Treatment should not be delayed if lumbar puncture is contraindicated. Appropriate IV antimicrobial therapy should be applied to cover all likely causative organisms without delay. A third-generation cephalosporin is commonly recommended with an excellent response against *H. influenzae, N. meningitidis,* and *S. pneumoniae.* Duration of antibiotic treatment should depend on the causative organism. Antibiotic treatment should be continued for 7 days for CNS infection with *H. influenzae* type b and *N. meningitidis*; 10 to 14 days for *S. pneumonia;* and a minimum of 2 weeks for gram-negative, group B *Streptococcus, E. coli*, and *L. monocytogenes.* Acyclovir should be administered promptly if HSV encephalitis is suspected at a dose of 60 mg/kg/day divided into three doses for 21 days. PCR should be obtained prior to discontinuing acyclovir. If the PCR remains positive, then therapy should be continued with weekly follow-up of CSF PCR until the PCR is found negative.

Beneficial effects of steroids are found in patients diagnosed with acute meningitis to reduce the inflammatory response, which can lead to tissue damage and worsening neurologic outcome such as hearing loss. Empiric use of dexamethasone at the dose of 0.15 mg/kg/dose four times a day is recommended for the duration of 2 to 4 days, prior or up to 12 hours after the first dose of antibiotics. However, routine administration of steroids in acute meningitis is not recommended.

Children diagnosed with CNS infection associated with *H. influenzae* or *N. meningitidis* should be isolated for the first 24 hours, commencing antibiotic treatment to prevent spread of infection. Close contact of all children with meningococcal meningitis should receive prophylactic treatment, and contacts of those with *H. influenzae* should receive ceftriaxone or rifampicin. Unvaccinated children less than 5 years of age also should be vaccinated against *H. influenzae* as soon as possible.

Sequelae of meningitis include hydrocephalus, mental retardation, epilepsy, and hearing loss. Intracranial pressure can be raised because of cerebral edema, cerebral infarction, cerebral venous thrombosis, obstructive hydrocephalus, and syndrome of inappropriate antidiuretic hormone secretion (SIADH) in children diagnosed with CNS infection. Therefore raised intracranial pressure should be recognized and treated promptly to prevent cerebral herniation and death.

FULMINANT ENCEPHALOPATHIES OF INFANCY AND CHILDHOOD

Several inflammatory disorders may first manifest with fever, depressed consciousness, seizures, meningeal signs, and CSF pleocytosis in the absence of infection.

Acute Disseminated Encephalomyelitis (ADEM)

ADEM is an immune-mediated inflammatory disorder of the CNS. The diagnosis is often made in the setting of defined viral infection or immunization. The age of presentation is usually between ages 5 and 8 years in children. ADEM is classically defined as a monophasic disorder. Approximately 70% of patients present with the clinical history of recent infection or immunization. The initial phase is often described by malaise, headache, and nausea and vomiting. The progression of the clinical symptoms is often fast and progresses into meningeal signs and drowsiness within a few days. Therefore ADEM is acknowledged as a rapid-onset encephalopathy associated with a combination of multifocal neurologic symptoms. Frequent neurologic symptoms include unilateral or bilateral **cortical** signs, ataxia, seizures, impairment of speech and swallow, visual loss, ataxia, and change in mental status ranging from lethargy to coma. In children, headache and fever are reported often. Seizures are seen rarely in adult patients, whereas they are more common in younger children. Seizures will often present with focal motor seizures. Status epilepticus is reported in more than 80% of patients. Peripheral nervous system involvement is rare in children presenting with ADEM. However, peripheral nervous system and CNS involvement is reported in approximately 50% of the adult patients presenting with ADEM. Neuroimaging findings are essential for the diagnosis of ADEM. Most frequent MRI abnormalities include patchy, increased fluid attenuation inversion recovery (FLAIR) signals. Lesions reported in ADEM are often asymmetric and seen in multiple distributions involving subcortical and central white matter, cortical gray–white matter junction, brain stem, cerebellum, and spinal cord. Additionally involvement of the thalamus and basal ganglia is seen. Large demyelinating lesions may extend into the corpus callosum. In ADEM, gadolinium-enhancing lesions may correlate with inflammation. Gadolinium-enhancing lesions can be seen in 30% to 100% of the patients. The enhancement pattern may vary from gyral to spotty to nodular enhancements. Meningeal enhancement is not expected. Spinal cord involvement can occur in only 10% to 30% of the patients. A variable enhancement pattern can be seen in nodular patterns as well. Four different patterns of MRI abnormalities are described in ADEM as follows:

1. Small lesions with diameters less than 5 mm.
2. Large **single** lesion surrounded by perilesional edema and mass effect.
3. Symmetric **bithalamic** involvement.
4. Acute hemorrhagic encephalomyelitis.

Based on the clinical history and neuroimaging findings, the differential diagnosis should include brain tumor, Schilder disease, brain abscess, and multiple sclerosis. Symmetric **bithalamic** involvement should raise the concern for Japanese B encephalitis, cerebral venous thrombosis, hypernatremia, and inborn error of metabolisms affecting energy metabolism such as organic aciduria or infantile bilateral striatal necrosis as a result of mitochondrial encephalomyopathy.

The treatment approaches for ADEM include steroids, IV immunoglobin (IVIG), or plasmapheresis. High-dose steroid treatment is recommended as IV methylprednisolone (10/30 mg/kg/day up to a maximum of 1 g/day) or dexamethasone (1 mg/kg) for 3 to 5 days. Oral steroid taper is recommended for 4 to 6 weeks. Full recovery is reported in 50% to 80% of the patients if treatment continues with oral steroid taper. IVIG should be used at the dose of 1 to 2 g/kg as a single dose or over 3 to 5 days. IVIG is recommended in the failure of IV pulse steroid therapy or in the cases of recurrent demyelination. In a small number of case series, the use of plasma exchange transfusion is reported for the children diagnosed with ADEM. Plasma exchange transfusion is beneficial to remove autoantibodies that might trigger the immune-mediated inflammatory response.

Multiple Sclerosis (MS)

Pediatric MS is a chronic inflammatory and demyelinating disease of the CNS. Fewer than 10% of individuals with multiple sclerosis experience the first clinical demyelinating event before the age of 18. Although it is rare, 20% of pediatric multiple sclerosis is diagnosed before the age of 10 years. Clinical presentation of pediatric multiple sclerosis includes visual loss, gait disturbance, motor weakness, and sensory changes. Transverse myelitis, cerebellar and brain stem involvement, and optic neuritis also could occur as isolated events. Seizures and mental status changes can occur in children; however, they are atypical signs. The relapsing-remitting course is the main clinical presentation in pediatric patients diagnosed with multiple sclerosis, reaching to 85% to 100% of the cases. Approximately one-third of the children who received the diagnosis of ADEM later received the diagnosis of multiple sclerosis.

Neuroimaging findings are essential for the diagnosis of multiple sclerosis. The presence of silent lesions in two of the four locations including periventricular, infratentorial, spinal cord, and juxtacortical regions are characteristic for multiple sclerosis in addition to the presence of **one-sided** gadolinium-enhancing and nonenhancing lesion. If the initial event does not meet the criteria for multiple sclerosis, then subsequent clinical attacks or serial MRI findings when showing new lesion support the diagnosis of multiple sclerosis.

CSF analysis can help to establish a diagnosis of multiple sclerosis. Oligoclonal band presence can occur in more than 90% of children diagnosed with multiple sclerosis. On the other hand, oligoclonal band presence is reported in 5% to 30% of children diagnosed with ADEM. Pericytosis can occur in up to 66% of the children, not exceeding **60 cell/mm^3**. Cytology and flow cytometry are essential to rule out malignancy.

Postinfectious Cerebellitis

Postinfectious cerebellitis can present with acute and profound cerebellar dysfunction, often after the resolution of a trivial infectious illness. In young children the presence of fewer encephalopathy seizures and progressive clinical course should raise the red flag for a differential diagnosis for vasculitis; infectious processes such as bacterial or viral meningitis; other autoimmune or immune-mediated diagnoses associated with autoantibodies such as N-methyl-D-aspartate (NMDA), against NMDA receptors, GAD, and so forth; CNS system lymphoma; inborn error of metabolism such as mitochondrial encephalomyopathy; and Aicardi-Goutières syndrome.

Neuromyelitis Optica (NMO)

NMO (Devic disease) is associated with optic neuritis and necrotizing myelitis occurring either simultaneously or in succession, often without CSF oligoclonal protein bands and often accompanied by cerebral white matter demyelinating plaques. Antimyelin oligodendrocyte glycoprotein (anti-MOG)–associated disease reported in children almost resembles the clinical features of multiple sclerosis. MOG is expressed on the outer myelin membrane.

Spinal cord and optic nerve involvements are seen predominantly with this diagnosis. Rarely brain and brain stem involvement can occur. The antibody against the AQP4 protein was identified with this syndrome. This protein is essential for the formation of the blood–brain barrier, and is expressed in astrocytes. Antibody binding astrocytes affect the function and therefore change in the blood–brain barrier formation, which triggers inflammation that promotes the demyelination process. In the presence of negative AQP4 testing, the testing should be repeated 6 months later.

Acute Toxic Encephalopathy

Acute toxic encephalopathy is more common in children younger than 2 years and may be preceded by banal infections, and it causes cerebral edema without inflammation. The CSF is under high pressure, but its composition is normal. **Acute hemorrhagic encephalitis** is the least common postinfectious and postvaccinal disorder. The pathologic process consists of small-vessel necrotizing vasculitis of gray and white matter with circulating atypical lymphocytes and albuminuria. The CSF pleocytosis occurs at the expense of polymorphonuclear cells. **Serum sickness** occurs as an adverse drug reaction, accompanied by CSF polymorphonuclear, lymphocytic, or eosinophilic pleocytosis; elevated protein; and, sometimes, peripheral eosinophilia. Numerous immune-modulating agents can cause a similar picture. CT is usually normal. **Systemic lupus erythematosus** occasionally presents with aseptic meningitis, epilepsy, or psychosis. **Behçet disease** also may present with meningitis or seizures caused by vasculitis in association with orogenital ulcers and uveitis. **Metabolic encephalopathies** are an important consideration even when acute encephalopathy presents without preexisting evidence of an abnormal neurologic substrate. Among these, organic acidemias, Leigh syndrome (subacute necrotizing encephalopathy), aminoacidopathies, urea cycle disorders, fatty acid oxidation defects, and mitochondrial encephalomyopathy with ragged red fibers and strokelike episodes (MELAS) must be considered. Analysis of serum glucose, carnitine metabolites, amino acids, ammonia, creatine kinase and lactate; of urinary ketones and other organic acids; and of CSF amino acids, lactate, and pyruvate constitute an effective initial screening strategy. A dietary trigger may sometimes be identified, as well as a mild prior infection. In the neonate, prompt retrieval of the cursory newborn screening results is mandatory, although not all disorders are screened in all locations (for a US listing, consult http://genes-r-us.uthscsa.edu/resources/newborn/state.htm).

PEDIATRIC STROKE

Stroke in children can be ischemic, hemorrhagic, or both. Ischemic stroke is more frequently caused by occlusion of the arteries, but it also may be secondary to venous occlusion of cerebral veins or sinuses. On the other hand, hemorrhagic stroke occurs as the result of bleeding into the site of acute ischemic stroke. In children, approximately 50% of all strokes are arterial ischemic strokes.

Approximately 10% to 25% of children diagnosed with stroke may die, and approximately 25% may have a recurrence. In children, clinical presentations of stroke may vary based on the age groups. Arterial ischemic strokes more often present with focal neurologic deficit, such as hemiparesis, which is the most common focal manifestation accounting for up to 94% of the cases. On the other hand, hemorrhagic strokes present more often with headache or alteration of mental status compared with arterial ischemic strokes. Seizures can occur in both ischemic and hemorrhagic strokes. Seizures are accounted in approximately 50% of the children with strokes. Younger children often present with nonspecific clinical symptoms such as irritability, feeding difficulties, or vomiting. Older children may have more specific neurologic deficits, particularly focal neurologic signs such as hemiparesis, speech difficulties, and visual deficits.

The underlying etiology is more diverse, and risk factors might be multiple in neonates and children compared with adults. **Fetal stroke** is rare and may be the consequence of maternal alloimmune thrombocytopenia, intrauterine cocaine exposure or trauma, or evolving into porencephaly. In the **neonate**, cardiovascular malformations, elevated plasma homocysteine, polycythemia, factor-V Leiden mutation, deficiency of protein C or protein S, prothrombin mutation, placental embolism, and institution of extracorporeal membrane oxygenation are associated with stroke. Typically, the signs of hemispheric infarction are short-lived (except when complicated by seizures) and do not manifest again until about 6 months of age, when hemiparesis becomes clinically detectable. Transthoracic (as opposed to transesophageal) echocardiography is sufficient to diagnose most cardiac malformations, including persistent foramen ovale. **Older children** also are susceptible to stroke from cardiogenic emboli. In addition, Fabry disease (associated to skin angiokeratomas and neuropathy); moyamoya disease (caused by dysplastic large intracranial vessels leading to compensatory proliferation of malformed capillaries), which is a common entity in both Asian children and in patients with sickle cell disease; and arterial dissection (as the consequence of neck trauma) are all causes of childhood stroke. Children with sickle cell disease are particularly prone to recurrent "silent" infarcts (generally affecting the deep frontal white matter) starting from infancy and causing intellectual decline or poor scholastic achievement. When the medial cerebral artery flow velocity is elevated beyond 200 cm/s in transcranial Doppler measurements, the risk of stroke is very significant unless transfusions are instituted. Conditions mimicking stroke include MELAS (in older children) and alternating hemiplegia of childhood (with onset during infancy); the latter is sometimes caused by a disorder of energy metabolism.

VENTRICULOPERITONEAL SHUNT MALFUNCTION

Permanent drainage of CSF is accomplished by ventriculojugular, ventriculoatrial, ventriculoureteral, or, most commonly, ventriculoperitoneal shunt. The most common cause of congenital or infantile-onset hydrocephalus is aqueductal stenosis, followed by late sequelae of intracranial hemorrhage or infection. Proximal shunt malfunction is caused by either disconnection or obstruction of the intracranial portion of the shunt by hemorrhage or protein. Distal shunt fracture or tip occlusion with viscous perforation or penetration through the retroperitoneal or abdominal fascia also may occur. Complete malfunction in the infant manifests as irritability, feeding difficulties, an enlarged head, and a tense fontanelle. In the older child, it first causes headache, vomiting, and progressive depression of consciousness. Seizures may seldom occur and they suggest shunt infection. An infected shunt additionally causes fever but rarely local signs of infection. Partial shunt malfunction is insidious, develops over weeks or months, and causes poor cognition (first manifested as school difficulties), papilledema, sixth nerve and upgaze palsies, hyperreflexia, and lower extremity hypertonicity. The evaluation involves a radiographic shunt series to assess the continuity and position of the system, a head CT to determine ventricular size (most helpful when prior scans are available for comparison), and tapping of the shunt reservoir by a neurosurgeon with measurement of the pressure if distal malfunction is suspected. All CSF samples should be routinely analyzed and cultured. If malfunction cannot be excluded, then admission for observation is warranted. When it is suspected or confirmed, urgent neurosurgical consultation is required. Infected shunts should generally be removed as soon as infection is found and temporary ventriculostomy considered. "Overshunting" refers to low CSF pressure caused by excess drainage. It also may cause subdural hematoma and postural headaches that are alleviated when the patient is in a supine position.

TUMORS

The mode of presentation of brain tumors depends on volume and location, infiltration of brain and meninges, and development of hydrocephalus. In infancy, they may cause irritability, failure to thrive, developmental arrest and regression, poor feeding, vomiting, and macrocephaly. In childhood, they may not produce localizing neurologic signs but cause progressive and recurrent episodes of headache, ataxia, and vomiting and a rapid increase in head circumference. **Supratentorial hemispheric** tumors, most commonly low-grade astrocytomas and malignant gliomas, may produce focal neurologic deficits and seizures. **Supratentorial midline** tumors such as low-grade gliomas, craniopharyngiomas, and pineal tumors may compress the optic chiasm producing visual disturbances; may affect the hypothalamus altering endocrine function, appetite, and behavior; and may cause Parinaud syndrome or obstructive hydrocephalus. **Infratentorial** tumors cause a variety of symptoms: diffuse brain stem glioma causes cranial neuropathies and long tract signs, and cerebellar astrocytomas, medulloblastomas, and ependymomas produce ataxia, hydrocephalus, and vomiting. On occasion, highly inflammatory demyelinating lesions may be difficult to differentiate from tumors and brain biopsy is recommended. **Neuroblastomas** are extraneural tumors (most commonly abdominal) that in two-thirds of cases are associated with neurologic complications such as metastasis, carcinomatous meningitis, and paraneoplastic opsoclonus-myoclonus. The latter causes erratic, conjugate eye movements ("dancing eyes") and irritability. Emergency **management** of brain tumors includes CT followed by staging MRI including the spine for tumors that are suspected to expand multifocally. **Dexamethasone**, administered **at 0.1 mg/kg four times a day**, relieves symptoms caused by peritumoral edema. Neurosurgical consultation for biopsy, resection, or relief of hydrocephalus must be obtained.

HEAD INJURY

Earlier recognition of a head injury is critical for early intervention and overall outcome. The child's appearance, work of breathing, and color will reveal potentially the underlying pathology. Primary survey of airway, breathing, circulation, and disability should be assessed rapidly for appropriate interventions for potential life-threatening airway or polytrauma issues. A brief history is important to identify the causes of injury and rule out nontraumatic injuries. Glasgow Coma Score is applied to determine the severity of head injury; a score of 13 to 15 is considered mild, 9 to 12 is moderate, and 3 to 8 is severe neurologic injury. After the primary examination, a secondary survey requires evaluation for the mechanism of injury, head examination, palpation for hematomas if present, examination of fontanels, and examination of the skull for possible skull fractures. The presence of periauricular bruising (Battle sign) may indicate basilar skull fracture. The presence of ear bleeding and periorbital bruising (raccoon eyes) are other clinical signs of a basilar skull fracture. Pupillary size and reactivity and funduscopic examination are other clinical features to be examined. Systemic neurologic examination also is essential to identify the severity of trauma.

Initial management of minor accidental head trauma requires establishing the likelihood of cerebral injury and the need for CT scanning of the head. In general, children with a normal examination who have fallen out of bed onto a hard surface, who wore protective equipment such as a helmet, or who were injured more than 6 hours prior to the examination have not sustained cerebral damage. Similarly, brief amnesia, headache, vomiting up to three times, and scalp laceration (alone or in combination) do not suggest brain injury. **Diagnosis** of suspected brain injury relies on CT scan. Skull radiographs are not sufficient for diagnosis. **Management** of suspected brain injury with normal CT includes admission to the hospital for a 24- to 48-hour observation period. The neurologic status should be assessed periodically.

A CT demonstrating hemorrhage or significant contusion must be repeated in 6 to 12 hours, along with prompt evaluation of coagulation. In the presence of severe head trauma, immediate management and resuscitation should include airway management and oxygenation, maintaining circulation, applying fluid resuscitation for the treatment or prevention of hypertension, and temperature regulation to eliminate hypothermia. Head position should be aligned at 30 degrees elevation to prevent secondary injury and to improve venous drainage.

Anticonvulsant drug may be administered for seizure prophylaxis when CT is abnormal, and neurosurgical consultation must be considered. Neurosurgical involvement may be required in the presence of hematoma, midline shift, and subdural or epidural collections. Extraventricular drain placement and intracranial pressure monitoring are required in the presence of a midline shift to prevent herniation. Decompressive craniotomy is not recommended as an early intervention strategy. Pharmacologic therapy should include sedation or analgesia, seizure prophylaxis with fosphenytoin or levetiracetam, and hyperosmolar therapy with application of mannitol or hypothermic saline to decrease intracranial pressure through the osmotic pathways. Posttraumatic seizures could occur in 10% of the patients with traumatic brain injury. To prevent secondary injuries caused by increased metabolic demand and ischemic changes, prophylactic treatment is recommended. However, long-term prophylactic treatment is not recommended once the patient is stabilized in the absence of clinical or electrographic seizures.

CHILD ABUSE

"Shaken-baby syndrome" should be suspected in injured infants and children younger than 3 years of age. The history is usually vague, and trivial head trauma disproportionate to the degree of injury is commonly invoked by the perpetrators. Abused children may fail to thrive and are sometimes admitted to the hospital solely for that reason. While hospitalized, these children quickly grow and gain weight.

Extracranial lesions include finger marks over the chest and limbs, bruising, burns, lacerations, and skeletal fractures, particularly those involving the lateral ribs and metaphyses of long bones. The lesions may have been inflicted at different times, as manifested by a yellowish discoloration of the older skin lesions. **Intracranial injuries** are subdural hematoma, subarachnoid hemorrhage with a preference for the interhemispheric fissure, loss of gray–white matter differentiation caused by axonal shearing, cerebral contusion, skull fracture, and retinal hemorrhages. Layering of subdural blood is indicative of trauma of different ages after coagulopathy has been excluded. **Clinical presentation** includes lethargy, irritability, seizures, meningeal signs, vomiting, poor feeding, apnea, a bulging fontanelle, and coma.

The **differential diagnosis** includes the retinal hemorrhages seen in up to 40% of vaginally delivered newborns (which resolve within 1 month), coagulopathy, sepsis, osteogenesis imperfecta (with blue sclerae, dental anomalies, short stature, and angulation of healed fractures), glutaric aciduria type I (with developmental delay, hypotonia, cerebral opercular hypotrophy, and chronic subdural collections), Menkes disease (in males), benign subdural fluid collections of infancy (usually bifrontal), and accidental trauma.

The **diagnosis** must be parsimoniously pursued, and the legal authorities alerted; it requires head CT scanning including bone windows, a radiographic skeletal survey, fundoscopy after mydriasis, coagulation profile (platelet count, prothrombin time [PT], partial thromboplastin time [PTT]), urinary organic acids, and serum copper (in males). Photographs of all visible injuries should be taken. Cerebral gradient EchoMRI aids with the identification of hemorrhage of different ages. Lumbar puncture performed to evaluate cases confounded with sepsis reveals a bloody fluid. Ophthalmologic consultation should document any retinal findings.

BRAIN DEATH

Determination of brain death in a child younger than 1 year of age represents a special challenge because the developing brain possesses a greater potential for recovery than does the adult brain. **Requisites** for the diagnosis of brain death include knowing the cause of coma, documentation of normothermia, normotension, and a normal metabolic and toxicologic profile, including the absence of prescribed agents that depress the nervous system. **Examination** must reveal coma, apnea, midpositioned or dilated unreactive pupils, absence of oculocephalic and caloric reflexes, absent corneal reflexes, absent gag reflex, flaccidity, and absence of spontaneous movements. In preterm infants before the 32nd gestational week, most brain stem reflexes remain undeveloped and therefore may not be assessed. The respiratory drive in response to sustained apnea also may develop as late as the 33rd week. Structural lesions in the posterior fossa that may resemble brain death include tumors, subdural hematoma, and Dandy-Walker and Chiari malformations and should be ruled out by imaging. **Adjunctive** diagnostic methods include radioisotopic cerebral blood flow determination, cerebral angiography, and EEG. In neonates, however, cerebral flow may persist after brain death, and it is only of diagnostic value when absent. Age-related brain death **criteria** may be locally legislated and may include:

1. *For patients over 1 year:*
   - Two examinations spaced 12 to 24 hours
   - EEG and cerebral blood flow determinations are optional
2. *For patients 2 months to 1 year:*
   - Two examinations and EEGs 24 hours apart *or*
   - One examination with an EEG and a cerebral blood flow study
3. *For patients 7 days to 2 months:*
   - Two examinations and EEGs 48 hours apart.

The latter criteria may be extended to term newborns younger than 7 days of age, but consensus has not been reached. In anencephaly, adjunctive techniques such as EEG and cerebral blood flow studies are not needed, and they may be impractical for anatomic reasons; the diagnosis is therefore clinical.

Dementia

Memory dysfunction may be variable in its presentation and ranges from the highly functioning senior citizen complaining of forgetfulness to the patient brought in by a relative for bizarre behavior and confusion. **Amnesia** is defined as a pure loss of memory without other cognitive dysfunction. **Dementia** implies chronic, progressive cognitive loss including chronic loss of memory to a degree sufficient to interfere with occupational or social performance. Dementia should not be confused with **delirium,** which is an acute, global disorder of thinking and perception characterized by impaired consciousness and inattention (see Chapter 8). **Retrograde amnesia** refers to loss of memory for events before a specific point in time. **Anterograde amnesia** is the inability to lay down new memory. Memory is often categorized into **immediate recall** (seconds), **short-term memory** (minutes to hours), and **long-term memory** (days to years), with short-term memory the most vulnerable to pathologic processes, both in acute amnestic states and in dementia syndromes. The hippocampi and parahippocampal structures, and dorsomedial thalamus along with the dorsolateral prefrontal cortex, have been implicated in short-term memory function. Verbal memory is mediated predominantly by the left hemisphere, and visuospatial memory is mediated by the right hemisphere.

The differential diagnosis of dementia can be categorized as follows:

V (vascular): cerebral infarction, multiple strokes, diffuse white-matter ischemia, bilateral thalamic infarctions, amyloid angiopathy

I (infectious): syphilis, chronic meningitis (tubercular or fungal), AIDS, progressive multifocal leukoencephalopathy, herpes simplex encephalitis, Creutzfeldt-Jakob (CJD) disease, subacute sclerosing panencephalitis, Whipple disease

T (traumatic): subdural hematoma, dementia pugilistica, head injury

A (autoimmune): central nervous system (CNS) vasculitis, multiple sclerosis, systemic lupus erythematosus (SLE), Hashimoto encephalopathy

M (metabolic/toxic): renal failure, hepatic failure, hypothyroidism, hypercalcemia, benzodiazepine and other tranquilizer intoxication, chronic alcohol use (Wernicke-Korsakoff syndrome), vitamin B_{12} deficiency, nicotinic acid deficiency (pellagra), lead exposure, carbon monoxide exposure

I (idiopathic/inherited): Alzheimer's disease (AD), Huntington disease (HD), Parkinson disease dementia (PDD), dementia with Lewy bodies (DLB), frontotemporal dementia (FTD), progressive supranuclear palsy (PSP), cortical basal ganglionic degeneration (CBD), transient global amnesia (TGA)

N (neoplastic): brain tumor, paraneoplastic limbic encephalitis, meningeal carcinomatosis, postradiation effects

S (seizure, psychiatric, structural): complex partial seizure, postictal state, depression (pseudodementia), normal-pressure hydrocephalus

EXAMINATION OF THE DEMENTED PATIENT

Dementia can be screened for with the standardized Mini-Mental State Examination (MMSE). A score less than 28 of 30 in a person with 12 or more years' education should be cause for concern. The MMSE score also can be used to monitor the patient over time.

1. **Higher Cortical Function**
   a. Alertness and attentiveness

   Have the patient count backward from 20 to 1 or recite the months of the year backward. Serial sevens (serially subtracting 7 from 100) also can be used, but the test may be influenced by education level.

   b. Aphasia

   Check for the following:
   (1) Fluency

   Listen for effortful, nonfluent speech with loss of grammar and syntax, not just word-finding difficulties.

   (2) Naming

   Anomia is a nonspecific finding common to many types of aphasia but may be the only language function affected in AD.

   (3) Auditory comprehension of single and multistep commands

   For example, use commands such as "show two fingers" or "with your eyes closed, tap your right knee with two fingers of your left hand."

(4) Repetition of unfamiliar phrases

When testing repetition, prepositional phrases such as "no ifs, ands, or buts" may be more challenging, but they may be overlearned, practiced utterances.

(5) Reading aloud

(6) Writing

Have the patient write a spontaneous sentence of their own initiative, or if they cannot do so, offer a topic such as "please write a sentence about the weather."

(7) Listen for phonemic paraphasias (substitution of one phoneme for another within a word, e.g., "cable" for "table") or semantic paraphasias (substitution of one semantically related word for another, e.g., "door" for "window").

c. Memory

Check for immediate recall by asking the patient to repeat number strings (digit span). Reciting fewer than six numbers forward or four numbers backward is generally abnormal in persons with 12 years' education. Check short-term memory by asking the patient to repeat three words and then to recall them after 5 minutes. Orientation can be tested by asking the current date, month, and year. Long-term memory and fund of knowledge can be tested by asking about patient family members' phone numbers or birthdates, and by asking the patient to name present and past presidents, governors, mayors, musicians, actors, or sports players. Be sure to take into account education level and interests (the patient may follow sports but not politics, or vice versa).

d. Calculations

Ask the patient to do two-digit addition or multiplication, based on his or her education level, or to tell you how many quarters are in $1.75.

e. Hemineglect

Have the patient bisect a horizontal line. Average deviation from the true midline greater than 10% on six lines is abnormal. Ask the patient to perform a target cancellation task (e.g., to circle all letter "a's" in an array of letters); look for left–right asymmetry in targets missed.

f. Apraxia

Apraxia is impairment of the execution of a learned or imitated movement in the absence of weakness, sensory loss, or incoordination. Ask the patient to pantomime or imitate striking a match or opening a lock with a key. Abnormal performance on this task (ideomotor apraxia) may be seen in AD and other dementias. In more severe dementia, inability to use real objects in a sequence of acts may be seen (ideational apraxia), for example, inability to put on and button a shirt.

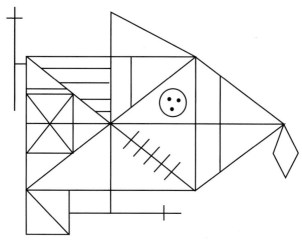

FIG. 28.1 Rey complex figure.

g. Drawing

Have the patient copy a complex figure, for example, interlocking pentagons or the Rey complex figure shown in Fig. 28.1. Dyspraxia for drawing (constructional apraxia) may be found in dementia. Evidence of hemineglect also may be picked up by this test (e.g., the left side of the drawing is incomplete or less organized than the right).

2. **Motor**

Look for signs of hemiparesis that may suggest a focal lesion such as subdural hematoma, stroke, or tumor. Adventitial movements such as myoclonus, chorea, and tremor may accompany degenerative dementias, particularly in the later stages. Signs of parkinsonism should suggest DLB, PSP, or PDD, but it also may be seen in AD or in patients treated with neuroleptics.

3. **Coordination and gait**

Ataxia may be present with Wernicke-Korsakoff syndrome. A magnetic gait, characterized by hesitancy and shuffling in initiation of gait and difficulty in turning 180 degrees, is seen in normal-pressure hydrocephalus (triad of urinary incontinence, gait dysfunction, and dementia).

4. **Signs of frontal lobe dysfunction**

Frontal lobe dysfunction may produce a disinhibition of motor and behavioral functions, signaled by the appearance of frontal release signs such as persistent blinking when the examiner taps the forehead just above the bridge of the nose

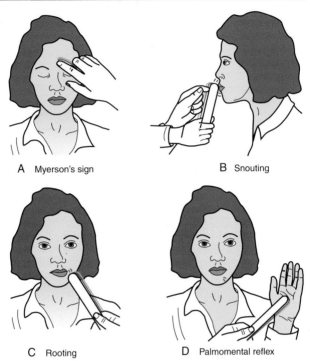

A Myerson's sign

B Snouting

C Rooting

D Palmomental reflex

FIG. 28.2 Frontal release signs. (A) Myerson sign. Patient displays persistent blinking (does not habituate) to repeated taps to the brow above the bridge of the nose. (B) Snouting. Patient purses lips reflexively in response to tapping with a pen or tongue blade. (C) Rooting. Patient's lips and mouth deviate toward a light scratch to the side of the mouth. (D) Palmomental reflex. Patient's chin twitches when the palm is scratched.

(Myerson or glabellar sign) or the snout, root, grasp, and palmomental reflexes (Fig. 28.2), although these responses are not always caused by disturbances of the frontal lobes. Other tests that may indicate frontal lobe dysfunction are the go-no-go test, in which the examiner gives the patient two different tasks to perform in response to two different cues (e.g., "If I show you one finger then you show me two, and if I show you two fingers then you show me none"), or the Luria three-step hand motion sequence.

PRIMARY NEURODEGENERATIVE DISORDERS

Alzheimer's Disease

AD is the most common neurodegenerative dementia, representing about 60% to 80% of patients with dementia. AD is among the top few leading causes of death in the United States, and the number of patients in the United States with AD is expected to increase to more than 13 million by 2050. AD is a relatively homogeneous disorder pathologically, marked by deposition of β-amyloid–containing neuritic plaques, and neurofibrillary tangles, and synaptic and ultimately neuronal losses.

Risk Factors

The most important risk factor for AD is age. AD is uncommon before age 60, and the prevalence doubles approximately every 5 years from age 60 to 90, becoming as high as 50% of individuals over age 85 to 90. A small percentage of AD (<1%) is attributable to autosomal dominant inherited mutations in amyloid precursor protein or presenilin genes, and it tends to present at an earlier age. The vast majority of AD is sporadic, although in late-onset disease, the e4 allele of the apolipoprotein E (ApoE) gene is an established risk factor, or susceptibility allele for AD. About one-third of the population has one or two ApoE e4 alleles, but about two-thirds of persons with AD have one or more ApoE e4 alleles. Because many persons with AD have no e4 alleles, and some elderly people even with two e4 alleles do not have AD, ApoE genotyping is not routinely done because of its lack of predictive power. Although most AD is considered sporadic, in that it is not autosomal dominantly inherited, there are an increasing number of genes, currently numbering over 30, for which variants each yield additional risk.

Clinical Presentation

The most common cardinal feature of AD is the insidious onset of **memory loss,** with associated slowly progressive decline in other cognitive domains. However, atypical presentations of AD may include primary symptoms of language or visuospatial dysfunction. Patients and family members may not have clear recollection of the onset of cognitive decline caused by slow progression, and may sometimes report incorrectly sudden onset of symptoms, tied to a medical or psychological stressor, or a peculiar signal event, such as getting lost, confused during a family event or travel, or leaving a pot on the stove. A careful history, with specific attention paid to changes in performance status, may elicit the more protracted course of cognitive and functional decline. It is important to confirm the history with one or more informants because patients with memory loss often lack insight into the extent of their impairment. Memory loss is initially manifest as forgetfulness for new information, such as names or recent events, but with progression of the disease more remote memories also are lost. Initial **language decline** may be characterized by dysnomia or reduced conversational output. Language may become progressively dysfluent, with eventual compromise of comprehension, and in later stages can progress to mutism. **Visuospatial disorientation** may initially present as having worsening ability at directions. Driving ability may become impaired, and, with progression of the disease, patients can become disoriented in previously familiar locations. Other aspects of cognitive decline often seen in early AD include **difficulty with calculations** (often manifest as difficulty handling money or financial affairs), **executive dysfunction** (with impaired organizational skills and impaired judgment), and praxis (including difficulty with television remote control or cell phone use). In contrast to the progressive cognitive deficits, social and interpersonal skills are often relatively preserved, although with disease progression these functions also may be compromised. **Behavioral changes** and **perceptual disorders** are also characteristic of AD. Delusions are common, often manifesting as paranoia, including delusions of theft, or infidelity. Behavioral disturbances such as disinhibition, agitation, wandering, and sleep disturbance are more common in advanced stages of AD and can lead to significant strain on caregivers. These symptoms, in combination with the progressive loss of basic independent skills such as feeding, bathing, and toileting, often lead to placement of late-stage AD patients in nursing homes. Survival of patients with AD is variable, but life expectancy can be shortened because of complications of severe cognitive decline, including aspiration pneumonia, decubitus skin ulcers, and urinary tract infections.

Diagnosis

The diagnosis of AD can be made clinically, but it may be supported by structural or functional brain imaging and cerebrospinal fluid (CSF) analysis. Criteria include a gradual onset and continuing decline of cognitive function from a previously higher level, resulting in impairment of social and occupational function, usually with impairment of more than one domain, usually recent memory and one other cognitive domain (including language, praxis, visuospatial function, attention, and executive function), and that these deficits are not caused by any other psychiatric, neurologic, or systemic diseases and do not occur exclusively in the setting of delirium. A thorough history should include full functional and psychiatric assessments. Outside of mental status testing, most AD patients will have a relatively normal neurologic examination, and any major or lateralizing abnormalities should be more fully investigated. Many AD patients in the later stages will exhibit some degree of paratonia or extrapyramidal rigidity. A thorough general examination should be performed to exclude any evidence of systemic disease that could be contributing to cognitive impairment. Routine blood work and ancillary tests to rule out other treatable disorders should be done. Structural brain imaging using magnetic resonance imaging (MRI) or computed tomography (CT) should always be performed to rule out structural abnormalities such as tumors, strokes, or hydrocephalus.

Functional neuroimaging studies such as position emission tomography (PET) or single-photon emission computed tomography (SPECT) showing characteristic bilateral temporoparietal hypometabolism is supportive. Molecular imaging using amyloid-binding ligands can be helpful, particularly to exclude AD, because positive findings are common in persons over ages 60 to 65 (and may occur in up to 25% of such individuals). CSF analysis is frequently performed, particularly in patients presenting with cognitive decline before age 65, and it is done both to rule out infectious, inflammatory, or neoplastic disorders, and to diagnose AD through the biomarkers Abeta42, tau, and phospho-tau.

Treatment

There are no curative or disease-modifying treatments currently available for AD, but there are a number of medications that have been shown to have modest but significant symptomatic benefit. In mild-to-moderate AD, these include the centrally acting cholinesterase inhibitors donepezil (Aricept), rivastigmine (Exelon), and galantamine (Razadyne), which inhibit breakdown of acetylcholine in brain synapses. Enhancement of CNS cholinergic tone has beneficial cognitive effects. Dosages of these medications are included for symptomatic treatment of memory dysfunction in mild, moderate, and severe AD:

Donepezil 5 mg qhs, which may be increased to 10 mg each night at bedtime (qhs) in 4 weeks, as tolerated, and in more severe disease up to 23 mg extended release (ER) daily

Rivastigmine 4.6 mg/day transdermal patch daily, which may be increased to 9.5 mg/day patch after 4 to 6 weeks, and in more severe disease up to 13.3 mg/day patch daily

Galantamine ER 8 mg every morning (qam), which may be increased to 16 mg ER daily, and then to 24 mg ER daily in more severe disease

Side effects of procholinergic therapy may include gastrointestinal symptoms such as nausea, diarrhea, and weight loss, and

TABLE 28.1	Medications That May Be Associated With Memory Impairment

Anticholinergic medications (e.g., scopolamine)
Antihistamines (e.g., diphenhydramine)
Benzodiazepines
Benzodiazepine agonists (e.g., zolpidem)
Barbiturates
Muscle relaxants (e.g., carisoprodol)
Interferons
Anticonvulsants (some at high doses)
Antipsychotics (rarely)

common leg cramps, disturbing dreams, or syncope. For treatment of moderate-to-severe AD, the medication memantine (Namenda), an *N*-methyl-D-aspartate (NMDA) receptor antagonist, may provide symptomatic benefit, whether alone or together with a cholinesterase inhibitor. **Start memantine at 7 mg extended release (XR) daily, and increase weekly by 7 mg to a target dose of 28 mg XR daily**. Other agents also may be particularly useful for treating other symptomatic and behavioral manifestations of AD (Table 28.1). The selective serotonin reuptake inhibitors (SSRIs) are helpful for treatment of concomitant depression and sleep disturbances. The atypical antipsychotics also are often used to treat behavioral disturbances and hallucinations, but these agents must be used with caution in the elderly because of the risk of sedation and extrapyramidal side effects, and they carry the warning that they may cause a small risk of increased mortality.

Lewy Body Dementias
Diffuse Lewy Body (DLB) Disease

DLB is the second most common neurodegenerative dementia. This dementing disorder is marked by development of three features: spontaneous parkinsonism, visual hallucinations (typically well formed), and **fluctuations in level of consciousness.** The cognitive impairment is characterized by varying degrees of memory impairment, executive dysfunction, spatial disorientation, visuospatial impairment, apathy, and bradyphrenia (slowed thought processes). Misidentification errors, in which patients fail to recognize once familiar people such as friends and family, often occur. DLB patients may not recognize their own reflection in a mirror and may develop Capgras syndrome, in which they do not recognize a spouse but instead develop a fixed belief that the spouse has been replaced by an identical-appearing impostor. Fluctuations can be a striking hallmark of DLB, in which some periods of time include relatively intact cognition, whereas other periods may be marked by significant confusion and hypersomnolence. Neuropsychiatric features of the disorder include visual hallucinations that are often well formed and vivid, whereas auditory or other types of hallucinations are less common. If parkinsonism is present for more than 1 year prior to cognitive symptomatology, then by convention, the diagnosis is PDD (see the following section), whereas development of parkinsonism within 1 year of cognitive change, or subsequently, is by convention diagnosed as DLB. Parkinsonism in DLB may be more symmetric, less dopa-responsive, and less frequently marked by rest tremor than in PD. Rapid eye movement **(REM) sleep behavior disorder** (RBD), in which there is a loss of muscle atonia during REM sleep, with associated dream enactment, including talking in sleep, and complex motor movements, is common in DLB (and PD) and may occur years before cognitive or motor change. RBD may lead to falling out of bed, or injuries to bed partners. Autonomic dysfunction, including orthostatic hypotension, syncope, impotence, urinary incontinence, and constipation, also may be present. Structural neuroimaging typically shows atrophy, often parietal and/or frontal, but usually shows less temporal atrophy than in AD. Functional neuroimaging, by SPECT or fluorodeoxyglucose (FDG)-PET, may be similar to that seen in AD, but additionally it may show occipital hypoperfusion or hypometabolism and less involvement of the temporal lobes. The histopathologic hallmark of DLB is the presence of Lewy bodies, which are intraneuronal inclusions composed of α-synuclein aggregates, in the brain stem, limbic, and neocortical regions. As in AD, there are no disease-modifying treatments available yet for DLB, and management is targeted toward symptomatic treatment. Cholinesterase inhibitors may have slightly more cognitive and behavioral efficacy in DLB than in AD. Patients with DLB may have significant psychosis, but are often exquisitely sensitive to neuroleptic medications, developing increased parkinsonism. Quetiapine is generally best tolerated, rarely causing extrapyramidal symptoms, but sometimes causing significant sedation. Carbidopa/levodopa may sometimes improve the parkinsonism (gait disorder and rigidity) but may exacerbate hallucinations or agitation. **RBD also may respond to carbidopa/levodopa, or to clonazepam 0.25 mg to 1 mg qhs**.

Parkinson Disease Dementia (PDD)

Patients with Parkinson disease are at risk for developing cognitive impairment that is similar in character to that seen in DLB. PDD is differentiated from DLB by the **time course of the onset of dementia,** which appears early in DLB and later, if at all, in PD, although there may be some overlap. Overlap also is present in the histopathology of these disorders, which are both characterized by the presence of Lewy bodies in the cerebral cortex. Symptomatic treatment is similar to that of DLB.

Frontotemporal Dementia (FTD)

First described in 1892 by Arnold Pick, FTD comprises a set of neurodegenerative syndromes characterized by circumscribed atrophy of the frontal and/or temporal lobes. Unlike AD, which is a molecularly and pathologically pathologic single entity, FTD is a clinical entity with multiple molecular pathologic causes, including disorders with TDP-43, tau, or other molecular abnormalities. Common aspects linking FTD include the structural presence of focal, severe frontal, and/or temporal atrophy, and the corresponding clinical features of behavior and/or language disturbance. Commonly, FTD presents as either a behavior-dominant or a language-dominant syndrome, with language-dominant presentations further subdivided into primary nonfluent aphasia, logopenic aphasia, or semantic dementia (SD), in which the primary defect is in comprehension and word meaning. Memory may be affected in FTD, but typically less obviously than in AD, and relative preservation of visuospatial ability is common; patients may be able to navigate and drive without difficulty. FTD prevalence is much lower than AD or DLB, usually representing only about 3% to 10% of overall dementia patients. However, FTD usually presents at younger ages than AD (typically under age 60), so it is relatively more common in this age group. A significant proportion of FTD cases develop motor neuron disease, particularly those with TDP43 pathology, which has been termed "ALS-dementia." DLB can present as an FTD-like illness, and the tau-related disorders, PSP, and CBD, are sometimes classified as part of the FTD family of disorders.

BEHAVIORAL FRONTOTEMPORAL DEMENTIA

This syndrome is characterized by early **progressive personality change** and **early decline in social interpersonal conduct.** Emotional blunting, impairment in personal conduct, and early loss of insight into these changes also are cardinal features of the disease. Associated behavioral changes such as decline in grooming and personal hygiene, disinhibition, mental inflexibility, hyperorality and hypersexuality (Klüver-Bucy syndrome), perseveration, and utilization behavior (unrestrained exploration of objects in the environment) are supportive of the diagnosis. Alterations in speech and language also are frequently seen, with decreased spontaneous speech, stereotypy, perseveration, echolalia, and mutism. Neuroimaging showing marked frontal and anterior temporal atrophy, hypometabolism, and/or hypoperfusion is part of the diagnostic criteria.

PRIMARY PROGRESSIVE APHASIA (PPA)

The core diagnostic feature of PPA is the insidious onset and gradual progression of **loss of speech fluency,** with associated **anomia, phonemic paraphasias,** and **agrammatism** (inappropriate word order and simplified sentence structure). Word meaning is preserved early in the disease, but stuttering, oral apraxia, impaired repetition, alexia, and agraphia are often present. With time, patients become mute and develop behavioral changes. Imaging reveals early left (dominant) perisylvian atrophy, which is usually more anterior than posterior.

SEMANTIC DEMENTIA (CD)

In SD, the language disorder is characterized by **fluent but empty spontaneous speech with loss of word meaning.** SD patients often present with word-finding difficulties and exhibit anomia, which stems from a fundamental loss of semantic knowledge about the item, leading to deficient object recognition with the associated naming defect. Semantic paraphasias are often present. Neuroimaging shows structural and/or metabolic changes of the left (dominant) anterior temporal lobe. With disease progression, more anterior language deficits and behavioral changes become evident.

PROGRESSIVE SUPRANUCLEAR PALSY (PSP)

PSP is characterized by supranuclear eye movement dysfunction including **vertical gaze palsy** (especially downgaze) and horizontal gaze abnormalities, **axial rigidity,** and **postural instability.** Progressive cognitive impairment mainly involving frontal lobes, with distractibility, inattention, and impulsivity, commonly evolves during the course of the illness. PSP motor symptoms may have minimal response to treatment with levodopa.

CORTICAL BASAL GANGLIONIC DEGENERATION (CBD)

The clinical syndrome of CBD is progressive cognitive impairment with associated **asymmetric rigidity, apraxia, cortical sensory loss,** and **pyramidal dysfunction.** Patients may manifest the phenomenon of alien limb, in which the limb seems to move without voluntary control, but this feature is not essential to the diagnosis. Myoclonus and focal limb dystonia are associated clinical features. Like PSP, this syndrome is poorly responsive to levodopa treatment, and management is supportive.

Treatment of Frontotemporal Dementia Syndromes

As in AD, there are no treatments yet that affect the course of FTD. Treatment is symptomatic and focuses mainly on modulation of

TABLE 28.2 Medications Commonly Used to Treat Symptoms Associated With Dementia

Symptom	Medication	Starting Dose	Typical Effective Dose
Agitation, disinhibition, wandering, psychosis, or other severe behavioral symptoms	Quetiapine	12.5 mg QD	25–200 mg/day (divided BID or TID)
	Risperidone	0.25 mg QD	0.5–4 mg/day (divided BID or TID)
	Olanzapine	2.5 mg QD	2.5–20 mg/day (divided BID or TID)
	Haloperidol	0.5 mg PRN	0.5–3 mg/day (divided BID or TID)
Depression or emotional lability	Sertraline	25 mg QD	50–200 mg QD
	Paroxetine	5 mg QD	10–60 mg QD
	Escitalopram	5 mg QD	10–20 mg QD
	Citalopram	10 mg QD	10–60 mg QD
	Fluoxetine	10 mg QD	10–40 mg QD
Anxiety or obsessive/compulsive behavior	SSRI	(See previous antidepression agents)	
	Lorazepam	0.25 mg QD	0.5–3 mg/day (divided BID or TID)
	Buspirone	5 mg QD	5–20 mg/day (divided BID or TID)
Insomnia	Trazodone	25 mg qhs	50–200 mg qhs
	Zolpidem	5 mg qhs	5–10 mg qhs
	Melatonin	3 mg qhs	3–12 mg qhs

BID, Two times a day; *PRN,* as needed; *QD,* daily; *qhs,* each night at bedtime; *SSRI,* selective serotonin reuptake inhibitor; *TID,* three times a day.

the behavioral syndrome to improve functional status and caregiver burden (Table 28.2). Evidence suggests that cholinesterase inhibitors or memantine are not useful for FTD.

Huntington Disease

HD is marked by hyperkinetic movements and neuropsychiatric impairment. Cognitive impairment seen early in HD tends to be mild, marked by forgetfulness and concentration difficulty. With time, more severe memory decline, learning difficulty, slowing of information processing, executive dysfunction, language decline, and apraxias may become evident, progressing to terminal bedridden mute state. Associated neurobehavioral changes such as agitation, depression, social withdrawal, impulsivity, outbursts, obsessive-compulsive behaviors, and sleep disturbances are common. There is no specific treatment for the disease, but symptomatic treatment is helpful for behavioral symptoms, including typical or atypical neuroleptics such as **haloperidol, quetiapine,** or **risperidone,** although these drugs carry a warning of possible increased mortality. Depression and obsessive-compulsive behaviors may respond to fluoxetine, paroxetine, or other SSRI medications.

OTHER DEMENTIA DISORDERS

Vascular Dementia

Progressive cognitive impairment may occur as a result of strokes or cerebrovascular disease. With better control of hypertension, and decreasing incidence of strokes, vascular cognitive impairment (VCI) is less common. Vascular dementia (VaD), was described by the National Institute of Neurological Disorders and Stroke-Association International pour la Recherché et l' Enseignement en Neurosciences (NINDS-AIREN) criteria as consisting of cognitive decline consisting of impairment of memory plus two additional cognitive domains, with **evidence of significant cerebrovascular disease** on neurologic examination and imaging, and a **relationship between the dementia and the cerebrovascular disease.** The strokes observed with neuroimaging must be relevant to the diagnosis of dementia, including multiple infarcts such as multiple basal ganglia and white matter lacunes; strategically placed infarcts, for example, in the thalamus, anterior limb of the internal capsule, or medial temporal lobes; or extensive periventricular white matter lesions. The relationship between onset of cognitive decline and cerebrovascular disease can be inferred by either abrupt onset, onset within 3 months of a recognized stroke, or a fluctuating, stepwise progression of cognitive deficits. In general, VaD patients show greater impairment of executive functioning with relatively less memory and visuospatial impairment than AD patients, possibly caused by increased involvement of subcortical structures in VaD. Neurologic examination often reveals deficits compatible with previous infarcts. Documenting infarcts on neuroimaging is essential to the diagnosis. Histopathology reveals atherosclerotic and microvascular ischemic changes in addition to infarcts. It is now recognized that many cases in which vascular insult is contributory toward dementia, the dominant pathology may still be AD (so-called "mixed dementia"). Preventive treatment focuses on reduction of modifiable risk factors for cerebrovascular disease, including hypertension, hyperlipidemia, and diabetes. Cholinesterase inhibitors may be helpful as well.

Normal Pressure Hydrocephalus

The classic triad of **gait disturbance, urinary incontinence,** and **cognitive dysfunction** should prompt further evaluation for normal pressure hydrocephalus (NPH). NPH is a poorly understood condition in which communicating hydrocephalus develops in elderly patients without clear structural obstruction to CSF outflow. Typically the classic magnetic gait, characterized by small steps with feet dragging across the floor and shuffling, presents prior to cognitive change. The dementia seen in NPH tends to involve memory and executive function, with a slowing of cognitive processes thought to be related to subcortical dysfunction. The coexistence of urinary incontinence with gait disorder in patients without significant signs of dementia is particularly suspicious for NPH, whereas other dementia patients tend to develop incontinence and gait abnormalities late after dementia onset. Ventriculomegaly out of proportion to brain atrophy is the classic finding on neuroimaging studies, but this finding can be hard to assess in the setting of advanced atrophy. Other findings include evidence of diffuse periventricular white matter changes suggesting transependymal fluid flow. CSF analysis is essential, both to exclude other causes of hydrocephalus and to attempt to assess whether removal of a large volume of CSF is beneficial. The "large-volume tap" is best performed with videotaped observation of the patient before and after removal of 30 to 40 cc CSF. A transient postpuncture improvement in gait is supportive of the possibility of NPH. In some cases, continuous CSF drainage over 3 to 5 days' hospitalization is an alternate diagnostic test. In cases of true NPH, gait and urination may improve markedly with shunting, and reversal of cognitive changes also may occur.

Creutzfeldt-Jakob Disease

CJD is a rapidly progressive dementia typically affecting persons over age 50, with a duration from first symptoms to death often as short as weeks to months. CJD is a prion disorder, whose etiology is self-propagating misfolded prion protein. Most cases in the United States are sporadic, although about 10% to 15% are familial and caused by one of many known genetic mutations in the prion gene. Very rarely, CJD can be transmitted iatrogenically, through human growth hormone injections, or grafts, such as cadaveric dural grafts. A variant form of CJD occurred between 1995 and 2010, in about 200 younger persons worldwide, mostly from the United Kingdom in persons exposed to beef products from cattle infected with bovine spongiform encephalopathy (BSE), representing interspecies transmission of BSE to humans.

CJD, whether sporadic or familial, is marked by rapidly progressive dementia, myoclonus, and gait disorder. Typically the dementia may not so clearly involve memory, but it may affect cortical vision and behavior. Myoclonus may be spontaneous and provoked by startle. Gait disorder is typically ataxic, with cerebellar dysfunction, but pyramidal spasticity also is common.

Diagnosis may be strongly supported by brain MRI, which shows increased diffusion-weighted imaging (DWI) signal in the cortical gray matter (cortical ribbon sign) and deep nuclei (caudate and thalami), typically not evident on T2 imaging. Electroencephalography (EEG) may show a characteristic pattern of periodic, synchronous, sharp wave complexes, at about a 1-Hz frequency, although this may only occur later in the disease course. CSF analysis is essential, both to exclude other conditions and because biomarkers of tau protein, 14-3-3 protein, and the newer real-time quaking-induced conversion (RT-QuIC) assay have high sensitivity and specificity. The presence of a pleocytosis is evidence against prion disease. Brain biopsy may be helpful in some cases. The most common conditions mistaken for CJD are DLB and immune-mediated encephalitides. Brain biopsy or autopsy shows spongiform cortical degeneration, with neuronal loss, gliosis, and positive immunostaining for abnormal prion proteins. Unfortunately, there are no known treatments for CJD, other than symptomatic treatment.

Immune-Mediated Encephalitidies

Rapidly progressive dementia, often with headaches, seizures, and behavioral disturbance, may be the result of the immune-mediated encephalitides, including the syndrome of limbic encephalitis. It is sometimes termed "paraneoplastic encephalitis" because in some cases these disorders are tumor associated. Many of these disorders typically affect younger individuals. NMDA receptor encephalitis affects children and young adults, usually female. Voltage-gated potassium encephalitis typically affects older individuals. These disorders are treatable with immune therapies, including corticosteroids, intravenous (IV) immunoglobulin, and rituximab.

Vitamin B$_{12}$ Deficiency

Cobalamin (vitamin B$_{12}$) deficiency is now a rare cause of dementia, marked by neuropathic, psychiatric, and cognitive impairment, including problems with memory, information processing, irritability, depression, and psychosis. Diagnosis requires demonstration of low vitamin B$_{12}$ levels in the blood, together with elevated homocysteine and methylmalonic acid blood levels, indicating a functional deficiency in B$_{12}$. Treatment typically consists of parenteral **B$_{12}$ replacement of 1000 µg intramuscularly (IM) daily for 5 days, followed by maintenance therapy with 1000 µg IM monthly, or some cases oral treatment of 1000 µg daily.**

HIV-Associated Dementia (Aids Dementia Complex)

HIV-associated cognitive impairment is now an uncommon cause of dementia. It presents as a subcortical dementia, initially with slowed processing speed and mild memory impairment. The syndrome later progresses to involve multiple cognitive domains, including language, executive function, affect, and praxis. The standard treatment of HIV-associated dementia is highly active antiretroviral therapy (HAART) combined with aggressive treatment of affective symptoms (see more on neuro-AIDS in Chapter 22).

Wernicke-Korsakoff Syndrome

Wernicke-Korsakoff syndrome is a nutritional thiamine deficiency occurring in chronic alcoholics. The acute component (Wernicke encephalopathy) is characterized by inattentiveness, lethargy, truncal ataxia, and ocular dysmotility (nystagmus, horizontal with or without a vertical or rotary component; gaze palsy, horizontal or lateral rectus palsy, progressing to complete external ophthalmoplegia). Other signs of nutritional deficiency may be present, such as skin changes or redness of the tongue. If left untreated, the condition is fatal in 10% of patients. Treatment is **thiamine 100 mg IV or IM, daily for 3 days**. These patients also should be watched carefully for any signs of alcohol withdrawal or delirium tremens, or evidence of hepatic encephalopathy, which also may affect cognitive status. Although the ataxia, inattentiveness, and ocular dysmotility may resolve, the more purely amnestic Korsakoff syndrome persists in greater than 80% of patients. Korsakoff syndrome is characterized by moderate to severe anterograde amnesia and patchy long-term memory loss. Unlike patients with TGA, patients with Korsakoff syndrome are not distressed by their amnesia. Confabulation is often present. Even with good nutrition, the amnesia of Korsakoff syndrome rarely resolves. Histopathologic examination shows cell loss and degenerative changes in the dorsomedial thalami, the mamillary bodies, the periaqueductal midbrain, and the Purkinje cell layer of the cerebellar vermis.

Transient Global Amnesia

TGA is a rare transient disorder. Patients are typically over age 50, often with hypertension, or other vascular risk factors, but may be quite healthy. Typically, they are brought in by a relative or friend because they are "confused." On examination, there are no focal neurologic deficits. Cognitive function and language are intact, except for profound anterograde amnesia and retrograde amnesia for the preceding several hours or days. Patients typically appear agitated and will repeat the same question over and over, such as "What am I doing here?" The anterograde amnesia clears gradually after minutes to hours and usually resolves completely within 24 to 48 hours. A residual retrograde amnesia for the hours immediately surrounding the event is often permanent. TGA often appears in the setting of an emotional or physical stress. The pathophysiology is unknown; both epileptic mechanisms and vascular mechanisms have been proposed. MRI and EEG should be performed, but they are normal in TGA. The condition is self-limited, and there is no specific treatment. Recurrence occurs in less than one-fourth of the patients.

Muscles of the Neck and Brachial Plexus

Muscle	Action to Test	Roots[a]	Nerve
Deep neck	Flexion, extension, rotation of neck	C1, C2, C3, C4	Cervical
Sternocleidomastoideus	Rotation of head to contralateral shoulder	XI, C2, C3	Spinal accessory
Trapezius	Elevation of the shoulders	XI, C3, C4	Spinal accessory
Diaphragm	Inspiration	C3, C4, C5	Phrenic
Serratus anterior	Forward shoulder thrust	C5, C6, C7	Long thoracic
Rhomboideus minor	Adduction and elevation of scapula	C4, C5	Dorsal scapular
Levator scapulae	Elevation of scapula	C4, C5	Dorsal scapular
Supraspinatus	Abduction of arm (0–90 degrees)	**C5**, C6	Suprascapular
Infraspinatus	Lateral arm rotation	**C5**, C6	Dorsal scapular
Deltoideus	Abduction of arm (>30 degrees)	**C5**, C6	Axillary
Teres minor	Medial arm rotation	C4, C5	Axillary
Biceps brachii	Flexion of supinated forearm	**C5**, C6	Musculocutaneous
Brachialis	Flexion of pronated forearm	C5, C6	Musculocutaneous
Teres major	Medial rotation and adduction of arm	C5–C7	Subscapular
Latissimus dorsi	Adduction of arm	C6, **C7**, C8	Thoracodorsal
Flexor carpi ulnaris	Ulnar flexion of hand	C7, **C8**, T1	Ulnar
Flexor digitorum profundus (ulnar part)	Flexion of distal phalanx of fingers 4 and 5	**C8**, T1	Ulnar
Adductor pollicis	Adduction of thumb	C8, T1	Ulnar
Abductor digiti minimi manus	Abduction of little finger	C8, **T1**	Ulnar
Flexor digiti minimi brevis manus	Flexion of little finger	C8, **T1**	Ulnar
Interossei	Abduction (dorsal) or adduction (palmar) of fingers	C8, T1	Ulnar
Lumbricals 3 and 4	Flexion of proximal phalanges and extension of two distal phalanges (fingers 4 and 5)	C8	Ulnar

Muscle	Action to Test	Roots[a]	Nerve
Flexor digitorum superficialis	Flexion of middle phalanx fingers 2–5, flexion of hand	C7, **C8**, T1	Median
Pronator teres	Pronation of forearm	C6, C7	Median
Flexor carpi radialis	Radial flexion of hand	C6, C7	Median
Palmaris longus	Wrist flexion	C6, C7	Median
Abductor pollicis brevis	Abduction of thumb metacarpal	C7, C8, **T1**	Median
Flexor pollicis brevis	Flexion of proximal phalanx of thumb	C8, **T1**	Median
Opponens pollicis	Opposition of thumb	C8, **T1**	Median
Lumbricals 1 and 2	Flexion of proximal phalanx and extension of distal phalanges (fingers 2 and 3)	C8, **T1**	Median
Flexor digitorum superficialis	Flexion of middle phalanx fingers 2–5, flexion of hand	C7, C8, T1	Median
Pronator teres	Pronation of forearm	C6, C7	Median
Flexor carpi radialis	Radial flexion of hand	C6, C7	Median
Palmaris longus	Wrist flexion	C7, C8, T1	Median
Abductor pollicis brevis	Abduction of thumb metacarpal	C8, T1	Median
Flexor pollicis brevis	Flexion of proximal phalanx of thumb	C8, T1	Median
Flexor digitorum profundus (radial part)	Flexion of distal phalanx of fingers 2 and 3; flexion of hand	C7, C8	Median (anterior interosseous nerve)
Flexor pollicis longus	Flexion of distal phalanx of thumb	C7, C8	Median (anterior interosseous nerve)
Triceps brachii	Forearm extension	C6, **C7**, C8	Radial
Brachioradialis	Forearm flexion (with thumb pointing upward)	**C6**, C7	Radial
Extensor carpi radialis	Radial hand extension	**C6**, C7	Radial

Muscle	Action	Nerve roots	Nerve
Supinator	Forearm supination	**C6**, C7	Radial
Extensor digitorum	Extension of hand and phalanges of fingers 2–5	C7, **C8**	Radial (posterior interosseous nerve)
Extensor carpi ulnaris	Ulnar hand extension	C7, **C8**	Radial (posterior interosseous nerve)
Abductor pollicis longus	Abduction of thumb metacarpal	C7, **C8**	Radial (posterior interosseous nerve)
Extensor pollicis brevis and extensor pollicis longus	Thumb extension and radial wrist extension	C7, **C8**	Radial (posterior interosseous nerve)
Extensor indicis	Index finger extension and hand extension	C7, **C8**	Radial (posterior interosseous nerve)

aBoldface letters indicate primary innervation.

Muscles of the Perineum and Lumbosacral Plexus

Muscle	Action to Test	Roots[a]	Nerve
Iliopsoas	Hip flexion	L1, **L2**, **L3**	Femoral and L1, L2 and L3
Sartorius	Hip flexion and lateral thigh rotation	L2, L3	Femoral
Quadriceps femoris	Leg extension	L2, **L3**, **L4**	Femoral
Adductor longus	Thigh adduction	L2, **L3**, L4	Obturator
Adductor brevis	Thigh adduction	L2, L3, L4	Obturator
Adductor magnus	Thigh adduction	L3, L4	Obturator
Gracilis	Thigh adduction	L2, L3, L4	Obturator
Obturator externus	Thigh adduction and lateral rotation	L3, L4	Obturator
Gluteus medius and gluteus minimus	Thigh adduction and medial rotation	**L4**, **L5**, S1	Superior gluteal
Tensor fasciae latae	Thigh adduction	L4, L5	Superior gluteal
Gluteus maximus	Hip extension	**L5**, **S1**, S2	Inferior gluteal
Biceps femoris	Knee flexion (and assistance with thigh extension)	L5, S1, S2	Sciatic (trunk)
Semitendinosus	Knee flexion (and assistance with thigh extension)	L5, S1, S2	Sciatic (trunk)
Semimembranosus	Knee flexion (and assistance with thigh extension)	L5, S1, S2	Sciatic (trunk)
Tibialis anterior	Foot dorsiflexion and inversion	L4, **L5**	Deep peroneal
Extensor digitorum longus	Extension of toes 2–5 and foot dorsiflexion	**L5**, S1	Deep peroneal
Extensor hallucis longus	Great toe extension and foot dorsiflexion	**L5**, S1	Deep peroneal
Extensor digitorum brevis	Extension of toes	**L5**, S1	Deep peroneal
Peroneus longus and peroneus brevis	Foot eversion (and assistance with plantar flexion)	**L5**, S1	Superficial peroneal
Tibialis posterior	Foot plantar flexion and inversion	L5, S1	Tibial
Flexor digitorum	Foot plantar flexion and flexion of toes 2–4	S2, S3	Tibial
Flexor hallucis longus	Foot plantar flexion and flexion of terminal phalanx of great toe	S1, S2	Tibial
Gastrocnemius	Knee flexion and ankle plantar flexion	**S1** (S2)	Tibial
Soleus	Ankle plantar flexion	**S1** (S2)	Tibial
Perineal muscles and sphincters	Voluntary contraction of the pelvic floor	S2, S3, S4	Pudendal

[a]Boldface letters indicate primary innervation.

Brachial Plexus

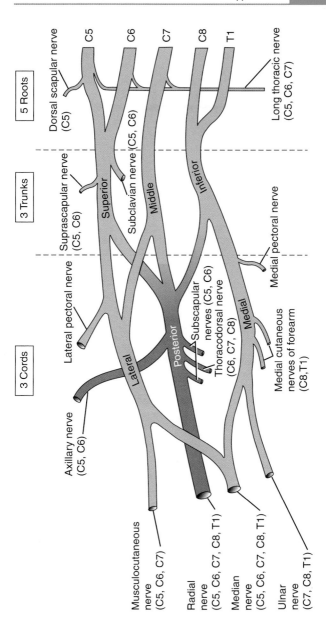

Lumbar Plexus

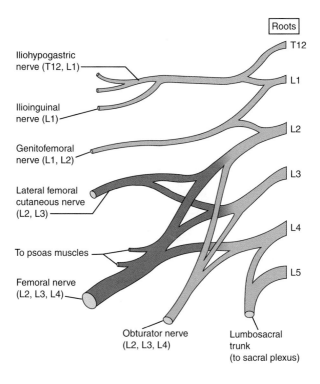

Roots

T12

L1

L2

L3

L4

L5

Iliohypogastric nerve (T12, L1)

Ilioinguinal nerve (L1)

Genitofemoral nerve (L1, L2)

Lateral femoral cutaneous nerve (L2, L3)

To psoas muscles

Femoral nerve (L2, L3, L4)

Obturator nerve (L2, L3, L4)

Lumbosacral trunk (to sacral plexus)

Sensory Dermatome Map

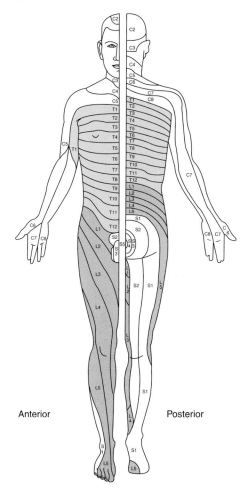

Anterior

Posterior

Surface Map of the Brain

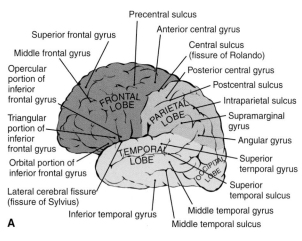

Superior frontal gyrus

Middle frontal gyrus

Opercular portion of inferior frontal gyrus

Triangular portion of inferior frontal gyrus

Orbital portion of inferior frontal gyrus

Lateral cerebral fissure (fissure of Sylvius)

Inferior temporal gyrus

Precentral sulcus

Anterior central gyrus

Central sulcus (fissure of Rolando)

Posterior central gyrus

Postcentral sulcus

Intraparietal sulcus

Supramarginal gyrus

Angular gyrus

Superior ternporal gyrus

Superior temporal sulcus

Middle temporal gyrus

Middle temporal sulcus

FRONTAL LOBE

PARIETAL LOBE

TEMPORAL LOBE

OCCIPITAL LOBE

A

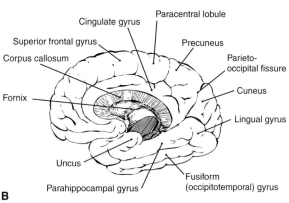

Cingulate gyrus

Superior frontal gyrus

Corpus callosum

Fornix

Uncus

Parahippocampal gyrus

Paracentral lobule

Precuneus

Parieto-occipital fissure

Cuneus

Lingual gyrus

Fusiform (occipitotemporal) gyrus

B

Nuclei of the Brain Stem

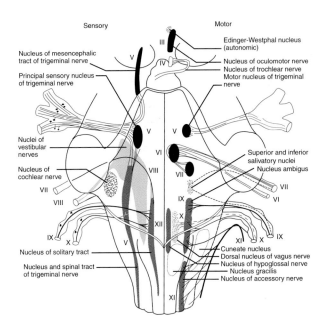

Sensory

Motor

III

V

IV

Edinger-Westphal nucleus
(autonomic)

Nucleus of oculomotor nerve
Nucleus of trochlear nerve
Motor nucleus of trigeminal
nerve

Nucleus of mesencephalic
tract of trigeminal nerve

Principal sensory nucleus
of trigeminal nerve

V

V

Nuclei of
vestibular
nerves

V

VI

VIII

Superior and inferior
salivatory nuclei
Nucleus ambigus

Nucleus of
cochlear nerve

VII

VII

IX

VII

VI

VIII

X

IX

IX

XII

XI

X

Nucleus of solitary tract

X

V

XI

X

IX

Cuneate nucleus
Dorsal nucleus of vagus nerve
Nucleus of hypoglossal nerve
Nucleus gracilis
Nucleus of accessory nerve

Nucleus and spinal tract
of trigeminal nerve

XI

Surface Anatomy of the Brain Stem

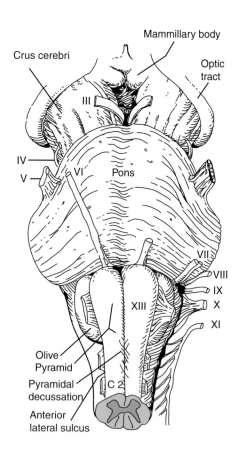

On-Call Formulary: Commonly Prescribed Medications in Neurology

Acetazolamide (Diamox)	**(Chapters 11, 14, 21)**
Indications	Pseudotumor cerebri, seizures, paroxysmal symptoms of MS
Actions	Carbonic anhydrase inhibitor, a weak diuretic that may reduce CSF volume and intracranial pressure
Side effects	Paresthesias, tinnitus, or hearing dysfunction, anorexia, nausea, vomiting, diarrhea, polyuria
Dose	250–500 mg two times a day
Acyclovir (Zovirax)	**(Chapters 5, 21)**
Indications	Herpes simplex encephalitis
Actions	Antiviral
Side effects	Local phlebitis, renal insufficiency, encephalopathy
Comments	Requires generous concurrent IV hydration to minimize risk of renal insufficiency
Dose	10 mg/kg IV over 1 h, every 8 h
Alprostadil (Edex)	**(Chapter 21)**
Indications	Erectile dysfunction in MS and spinal cord injury
Actions	Relaxes arterial smooth muscle, producing vasodilation, resulting in penile engorgement
Side effects	Hypotension, hematoma, ecchymosis, erectile pain, bleeding, headache, back pain, flulike symptoms, hypertension, sinusitis; rare: penile fibrosis, priapism
Comments	Avoid use in patients with history of sickle cell trait, leukemia, multiple myeloma, and in patients taking anticoagulants
Dose	2.5 to 40 μg intracavernous injection prior to intercourse

Amantadine (Symmetrel)	**(Chapter 25)**
Indications	Parkinson disease
Actions	Antiviral agent that also increases dopamine release, blocks dopamine reuptake, and stimulates dopamine receptors
Side effects	Livedo reticularis, ankle edema, confusion, hallucinations, insomnia
Comments	More effective for akinesia and rigidity, less effective for tremor; best used for 6 months to 1 year as monotherapy in patients with mild to moderate Parkinson disease; may delay need for initiation of levodopa
Dose	100–300 mg two times a day

Amitriptyline (Elavil)	**(Chapters 14, 17, 21)**
Indications	Neuropathic pain, migraine prophylaxis, depression
Actions	Inhibitor of membrane pump responsible for uptake of norepinephrine and serotonin, anticholinergic effects; unknown mechanism for action on neuropathy and migraine
Side effects	Drowsiness, paresthesias, urinary retention, dry mouth, dizziness, constipation, blurred vision, confusion, cardiac conduction block, arrhythmias; rare: seizures, MI, stroke, bone marrow suppression
Comments	Sedative effect may limit use for migraine and neuropathy to evening doses; monitor CBC
Dose	25–75 mg every day at nighttime for migraine and peripheral neuropathy; up to 150 mg daily in divided doses may be required for antidepressant effect

Amphotericin B (Amphocin, AmBisome, Abelcet)	**(Chapter 21)**
Indications	Fungal meningitis
Actions	Antifungal
Side effects	Fever, chills, nausea, headache, dyspnea, renal insufficiency, injection site reaction, muscle cramps, vomiting
Comments	Liposomal and lipid complex preparations (AmBisome and Abelcet) are available with better side effect profiles
Dose	1.5 mg/kg/day IV for 4–6 weeks

Ampicillin/sulbactam (Unasyn) (Chapter 6)

Indications	Bacterial meningitis
Actions	Combination antibacterial
Side effects	Rash, diarrhea, fungal superinfection
Dose	1.5 g (1 g ampicillin, 0.5 g sulbactam) IV every 6 h

Arginine vasopressin (Pitressin) (Chapters 9, 18)

Indications	Diabetes insipidus, refractory hypotension after brain death
Actions	Antidiuretic hormone analog
Side effects	Vasopressin infusion combined with free water administration can lead to dilutional hyponatremia
Comments	Causes renal free water retention and peripheral vasoconstriction
Dose	Acute diabetes insipidus: 6–10 U IV push, every 6 h; maintenance therapy for hypotension of diabetes insipidus: 1–4 U/h

Aspirin (Ecotrin, Ascriptin, Bayer) (Chapter 24)

Indications	Secondary stroke prevention
Actions	Platelet aggregation inhibitor
Side effects	Dyspepsia, GI bleeding
Comments	Reduces risk of recurrent stroke by 10%–20% compared with placebo
Dose	81 mg or 325 mg once a day

Aspirin/extended release dipyridamole (Aggrenox) (Chapter 24)

Indications	Secondary stroke prevention
Actions	Platelet aggregation inhibitor
Side effects	Headache, dizziness, nausea, abdominal pain, dyspepsia
Comments	Reduces risk of recurrent stroke by 10% compared with either agent alone, or 24% compared with placebo
Dose	25–200 mg twice a day

Atenolol (Tenormin) (Chapter 16)

Indications	Recurrent vasovagal syncope
Actions	Beta 1-adregenergic (cardiac-selective) blocker
Side effects	Bradycardia, lightheadedness, nausea, bronchospasm
Dose	50–100 mg PO daily

Atropine	**(Chapter 15)**
Indications	Reversal of edrophonium, reversal of organophosphate poisoning
Actions	Anticholinergic (muscarinic) antagonist
Side effects	Dry mouth, palpitations, dilated pupils, tremor
Comments	Caution in patients over 40; may precipitate acute glaucoma, convert pyloric stenosis to obstruction, or urinary retention in prostate hypertrophy
Dose	0.4 mg IV

Azathioprine (Imuran)	**(Chapter 15)**
Indications	Myasthenia gravis (long-term management)
Actions	Immunosuppressant
Side effects	Leukopenia, thrombocytopenia, nausea, vomiting, increased secondary infection risk
Comments	Adequate immunosuppression is reflected by mild decrease in white blood cell count and increase in mean corpuscular volume
Dose	100–250 mg/day

Baclofen (Lioresal)	**(Chapters 21, 25)**
Indications	Dystonia, spasticity of MS
Actions	γ-Aminobutyric acid agonist, antispasmodic
Side effects	Confusion, sedation, increased muscle weakness
Comments	Can be given via intrathecal pump for severe cases
Dose	10–20 mg three times a day (up to 240 mg/day in some cases)

Benztropine (Cogentin)	**(Chapter 25)**
Indications	Parkinsonism, extrapyramidal reactions
Actions	Anticholinergic
Side effects	Dry mouth, constipation, urinary retention, tachycardia, psychosis
Comments	Effective for Parkinsonian tremor
Dose	Start 0.5 mg once or twice daily, increase 0.5 mg a day every 5 days to a maximum of 6 mg a day

Bethanechol (Urecholine)	**(Chapter 21)**
Indications	Urinary retention caused by neurogenic atonic bladder
Actions	Cholinergic agonist that stimulates parasympathetic muscarinic receptors

Side effects	Cramps, nausea, diarrhea, lacrimation, hypotension, sweating
Comments	Antidote for overdose is atropine 0.6 mg IV
Dose	10–50 mg PO three to four times a day

Biperiden (Akineton) (Chapter 25)

Indications	Parkinsonism, extrapyramidal reactions
Actions	Anticholinergic
Side effects	Dry mouth, constipation, urinary retention, tachycardia, psychosis
Comments	Helpful for extrapyramidal reactions caused by neuroleptic agents
Dose	2 mg one to three times a day

Botulinum toxin (Botox) (Chapter 25)

Indications	Focal dystonia, blepharospasm
Actions	Neuromuscular blocking agent
Side effects	Increased muscle weakness
Comments	Antibody-mediated tolerance may develop over time
Dose	1.25–2.50 U per injection site

Bromocriptine (Parlodel) (Chapters 20, 25)

Indications	Parkinson disease, neuroleptic malignant syndrome, prolactinoma
Actions	Dopamine agonist
Side effects	Nausea, headache, dizziness, fatigue, vomiting
Comments	May delay the need for levodopa
Dose	2.5–10 mg three times a day

Cabergoline (Dostinex) (Chapters 22)

Indications	Prolactinoma
Actions	Dopamine agonist
Side effects	Orthostatic hypotension, nausea, dizziness, fatigue, increased libido
Comments	Not approved by the FDA
Dose	0.25–1.0 mg PO once or twice a week

Calcium gluconate (Chapter 8)

Indications	Hypocalcemia
Actions	Calcium replacement
Side effects	Bradycardia, syncope, chalky taste
Dose	10–20 mL (1–2 g) of 10% calcium gluconate IV in 100 mL D5W over 30 min

Capsaicin (Zostrix) (Chapter 18)

| Indications | Painful peripheral neuropathy |
| Actions | Topical analgesic; probable substance P mediator in sensory neurons |

Side effects	None significant
Comments	Now available without prescription
Dose	0.025% or 0.075% cream, apply topically three to four times a day

Carbamazepine (Tegretol)   (Chapters 21, 24, 26)

Indications	Partial and generalized seizures, trigeminal neuralgia, neuropathic pain
Actions	Reduces polysynaptic responses and blocks posttetanic potentiation
Side effects	Double or blurred vision, dizziness, drowsiness, vertigo, ataxia, GI upset, diarrhea, rare agranulocytosis, syndrome of inappropriate antidiuretic hormone, rash, hyponatremia, hypersensitivity; rare: cardiac arrhythmias, bone marrow suppression, cutaneous eruptions
Comments	Half-life of 10–35 h; drug levels needed for anticonvulsant use are 4–12 µg/mL; raises levels of phenytoin, lowers levels of valproate; monitor CBC, Na^{2+}
Dose	300–1600 mg daily in divided doses three to four times a day; usual starting dose is 200 mg three times a day; Tegretol XR (100 mg, 200 mg, or 400-mg caps) can be given twice a day

Ceftriaxone (Rocephin)   (Chapters 5, 8, 21)

Indications:	Bacterial meningitis, alternative for CNS Lyme disease
Actions	Antibacterial
Side effects	Diarrhea, LFT elevations
Dose	2 g IV every 12 h

Clindamycin (Cleocin)   (Chapters 6, 21)

Indications	Toxoplasmosis (with pyrimethamine) in patients with sulfa allergies
Actions	Antimicrobial
Side effects	Abdominal pain, colitis
Dose	600 mg IV or PO four times a day

Clonazepam (Klonopin)   (Chapter 25)

Indications	Tourette syndrome, tics, anxiety, seizures
Actions	Benzodiazepine sedative-hypnotic drug
Side effects	Sedation
Comments	May be habit forming
Dose	1–10 mg/day, divided, two to three times a day

Clopidogrel (Plavix)	**(Chapter 24)**
Indications	Secondary stroke prevention
Actions	Platelet aggregation inhibitor
Side effects	Dyspepsia, thrombotic thrombocytopenic purpura (rare)
Comments	Also reduces risk of fatal and nonfatal vascular events in patients with MI or peripheral vascular disease
Dose	75 mg once a day

Cyproheptadine (Periactin)	**(Chapter 14)**
Indications	Migraine prophylaxis
Actions	Serotonin and histamine antagonist
Side effects	Dizziness, drowsiness, decreased coordination
Comments	Second line of therapy; contraindicated with monoamine oxidase inhibitors, closed-angle glaucoma, pyloric or bladder obstruction
Dose	4–8 mg PO three times a day

Dantrolene (Dantrium)	**(Chapter 20)**
Indications	Neuroleptic malignant syndrome
Actions	Direct-acting skeletal muscle relaxant
Side effects	Pulmonary edema, thrombophlebitis
Comments	Approved by FDA for use in malignant hyperthermia; use in neuroleptic malignant syndrome described in medical literature
Dose	1–10 mg/kg IV every 4–6 h

Dexamethasone (Decadron)	**(Chapters 5, 7, 21, 23)**
Indications	Spinal cord compression, neoplasm or abscess of the brain or spinal cord, acute bacterial meningitis, MS acute relapses
Actions	Antiinflammatory agent
Side effects	Peptic ulcer disease, sodium and fluid retention, hypertension, hyperglycemia, myopathy, impaired wound healing, avascular necrosis of femoral or humeral heads, endocrine abnormalities
Comments	Reduces vasogenic edema but not cytotoxic edema
Dose	For spinal neoplasm: 100 mg IV bolus; for intracranial mass: 4–10 mg IV every 6 h

Diazepam (Valium)	(Chapters 4, 8, 21)
Indications	Seizures, anxiety, alcohol withdrawal
Actions	Benzodiazepine
Side effects	Sedation, hypotension, respiratory depression, paradoxical agitation
Comments	May be administered IV, PO, or rectally as a gel; patients with history of benzodiazepine use or ethanol abuse may have cross-tolerance, requiring higher doses; habit forming with chronic use
Dose	For ongoing seizure or status epilepticus: 5 mg IV push, repeat every 5 min up to 20 mg; for ongoing seizures at home, rectal gel 2.5 mg, 5 mg, 10 mg, or 20 mg via syringe; for agitation, anxiety, spasticity, or ethanol withdrawal: 2–10 mg PO or IV every 4 h

Diphenhydramine (Benadryl)	(Chapter 18)
Indications	Acute drug-induced dystonic reaction, insomnia
Actions	Antihistamine and anticholinergic
Side effects	Drowsiness, dizziness, dry mouth, urinary retention
Comments	Avoid use in elderly, confused patients: may have CNS side effects
Dose	For dystonic reaction: 50 mg IV or IM, may repeat after several minutes; for insomnia: 25–50 mg PO per day at night

Docusate sodium (Colace)	(Chapter 21)
Indications	Constipation
Actions	Stool softener
Side effects	Diarrhea, cramps, throat irritation, rash, electrolyte disorders
Comments	Contraindicated in bowel obstruction and undiagnosed abdominal pain
Dose	100 mg three times daily with meals

Donepezil hydrochloride (Aricept)	(Chapter 18)
Indications	Alzheimer's disease
Actions	Cholinesterase inhibitor
Side effects	Nausea, diarrhea
Comments	May promote GI bleeding in patients with peptic ulcer disease
Dose	5–10 mg PO per day

Doxycycline	**(Chapter 21)**
Indications:	Lyme disease
Actions	Antibacterial
Side effects	Anorexia, nausea, vomiting
Comments	For CNS Lyme disease doxycycline should be used only if there is isolated facial palsy with normal CSF
Dose	100 mg PO two times a day

Duloxetine (Cymbalta)	**(Chapter 17)**
Indications	Diabetic peripheral neuropathy
Actions	Selective serotonin and norepinephrine reuptake inhibitor
Side effects	Nausea, somnolence, dizziness, fatigue
Dose	60 mg PO daily

Edrophonium (Tensilon)	**(Chapter 15)**
Indications	Evaluation for myasthenia gravis
Actions	Short-acting anticholinesterase (cholinergic action)
Side effects	Nausea, bradycardia, arrhythmias
Comments	Atropine 0.4 mg should be kept at the bedside to reverse adverse cholinergic side effects
Dose	2 mg IV test dose, then 8 mg IV after 45 s

Enoxaparin	**(Chapter 15)**
Indications	DVT prophylaxis in immobilized hospital patients; thromboembolic stroke prevention
Actions	Anticoagulant (low-molecular-weight heparin)
Side effects	Hemorrhage
Comments	May be used as a bridge to oral anticoagulation when indicated in cardioembolic stroke
Dose	For DVT prophylaxis 40 mg SC daily; as bridge to Coumadin 1 mg/kg SC every 12 h

Ergotamine (dihydroergotamine [DHE] 45 IV or IM injection; with Caffeine: Cafergot, Wigraine)	**(Chapter 14)**
Indications	Migraine (abortive therapy)
Actions	Alpha-adrenergic/serotonin antagonist; cranial vasoconstrictor
Side effects	Precordial tightness, myalgias, paresthesias, nausea

Comments	DHE 45 may require pretreatment with metoclopramide 10 mg IV or IM and promethazine 50 mg IV as antiemetic; contraindicated in complicated migraine or patients with coronary artery disease
Dose	1 tablet PO at onset, then repeat every 30 min up to 6 tablets; alternatively, 1 suppository per rectum, may repeat one time; DHE 45: 1 mg IV or IM, repeat in 1 h if needed

Ethosuximide (Zarontin)   (Chapter 26)

Indications	Absence seizures
Actions	Anticonvulsant
Side effects	Drowsiness, GI upset, anorexia, headache, dizziness, hiccups
Comments	Pediatric population
Dose	250 mg PO per day (ages 3–6), 500 mg PO per day if over 6 years of age

Felbamate (Felbatol)   (Chapter 26)

Indications	Adjunctive therapy for Lennox-Gastaut syndrome
Actions	Anticonvulsant
Side effects	Aplastic anemia (can be fatal), hepatotoxicity, anorexia, headache, insomnia, somnolence
Comments	Use only with written informed consent because of risk of potentially fatal hepatotoxicity
Dose	400 mg PO three times a day, taper up to 3600 mg/day; in pediatric patients: begin 15 mg/kg/day

Fluconazole (Diflucan)   (Chapter 21)

Indications	Fungal meningitis (mild)
Actions	Antifungal
Side effects	Headache, rash, vomiting, elevated LFTs/hepatitis
Comments	Severe meningitis cases need to be treated with amphotericin
Dose	400–800 mg PO daily

Fludrocortisone (Florinef)   (Chapter 16)

Indications	Orthostatic hypotension
Action	Potent mineralocorticoid
Side effects	Volume overload, congestive heart failure, hypertension, edema
Comments	Lowest possible effective dose should be used
Dose	0.1 mg PO one to three times per day

Flumazenil (Romazicon)	**(Chapters 5, 10)**
Indications	Benzodiazepine overdose
Actions	Benzodiazepine antagonist
Side effects	Agitation, anxiety, dizziness
Comment	May precipitate seizures
Dose	0.5 mg IV

Folinic acid	**(Chapter 21)**
Indications	Adjunctive therapy in toxoplasmosis
Actions	Reduces hematologic toxicity of toxoplasmosis antimicrobials
Dose	10–20 mg PO every day

Foscarnet	**(Chapter 21)**
Indications	CMV retinitis, CMV CNS infection in HIV patients
Actions	Antiviral
Side effects	Renal impairment, electrolyte disturbances
Comments	Second-line therapy after ganciclovir for CNS infection
Dose	60 mg/kg IV every 8 h for 14 days

Fosphenytoin	**(Chapter 4)**
Indications	Status epilepticus
Actions	Anticonvulsant
Side effects	Nystagmus, ataxia, cardiac arrhythmias, hypotension
Comments	Phenytoin prodrug that is rapidly converted to phenytoin within minutes; causes less hypertension than IV phenytoin; can also be given IM
Dose	15–20 mg/kg IV load infused at 50 mg/min

Fresh frozen plasma	**(Chapter 5)**
Indication	Reversal of oral anticoagulant therapy in patients with acute intracranial hemorrhage
Actions	Replaces the essential vitamin K-dependent coagulation factors II, VII, IX, and X
Side effects	Fluid overload, congestive heart failure, allergic transfusion reaction, anaphylaxis, transfusion-related acute lung injury
Comments	Requires serial monitoring of INR to establish successful reversal of anticoagulation
Dose	15 mL/kg (usually 4–6 200-mL units)

Gabapentin (Neurontin)	**(Chapters 4, 21)**
Indications	Adjunctive therapy in adult epilepsy, neuropathic pain
Actions	Anticonvulsant
Side effects	Somnolence, dizziness, ataxia, fatigue, nystagmus, drowsiness, weight gain; rare: leukopenia
Comments	Useful for partial-onset seizures; renally cleared with no drug interactions, and very safe; FDA approved for painful diabetic peripheral neuropathy
Dose	Taper from 100–300 mg PO three times a day over a few days; average dose is 300–900 mg three times a day to a maximum of 1600 mg three times a day

Galantamine (Razadyne)	**(Chapter 28)**
Indications	Alzheimer's Disease
Actions	Cholinesterase inhibitor
Side effects	Nausea, vomiting, dizziness, drowsiness, loss of appetite, weight loss
Comments	Use is not recommended with severe hepatic or renal impairment. Use with caution in patients with bronchospasm or chronic obstructive pulmonary disease
Dose	Start 4 mg PO twice daily (BID) or the extended release (ER) formulation 8 mg PO once daily, to a maximum dose of 24 mg daily

Ganciclovir (Cytovene)	**(Chapter 21)**
Indications	CMV retinitis, CNS CMV infection in HIV patients
Actions	Antiviral
Side effects	Fever, leukopenia, thrombocytopenia diarrhea
Dose	5 mg/kg IV every 12 h

Glatiramer (Copaxone)	**(Chapter 21)**
Indications	Relapsing-remitting MS
Actions	Immune modulator
Side effects	Injection-site pain, systemic reaction with chest pain, vasodilation
Comments	Reduces frequency and severity of MS episodes; in 10% of patients, transient weakness, flushing, and palpitations may occur after injection
Dose	20 mg injected SC every day

Glycopyrrolate (Robinul)	**(Chapter 15)**
Indications	Control of secretions in myasthenia gravis or bulbar amyotrophic lateral sclerosis
Actions	Anticholinergic (antimuscarinic) agent
Side effects	Anticholinergic: decreased sweating, urinary retention, tachycardia, blurred vision
Dose	1–2 mg PO three times a day

Haloperidol (Haldol)	**(Chapters 8, 25)**
Indications	Psychosis, acute agitation, Tourette syndrome, Huntington disease
Actions	Antipsychotic neuroleptic butyrophenone
Side effects	Sedation, extrapyramidal effects (acute or with chronic use), galactorrhea, jaundice, neuroleptic malignant syndrome
Comments	Extrapyramidal effects may occur acutely or with chronic use
Dose	For agitation or acute psychosis: 2–10 mg IM, may repeat every hour; for chronic agitation or psychosis: 0.5–2 mg PO two to three times a day

Heparin	**(Chapters 6, 11, 24)**
Indications	Acute embolic or progressing stroke, transient ischemic attack
Actions	Antithrombin effect; acts in conjunction with antithrombin III
Side effects	Hemorrhage, thrombocytopenia
Comments	Monitor aPTT, usually to a target of 1.5 to 2 times control
Dose	20,000 units in 500 mL D5W at 20 mL/h (800 U/h maintenance, no bolus)

Hypertonic saline solution (2%, 3%, 23.4% sodium chloride-acetate solution)	**(Chapter 5)**
Indications	Control of elevated intracranial pressure, treatment of acute symptomatic hyponatremia
Actions	Reduces brain edema by shifting water from the intracellular to the intravascular fluid compartment
Side effects	Congestive heart failure, fluid overload, rebound hyponatremia and brain swelling after discontinuation

Comments	2% and 3% infusions are generally given to establish and maintain a state of hypernatremia (target sodium 150–155 mEq/L) and hyperosmolality (target osmolality 300–320 mOsm/L)
	Infusions should be slowly tapered over 48 h and sodium not allowed to fall >12 mEq/L over 24 h
	The anion is a 50:50 mixture of chloride and acetate to avoid hyperchloremic metabolic acidosis
	Highly concentrated 23.4% solution comes in 30-mL vials and is given as bolus therapy through a central line for acute ICP control
Dosage	2% and 3% solutions: 1 mL/kg/h
	23.4% solution: 0.5–2.0 mL/kg

Immune globulin (IVIG) (Chapters 17, 20, 21)

Indications	GBS, CIDP, myasthenia gravis, acute disseminated encephalomyelitis
Actions	Immunosuppressive
Side effects	Renal failure, aseptic meningitis, anaphylaxis, hyperviscosity syndrome, leukopenia
Comments	Hydrate patient well to avoid renal toxicity
Dose	For GBS: 0.4 g/kg IV per day for 5 days; for CIPD 0.4 g/kg IV weekly

Interferon β-1a (Avonex) (Chapter 21)

Indications	Relapsing-remitting MS
Actions	Cytokine, immune modulator
Side effects	Flulike symptoms, muscle ache, fevers, chills, liver function abnormalities, leukopenia, thyroid function abnormalities, depression
Comments	Reduces frequency and severity of MS episodes; use with caution in patients with depression or seizures
Dose	30 µg injected IM once a week

Interferon β-1a (Rebif) (Chapter 21)

Indications	Relapsing-remitting MS
Actions	Cytokine, immune modulator
Side effects	Flulike symptoms, muscle ache, fevers, chills, liver function abnormalities, leukopenia, thyroid function abnormalities, depression
Comments	Reduces frequency and severity of MS episodes; use with caution in patients with depression or seizures
Dose	22 µg or 44 µg injected SC three times weekly

Interferon β-1b (Betaseron) — (Chapter 21)

Indications	Relapsing-remitting MS
Actions	Antiviral, immunoregulatory agent
Side effects	Injection site pain and inflammation, influenza-like symptoms, headache
Comments	Reduces frequency and severity of MS episodes
Dose	0.3 mg (9.6 million IU [one vial]) SC every other day

Isoniazid — (Chapter 21)

Indications	Tuberculous meningitis
Actions	Antimicrobial
Side effects	Paresthesias, peripheral neuropathy
Comment	Need to give concomitant pyridoxine (vitamin B$_6$)
Dose	300 mg/day

Labetalol (Normodyne, Trandate) — (Chapters 5, 9)

Indications	Control of acute hypertension
Actions	Combined beta and alpha receptor antagonist
Side effects	Hypotension, bradycardia, bronchospasm
Comments	Arterial BP monitoring is recommended
Dose	For acute BP control: 10–80 mg IV push every 10–15 min, to a maximal total dose of 240 mg; for infusion 2–8 mg/min adjusted to target BP level

Lactulose — (Chapter 8)

Indications	Hepatic encephalopathy
Actions	Diarrheal, reduces ammonia-producing intestinal flora
Comments	Follow ammonia level as indicator of efficacy during treatment
Dose	15–45 mL two to four times per day

Lamotrigine (Lamictal) — (Chapters 21, 26)

Indications	Partial-onset or generalized epilepsy, neuropathic pain
Actions	Anticonvulsant
Side effects	Rash (including Stevens-Johnson syndrome), dizziness, ataxia, nausea, vomiting, somnolence, headache, insomnia; rare: bone marrow suppression, hepatic failure, pancreatitis

Comments	Dose must be reduced with concurrent phenytoin, carbamazepine, or phenobarbital; risk of rash is especially high when given with valproic acid, or in children; monitor CBC and LFTs
Dose	Start 50 mg PO per day for 14 days, then 50 mg two times a day for 14 days, up to 150–250 mg two times a day

Levetiracetam (Keppra) (Chapter 26)

Indications	Add-on for partial-onset seizures in adults
Actions	Antiepileptic
Side effects	Sedation, dizziness, behavioral, infection (mostly mild URIs)
Comment	Primarily renal excretion; no drug interactions; may help for primary generalized seizures also
Dose	1000–3000 mg daily divided twice a day; start at 500 mg twice a day

Levodopa-carbidopa (Sinemet, Sinemet Controlled Release [CR]) (Chapter 25)

Indications	Parkinson disease
Actions	Levodopa is converted to dopamine in the basal ganglia; carbidopa inhibits dopamine production (dopa decarboxylation) in the periphery
Side effects	Dyskinesias: dystonia, chorea; confusion, paranoia
Comments	Dosing highly dependent on clinical response; top number denotes milligrams of carbidopa, bottom number denotes milligrams of levodopa; controlled-release preparation may mediate on/off changes; available in 10/100, 25/100, 25/250, and 50/200 (CR)
Dose	Start with 25/100 tablets three times a day, taper up as clinically indicated

Lidocaine patch 5% (Lidoderm transdermal patch) (Chapter 17)

Indications	Postherpetic neuralgia
Action	Local anesthetic, inhibits sodium channels
Side effects	Local skin irritation
Comment	Apply only to intact skin
Dose	Apply to cover painful areas, may use up to three patches at a time, for up to 12 h daily

Lorazepam (Ativan)	**(Chapters 4, 8)**
Indications	Ongoing seizure or status epilepticus, anxiety
Actions	Benzodiazepine sedative, anxiolytic; anticonvulsant
Side effects	Drowsiness, respiratory depression
Comments	Habit forming
Dose	For status epilepticus: 0.1 mg/kg IV given versus repeated 2-mg boluses; for anxiety 0.5–2 mg PO two times a day

Mannitol (Osmitrol)	**(Chapters 9, 12)**
Indications	Increased ICP
Actions	Osmotic diuretic
Side effects	Hypotension, dehydration, hyponatremia, hyperosmolar renal tubular damage, CHF exacerbation
Comments	Rebound intracranial hypertension with prolonged administration; monitor serum osmolality, electrolytes, and fluid balance
Dose	0.25–1.5 g/kg of 20% solution (20 g per 100 mL), repeat every 1–6 h according to ICP values and clinical exam

Meclizine (Antivert)	**(Chapter 13)**
Indications	Benign positional vertigo, labyrinthitis
Actions	Antihistamine
Side effects	Drowsiness, dry mouth, blurred vision
Comments	Efficacy in about 50% of patients
Dose	12.5–25 mg PO three times a day

Memantine (Namenda)	**(Chapter 27)**
Indications	Moderate to severe Alzheimer's disease
Actions	NMDA antagonist
Side effects	Dizziness, headache, constipation, confusion
Comments	Generally used in combination with a cholinesterase inhibitor
Dose	Start memantine at 5 mg daily and increase by 5 mg weekly to a target dose of 10 mg twice a day

Methylphenidate (Ritalin)	**(Chapter 21)**
Indications	Narcolepsy, attention deficit disorder, fatigue, and lassitude of MS
Actions	Stimulant
Side effects	Dependency, nervousness, insomnia, nausea, anorexia, abdominal pain, dyskinesia, rash, BP changes, seizures, arrhythmias, angina; rare: leukopenia, thrombocytopenic purpura, toxic psychosis, cutaneous eruptions

| Comment | Second-line therapy for lassitude of MS |
| Dose | 5–15 mg up to three times; last dose before 6 p.m. |

Methylprednisolone (Solu-Medrol)   (Chapters 11, 14, 20, 21)

Indications	Traumatic spinal cord injury, MS relapse, inflammatory optic neuritis, pseudotumor cerebri
Actions	Antiinflammatory/immunosuppressive agent
Side effects	Peptic ulcer disease, sodium and fluid retention, hypertension, hyperglycemia, psychosis, insomnia, increased appetite, myopathy, impaired wound healing, avascular necrosis of femoral or humeral heads, endocrine abnormalities
Comments	Stronger mineralocorticoid effect than dexamethasone or prednisone
Dose	For MS and inflammatory optic neuritis: 1 g IVSS per day for 5–10 days, followed by prednisone taper; for traumatic cord injury: 30 mg/kg IV bolus over 15 min, then 45-min pause, and then 5.4 mg/kg/h continuous IV infusion over the next 23 h; for pseudotumor cerebri: 250 mg IVSS four times a day

Methysergide (Sansert)   (Chapter 14)

Indications	Migraine prophylaxis
Actions	Serotonin antagonist
Side effects	Retroperitoneal and pleuropulmonary fibrosis, nausea, vomiting, drowsiness, insomnia, hallucinations
Comments	Should not be used for 2–6 months after 6 months of use
Dose	2 mg PO one to three times a day

Midazolam (Versed)   (Chapters 4, 15)

Indications	Agitation while on ventilator, refractory status epilepticus
Actions	Short-action benzodiazepine sedative-hypnotic
Side effects	Drowsiness, respiratory depression, hypotension
Comments	Rapid acting, with very short half-life
Dose	For sedation: 1–2 mg IV/IM every 30–60 min; for status epilepticus: 0.1–0.3 mg/kg IV push load, then maintenance of 0.05–0.4 mg/kg/h

Midodrine (ProAmatine)	**(Chapter 16)**
Indications	Orthostatic hypotension
Actions	Alpha receptor agonist
Side effects	Supine hypertension, paresthesias, pruritus
Comments	Last dose should be given no later than 6 p.m. to avoid nocturnal supine hypertension
Dose	10 mg PO three times per day

Mitoxantrone (Novantrone)	**(Chapter 21)**
Indications	Relapsing and progressive MS
Actions	Chemotherapeutic agent breaks DNA in actively dividing cells
Side effects	Dose-dependent cardiotoxicity, CHF, arrhythmias, hepatotoxicity, serious infections, myelosuppression, hypotension, nausea, diarrhea, constipation, dyspnea, elevated alkaline phosphatase, urine discoloration, cough; menstrual irregularities, amenorrhea, fatigue, anorexia, alopecia, urinary tract infection; rare: anaphylaxis, secondary leukemia, interstitial pneumonitis, renal failure, hemorrhage, tissue necrosis caused by extravasation
Comments	Used primarily for MS patients who have experienced disease progression despite treatment with interferon-β or glatiramer acetate; monitor left ventricular function every 6 months, check CBC and LFTs prior to each dose and check CBC 14 days after each dose
Dose	12 mg/m^2 every 3 months for up to 2 years; cumulative lifetime total dose 140 mg/m^2; alternative schedule 5 mg/m^2 every month

Modafinil (Provigil)	**(Chapter 21)**
Indications	Narcolepsy, fatigue in MS, abulia
Actions	Stimulant
Side effects	Headache, nausea, diarrhea, dry mouth, anorexia
Comments	May impair thinking or motor skills
Dose	100–200 mg PO once to twice a day

Naloxone (Narcan)	**(Chapter 5)**
Indications	Suspected narcotic coma
Actions	Narcotic antagonist

Side effects	Nausea, vomiting, may precipitate withdrawal in narcotic addicts
Comments	Reversal of narcotic coma may wear off after 1–2 h
Dose	0.4–2.0 mg IV, IM, or SC every 5 min to a maximum dose of 10 mg

Naratriptan (Amerge)   (Chapter 14)

Indications	Migraine (abortive therapy)
Actions	Selective serotonin agonist
Side effects	Paresthesias, dizziness, drowsiness, fatigue, throat tightness
Comments	Longer duration of action than other triptans, but slower onset and lower efficacy rate; contraindicated in patients with coronary artery disease
Dose	1 mg or 2.5 mg, may repeat after 4 h, maximum 5 mg daily

Natalizumab (Tysabri)   (Chapter 21)

Indications	Relapsing MS
Actions	Inhibits leukocyte trafficking by binding to $\alpha4\beta1$-integrin expressed on the cell surface of activated lymphocytes
Side effects	Hypersensitivity reaction, anaphylaxis, headache, infusion reaction, fatigue, depression, arthralgia, infections, pharyngitis, rash, menstrual irregularities; rare: progressive multifocal leukoencephalopathy, serious infections
Comments	Withdrawn from market
Dose	300 mg IV every month

Neomycin   (Chapter 8)

Indications	Hepatic encephalopathy
Actions	Antibiotic to reduce ammonia-producing bacteria in the intestines
Side effects	Nausea, diarrhea
Dose	2–4 g/day PO

Neostigmine (Prostigmin)   (Chapter 15)

Indications	Myasthenia gravis
Actions	Acetylcholinesterase inhibitor
Side effects	Abdominal cramps, diarrhea, salivation, fasciculations
Comments	Has longer duration of action than does pyridostigmine

Dose	15–90 mg PO four times a day; 0.5–1.0 mg IV or IM every 2–3 h

Nicardipine (Cardene) (Chapters 5, 9)

Indication	Control of acute hypertension
Actions	Dihydropyridine calcium channel blocker
Side effects	Hypotension, reflex tachycardia
Comments	Continuous arterial BP monitoring is recommended
Dose	5–15 mg/h as a continuous IV infusion

Nimodipine (Nimotop) (Chapter 24)

Indications	Subarachnoid hemorrhage
Actions	Calcium-channel blocker with CNS penetration
Side effects	Hypotension
Comments	Reduces the frequency of delayed ischemia from vasospasm by 30%
Dose	60 mg every 4 h for 21 days

Oxcarbazepine (Trileptal) (Chapters 21, 26)

Indications	Monotherapy or add-on for partial-onset seizures in adults; add-on for children ages 4 years or older; neuropathic pain
Actions	Antiepileptic; sodium-channel blocker
Side effects	Dizziness, sedation, nausea, vomiting, diplopia, rash, fatigue, acne, alopecia, hyponatremia; rare: angioedema, bone marrow suppression, cutaneous eruptions
Comment	Similar to carbamazepine but fewer side effects and drug interactions; active ingredient is the 10-monohydroxy metabolite; monitor CBC, Na^{2+}, LFTs
Dose	300–to 3600 mg a day divided in two doses (usually need 150% of carbamazepine dose)

Oxybutynin (Ditropan) (Chapter 21)

Indications	Bladder spasticity (e.g., in MS)
Actions	Smooth muscle antispasmodic, antimuscarinic
Side effects	Palpitations, decreased sweating, dry mouth, dizziness, urinary retention, constipation
Comments	Contraindicated in patients with obstructive uropathy
Dose	5 mg PO three to four times daily

Pemoline (Cylert) (Chapter 21)

Indications	Narcolepsy, abulia after brain injury, attention deficit disorder

Actions	CNS stimulant
Side effects	Insomnia, anorexia, weight loss, seizure, dyskinesias, hallucinations, rare aplastic anemia
Comments	Contraindicated in patients with impaired hepatic function
Dose	18.75 mg PO every day, taper weekly as indicated up to maximum of 75 mg/day

Penicillamine (Cuprimine) (Chapter 25)

Indications	Wilson disease
Actions	Copper chelator
Side effects	Lupus-like rash, polyarteritis, leukopenia, thrombocytopenia, epigastric pain, nausea, diarrhea, nephrotic syndrome, tinnitus, neuropathy
Comments	May precipitate myasthenia gravis
Dose	125–1000 mg/day, divided, two to four times a day

Pentobarbital (Chapters 4, 9)

Indications	Status epilepticus, increased intracranial pressure
Actions	Anticonvulsant, sedative
Side effects	Respiratory suppression, sedation, hypotension
Comments	EEG monitoring indicated; hypotension may require pressors; levels of 25–35 mg/L are generally sufficient to control intracranial pressure; levels of <5 mg/L are compatible with a clinical diagnosis of brain death
Dose	5–20 mg/kg IV load, 1–4 mg/kg/h maintenance

Pergolide (Permax) (Chapter 25)

Indications	Parkinson disease
Actions	Dopamine agonist
Side effects	Nausea, headache, dizziness, fatigue, vomiting
Comments	May delay onset or reduce required dose of levodopa
Dose	0.75–3.0 mg/day, divided, three to four times a day

Phenobarbital (Luminal) (Chapter 4)

Indications	Epilepsy, status epilepticus
Actions	Anticonvulsant

Side effects	Sedation, respiratory suppression, hypotension, behavioral changes, hyperactivity
Comments	For chronic therapy, therapeutic range is 20–40 µg/mL; lowers levels of phenytoin, carbamazepine, and valproate
Dose	For status epilepticus: 10–20 mg/kg IV load infused at 100 mg/min; for epilepsy 60 mg PO two to three times a day; for pediatric patients: 3–6 mg/kg/day

Phenoxybenzamine   (Chapter 17)

Indications	Reflex sympathetic dystrophy
Actions	Systemic alpha-adrenergic blocker
Side effects	Postural hypotension, tachycardia, impotence
Comments	Taper up dose until side effects occur
Dose	10 mg two times a day, tapering up to 120 mg/day

Phenylephrine (Neo-Synephrine)   (Chapter 5)

Indications	Low cerebral perfusion pressure
Actions	Alpha receptor agonist
Side effects	Reflex bradycardia, excessive hypertension
Comments	Intraarterial BP monitoring is recommended; can be used to raise BP in hemodynamically unstable ischemic stroke syndromes, or in patients with elevated ICP
Dose	10–200 µg/min titrated to desired BP target

Phenytoin (Dilantin)   (Chapter 4)

Indications	Epilepsy, status epilepticus
Actions	Anticonvulsant
Side effects	Nystagmus, ataxia, gingival hyperplasia, hirsutism, rash, adenopathy, LFT abnormalities
Comments	For chronic therapy, therapeutic range is 10–20 µg/mL; lowers levels of carbamazepine and valproate and increases or decreases phenobarbital level
Dose	Typical maintenance dose is 300 mg every day at night

Pimozide (Orap)   (Chapter 25)

Indications	Tourette syndrome
Actions	Piperidine antipsychotic
Side effects	Dry mouth, sedation, dyskinesias, akinesia, behavioral effects, prolongation of QT interval

Comments	None
Dose	Start with 1 mg PO two times a day, up to 2–10 mg/day in divided doses

Pramipexole (Mirapex) (Chapter 25)

Indications	Parkinson disease
Actions	Dopamine agonist
Side effects	Hallucinations, dizziness, somnolence, nausea
Comments	Can be used alone or in combination with levodopa
Dose	0.125 mg three times daily, increase weekly to a maximum of 1.5 mg three times a day

Prednisone (Chapter 11)

Indications	Temporal arteritis, Bell palsy
Actions	Antiinflammatory agent
Side effects	Peptic ulcer disease, sodium and fluid retention, hypertension, hyperglycemia, myopathy, impaired wound healing, avascular necrosis of femoral or humeral heads, endocrine abnormalities, increased susceptibility to infection
Comments	Initiate therapy as soon as diagnosis is suspected to avoid irreversible visual loss
Dose	100 mg PO per day, tapered slowly to alternate-day therapy over several weeks

Pregabalin (Lyrica) (Chapter 17)

Indications	Peripheral (diabetic) neuropathy, postherpetic neuralgia, central pain syndromes
Actions	Antinociceptive, antiseizure
Side effects	dizziness, somnolence, dry mouth
Dose	150–300 mg PO twice a day

Primidone (Mysoline) (Chapters 4, 25)

Indications	Generalized tonic-clonic epilepsy, essential tremor
Actions	Anticonvulsant
Side effects	Ataxia, vertigo, nausea, anorexia, vomiting, irritability, sedation
Comments	Second line of therapy; metabolized to phenobarbital
Dose	Start with 100–125 mg PO once a day, taper up to 250 mg three to four times a day

Propantheline Bromide (Pro-Banthine) (Chapter 15)

Indications	Control of secretions in myasthenia gravis
Actions	Antimuscarinic agent

Side effects	Anticholinergic: decreased sweating, urinary retention, tachycardia, blurred vision
Comments	None
Dose	15 mg PO four times a day

Propofol (Diprivan) (Chapters 4, 9)

Indications	Refractory status epilepticus, ICP control, sedation in setting of mechanical ventilation
Actions	Alkylphenol sedative-hypnotic agent
Side effects	Apnea, respiratory depression, hypotension, propofol infusion syndrome (metabolic acidosis, hypotension, renal failure), bloodstream infections
Comments	Should only be administered to patients who are intubated; continuous arterial BP monitoring is recommended; prolonged high dosages, particularly in children, are not recommended because of an increased risk of propofol infusion syndrome
Dose	For status epilepticus: 1–3 mg/kg loading dose, followed by 50–250 µg/kg/min; for sedation: 25–100 µg/kg/min

Propranolol (Inderal) (Chapters 14, 25)

Indications	Benign essential tremor, migraine prophylaxis
Actions	Nonspecific beta-adrenergic blocker
Side effects	Hypotension, bradycardia, bronchospasm, may mask symptoms of hypoglycemia, impotence
Comments	Avoid use in asthmatics and diabetics
Dose	For tremor: 40–240 mg PO per day, divided, three to four times a day; for migraine 20–40 mg/day

Protamine sulfate (Chapter 5)

Indications	Reversal of heparin-induced coagulopathy in patients with acute intracranial hemorrhage
Actions	1 mL of protamine sulfate neutralizes ~100 U of heparin
Side effects	Hypotension, allergic reaction
Comments	Requires PTT monitoring to assess adequacy of response
Dose	10–50 mg slow IV push

Psyllium (Metamucil) (Chapter 21)

Indications	Constipation
Actions	Increases stool bulk

Side effects	Diarrhea, constipation, cramps, bronchospasm, rhinitis, esophageal obstruction, bowel obstruction
Comments	Contraindicated in bowel obstruction and undiagnosed abdominal pain
Dose	1–2 teaspoons three times daily with meals

Pyridostigmine (Mestinon) (Chapter 15)

Indications	Myasthenia gravis
Actions	Acetylcholinesterase inhibitor
Side effects	Excess salivation, pulmonary secretions, diarrhea
Comments	Muscarinic side effects controlled by glycopyrrolate or propantheline bromide
Dose	Start at 30 mg PO three times a day, up to 120 mg every 3–6 h

Recombinant activated factor VII (NovoSeven) (Chapter 5)

Indications	Acute coagulopathic intracranial hemorrhage, spontaneous intracerebral hemorrhage
Actions	Promotes rapid hemostasis and clot formation by accelerating thrombin formation on the surface of activated platelets
Side effects	MI, cerebral infarction, venous thromboembolism, disseminated intravascular coagulation
Comments	Use for acute intracranial hemorrhage is currently investigational and considered off-label; cost is prohibitive, approximately $1 per microgram
Dose	40–80 µg/kg IV push over 1–2 min; doses may be rounded to the nearest 1.2-mg, 2.4-mg, or 4.8-mg vial

Riluzole (Rilutek) (Chapter 20)

Indications	Amyotrophic lateral sclerosis
Actions	Glutamate antagonist
Side effects	Malaise, abdominal pain, nausea, dizziness, circumoral numbness, liver function abnormalities
Comments	May extend survival 60–90 days and delay time to intubation; avoid use in patients with liver dysfunction
Dose	50 mg PO two times a day

Rivastigmine (Exelon)	**(Chapter 27)**
Indications	Alzheimer's dementia
Actions	Centrally acting cholinesterase inhibitor
Side effects	Nausea, dizziness
Comments	May be first-line or second-line therapy after donepezil
Dose	1.5 mg twice a day, increase to 6 mg twice a day over 4 weeks, as tolerated

Rizatriptan (Maxalt)	**(Chapter 14)**
Indications	Migraine (abortive therapy)
Actions	Selective serotonin agonist
Side effects	Weakness, fatigue, chest or throat pressure, dizziness, somnolence
Comments	Faster acting and slightly more effective than other triptans, but more likely to cause side effects; contraindicated in patients with coronary artery disease
Dose	5–10 mg, may repeat in 2 h, maximum 30 mg daily

Ropinirole (Requip)	**(Chapter 25)**
Indications	Parkinson disease
Actions	Dopamine agonist
Side effects	Syncope, hallucinations, dyskinesias, nausea, dizziness, somnolence, headache
Comments	May be used alone or in combination with levodopa
Dose	0.25 mg three times daily

Selegiline (Eldepryl)	**(Chapter 25)**
Indications	Parkinson disease
Actions	Monoamine oxidase B inhibitor: antioxidant
Side effects	Nausea, dizziness, confusion, hallucinations
Comments	Thought to slow progression of disease
Dose	Taper up to 5 mg PO two times a day

Senna (Senokot)	**(Chapter 21)**
Indications	Constipation
Actions	Increases peristalsis
Side effects	Nausea, bloating, cramps, flatulence, diarrhea, urine discoloration, melanosis coli; rare: cathartic colon, laxative abuse
Comments	Contraindicated in bowel obstruction and undiagnosed abdominal pain
Dose	6.6 mg sennosides, take 2–4 tablets at night

Sildenafil (Viagra)	**(Chapter 21)**
Indications	Erectile dysfunction in MS and spinal cord injury
Actions	Inhibits phosphodiesterase type 5, enhances effects of nitric oxide-activated increases in cGMP, resulting in penile engorgement
Side effects	Headache, flushing, dyspepsia, nasal congestion, dizziness, rash, priapism; rare: MI, stroke, sudden death, cardiac arrhythmia, hypotension, hemorrhage, hypersensitivity reaction, dyspnea
Comments	Avoid use in patients with history of coronary artery disease
Dose	25–100 mg 0.5–4 h prior to intercourse

Sumatriptan (Imitrex)	**(Chapter 14)**
Indications	Migraine (abortive therapy)
Actions	Selective serotonin agonist
Side effects	Coronary vasospasm; tingling; flushing; tightness in jaw, neck, and chest; dizziness; injection site reaction
Comments	Contraindicated in patients with coronary artery disease
Dose	6 mg SC, may repeat in 1 h, maximum 12 mg/day, six doses per month; 25 mg PO, may repeat up to 100 mg in 2 h

Tacrine (Cognex)	**(Chapter 18)**
Indications	Alzheimer's disease
Actions	Reversible cholinesterase inhibitor
Side effects	Nausea, vomiting, diarrhea, abdominal pain, fatigue, agitation, confusion
Comments	May improve cognitive scores in some patients
Dose	Start 10 mg PO three times a day, tapering up to 30 mg three times a day

Tadalafil (Cialis)	**(Chapter 21)**
Indications	Erectile dysfunction in MS and spinal cord injury
Actions	Inhibits phosphodiesterase type 5, enhances effects of nitric oxide-activated increases in cGMP, resulting in penile engorgement
Side effects	Headache, dyspepsia, back pain, myalgia, nasal congestion, flushing, limb pain, priapism; rare: angina, MI, stroke, hypotension, hypertension, syncope

| Comments | Avoid use in patients with history of coronary artery disease, effects may last up to 36 h, lower dose in patients with hepatic dysfunction |
| Dose | 5–20 mg prior to intercourse |

Temozolomide (Temodar)   (Chapter 22)

Indications	Newly diagnosed glioblastoma multiforme, refractory anaplastic astrocytoma
Actions	Cytotoxic alkylating agent which damages DNA in rapidly multiplying cells
Side effects	Leukopenia, thrombocytopenia, alopecia, nausea/vomiting, anorexia, headache, weakness
	Women and older patients are at higher risk for complications
	During concomitant phase, Bactrim must be given three times a week for *Pneumocystis carinii* prophylaxis, and CBC should be measured weekly
	Therapy should be suspended if absolute neutrophil count < 1,500/μL or platelets < 100,000/μL
Dosage	75 mg/m^2 PO daily concomitant with radiation treatment for 42 days, followed by maintenance therapy with 150–200 mg/m^2 PO daily for 5 days every 28 days over six cycles

Thiamine   (Chapters 4, 8)

Indications	Coma, thiamine deficiency neuropathy
Actions	Enzymatic cofactor in oxidative metabolism (thiamine pyrophosphate)
Side effects	None
Comments	Give with glucose in setting of coma to prevent Wernicke encephalopathy
Dose	For coma: 100 mg IV push; 100 mg PO or IM for 3 days

Tiagabine (Gabitril)   (Chapter 26)

Indications	Add-on for partial-onset seizures in adults
Actions	Antiepileptic; GABA-reuptake inhibitor
Side effects	Sedation, cognitive dysfunction, dizziness, nausea, vomiting, tremor, anxiety
Comment	Highly protein-bound
Dose	4–56 mg daily, divided two to four times a day

Ticlopidine (Ticlid)	**(Chapter 24)**
Indications	Secondary stroke prevention
Actions	Platelet aggregation inhibitor
Side effects	Neutropenia, diarrhea, rash, nausea, vomiting, thrombotic thrombocytopenic purpura
Comments	Check CBC every 2 weeks during the first 3 months of treatment
Dose	250 mg twice a day

Tissue plasminogen activator (t-PA)	**(Chapters 6, 24)**
Indications	Hyperacute ischemic stroke
Actions	Thrombolytic
Side effects	Intracerebral hemorrhage
Comments	Must be given within 3 h of stroke onset; increases chance of full recovery or minimal residual deficit at 3 months by 33%; patients with acute hemorrhage, uncontrolled hypertension (>180/105 mm Hg), or those on anticoagulant therapy should be excluded
Dose	0.9 mg/kg IV (10% IV push, then infuse the remaining 90% over 1 h), maximum dose 90 mg

Tolcapone (Tasmar)	**(Chapter 25)**
Indications	Parkinson disease
Actions	COMT inhibitor
Side effects	Fulminant hepatic failure (may be fatal), dyskinesias, nausea, sleep disorders, anorexia, somnolence
Comments	Should be reserved for patients with symptom fluctuations on levodopa who do not respond to other adjunctive agents; withdraw if no substantial benefit is seen after 3 weeks
Dose	100–200 mg three times daily

Topiramate (Topamax)	**(Chapters 21, 26)**
Indications	Add-on for partial-onset or primary generalized seizures, neuropathic pain
Actions	Antiepileptic, weak carbonic-anhydrase inhibitor
Side effects	Sedation, cognitive dysfunction, anorexia, dizziness, paresthesias, ataxia, renal stones, metabolic acidosis, visual disturbance, weight gain, agitation; rare: angle closure glaucoma, bone marrow suppression, cutaneous eruptions

Comment	Probably effective for all seizure types; mostly renal excretion; monitor CBC
Dose	Start 25–50 mg/day; maintenance 100–600 mg/day divided in two doses; 1–10 mg/kg/day in children; also available in sprinkles

Tramadol (Ultram) (Chapter 21)

Indications	Analgesia
Actions	Exact mechanism is unknown but parent compound and M1 metabolite bind opiate μ receptors; and parent compound also inhibits reuptake of norepinephrine and serotonin
Side effects	Dizziness, nausea, constipation, headache, somnolence, psychiatric disturbance, urinary retention, withdrawal symptoms; rare: seizures, respiratory depression, angioedema, cutaneous eruptions, serotonin syndrome, orthostatic hypotension, hallucinations
Comment	Useful for neuropathic pain; use with SSRIs or other antidepressants may trigger serotonin syndrome
Dose	50–100 mg three times daily

Trihexyphenidyl HCl (Artane) (Chapter 25)

Indications	Parkinson disease, idiopathic torsion dystonia
Actions	Anticholinergic
Side effects	Visual blurring, dry mouth, urinary retention
Comments	May be effective in treating parkinsonian tremor; botulinum toxin has largely replaced anticholinergics for the treatment of focal dystonias
Dose	1–15 mg PO per day, divided, three to four times a day

Valproic acid (Depakote, Depakene [syrup], Depacon [IV]) (Chapter 4)

Indications	Partial or generalized seizures, migraine prophylaxis
Actions	Anticonvulsant
Side effects	Nausea, weight gain, hair loss, tremor, hepatitis, agranulocytosis, thrombocytopenia, Stevens-Johnson syndrome

| Comments | Therapeutic range is 50–100 µg/mL; increases levels of carbamazepine, phenytoin, and lamotrigine |
| Dose | 250–2000 mg PO four times a day; 5–15 mg/kg IV every 6 h; loading dose for status epilepticus is 30–60 mg/kg IV |

Vardenafil (Levitra) (Chapter 21)

Indications	Erectile dysfunction in MS and spinal cord injury
Actions	Inhibits phosphodiesterase type 5, enhances effects of nitric oxide-activated increases in cGMP, resulting in penile engorgement
Side effects	Headache, flushing, rhinitis, dyspepsia, dizziness, nausea, arthralgias, elevated CPK, priapism; rare: anaphylaxis, angina, MI, cardiac arrhythmia, hypotension, hypertension
Comments	Avoid use in patients with history of coronary artery disease, lower doses in patients with hepatic dysfunction
Dose	5–20 mg 1 h prior to intercourse

Warfarin (Coumadin) (Chapters 6, 24)

Indications	Stroke prophylaxis in atrial fibrillation or other conditions predisposing to cardioembolism
Actions	Inhibits vitamin K-dependent clotting factors
Side effects	Hemorrhage, rash
Comments	Used for secondary stroke prevention in cardioembolic stroke and in large-vessel atherosclerosis when antiplatelet therapy has failed; used for primary stroke prevention in atrial fibrillation; close monitoring of prothrombin times (PT or INRs) required
Dose	Begin with 4 mg PO per day, with dose adjusted according to target PT/INR

Zolmitriptan (Zomig) (Chapter 14)

Indications	Migraine (abortive therapy)
Actions	Selective serotonin agonist
Side effects	Paresthesias, nausea, neck or chest tightness, dry mouth, somnolence
Comments	May be useful for keeping headaches away in patients with early recurrence after sumatriptan; contraindicated in patients with coronary artery disease
Dose	2.5 mg may repeat after 2 h, maximum 10 mg daily

Zolpidem (Ambien)	(Chapter 18)
Indication	Insomnia
Action	Sedative
Side effects	Confusion in the elderly
Comments	Do not use for benzodiazepine or ethanol withdrawal
Dose	5–10 mg at night

Zonisamide (Zonegran)	(Chapters 21, 26)
Indications	Add-on for partial-onset seizures in adults; neuropathic pain
Actions	Antiepileptic, weak carbonic anhydrase inhibitor
Side effects	Sedation, dizziness, anorexia, irritability, rash, kidney stones, psychiatric disturbance, withdrawal seizures; rare cutaneous eruptions, bone marrow suppression, heat stroke, pancreatitis
Comments	Sulfa drug; mostly renal excretion; may help for absence seizures and for other generalized seizures; monitor CBC
Dose	100–600 mg daily, divided twice a day

aPTT, Activated partial thromboplastic time; *BP*, blood pressure; *CBC*, complete blood count; *cGMP*, cyclic guanosine monophosphate; *CHF*, congestive heart failure; *CIPD*, chronic inflammatory demyelinating polyneuropathy; *CMV*, cytomegalovirus; *CNS*, central nervous system; *COMT*, catechol-*O*-methyltransferase; *CPK*, creatine phosphokinase; *CSF*, cerebrospinal fluid; *DVT*, deep vein thrombosis; *EEG*, electroencephalography; *FDA*, US Food and Drug Administration; *GABA*, γ-aminobutyric acid; *GBS*, Guillain-Barré syndrome; *GI*, gastrointestinal; *ICP*, intracranial pressure; *IM*, intramuscularly; *INR*, international normalized ratio; *IV*, intravenously; *LFT*, liver function test; *MI*, myocardial infarction; *MS*, multiple sclerosis; *NMDA*, *N*-methyl-ᴅ-aspartate; *PO*, by mouth; *PT*, prothrombin time; *PTT*, partial thromboplastic time; *SSRI*, selective serotonin reuptake inhibitor; *URI*, upper respiratory infection,

Index

Note: Page numbers followed by *f* indicate figures, *t* indicate tables, and *b* indicate boxes.